Evidence Report/Technology Assessment
Number 218

The Effectiveness and Risks of Long-Term Opioid Treatment of Chronic Pain

Prepared for:
Agency for Healthcare Research and Quality
U.S. Department of Health and Human
Services 540 Gaither Road
Rockville, MD 20850
www.ahrq.gov

Contract No. 290-2012-00014-I

Prepared by:
Pacific Northwest Evidence-based Practice Center
Oregon Health and Science University, Portland, OR
University of Washington, Seattle, WA

Investigators:
Roger Chou, M.D., FACP
Rick Deyo, M.D., M.P.H.
Beth Devine, Pharm.D., Ph.D., M.B.A.
Ryan Hansen, Pharm.D., Ph.D.
Sean Sullivan, Ph.D.
Jeffrey G. Jarvik, M.D., M.P.H.
Ian Blazina, M.P.H.
Tracy Dana, M.L.S.
Christina Bougatsos, M.P.H.
Judy Turner, Ph.D.

AHRQ Publication No. 14-E005-EF
September 2014

This report is based on research conducted by the Pacific Northwest Evidence-based Practice Center (EPC) under contract to the Agency for Healthcare Research and Quality (AHRQ), Rockville, MD (Contract No. 290-2012-00014-I). The findings and conclusions in this document are those of the authors, who are responsible for its contents; the findings and conclusions do not necessarily represent the views of AHRQ. Therefore, no statement in this report should be construed as an official position of AHRQ or of the U.S. Department of Health and Human Services.

The information in this report is intended to help health care decisionmakers—patients and clinicians, health system leaders, and policymakers, among others—make well-informed decisions and thereby improve the quality of health care services. This report is not intended to be a substitute for the application of clinical judgment. Anyone who makes decisions concerning the provision of clinical care should consider this report in the same way as any medical reference and in conjunction with all other pertinent information, i.e., in the context of available resources and circumstances presented by individual patients.

This report may be used, in whole or in part, as the basis for development of clinical practice guidelines and other quality enhancement tools, or as a basis for reimbursement and coverage policies. AHRQ or U.S. Department of Health and Human Services endorsement of such derivative products may not be stated or implied.

This report may periodically be assessed for the urgency to update. If an assessment is done, the resulting surveillance report describing the methodology and findings will be found on the Effective Health Care Program Web site at: www.effectivehealthcare.ahrq.gov. Search on the title of the report.

This document is in the public domain and may be used and reprinted without permission except those copyrighted materials that are clearly noted in the document. Further reproduction of those copyrighted materials is prohibited without the specific permission of the copyright holder.

Persons using assistive technology may not be able to fully access information in this report. For assistance contact EffectiveHealthCare@ahrq.hhs.gov.

None of the investigators have any affiliations or financial involvement that conflicts with the material presented in this report.

Suggested citation: Chou R, Deyo R, Devine B, Hansen R, Sullivan S, Jarvik JG, Blazina I, Dana T, Bougatsos C, Turner J. The Effectiveness and Risks of Long-Term Opioid Treatment of Chronic Pain. Evidence Report/Technology Assessment No. 218. (Prepared by the Pacific Northwest Evidence-based Practice Center under Contract No. 290-2012-00014-I.) AHRQ Publication No. 14-E005-EF. Rockville, MD: Agency for Healthcare Research and Quality; September 2014. www.effectivehealthcare.ahrq.gov/reports/final.cfm.

Preface

The Agency for Healthcare Research and Quality (AHRQ), through its Evidence-based Practice Centers (EPCs), sponsors the development of systematic reviews to assist public- and private-sector organizations in their efforts to improve the quality of health care in the United States. These reviews provide comprehensive, science-based information on common, costly medical conditions, and new health care technologies and strategies.

Systematic reviews are the building blocks underlying evidence-based practice; they focus attention on the strength and limits of evidence from research studies about the effectiveness and safety of a clinical intervention. In the context of developing recommendations for practice, systematic reviews can help clarify whether assertions about the value of the intervention are based on strong evidence from clinical studies. For more information about AHRQ EPC systematic reviews, see www.effectivehealthcare.ahrq.gov/reference/purpose.cfm.

AHRQ expects that these systematic reviews will be helpful to health plans, providers, purchasers, government programs, and the health care system as a whole. Transparency and stakeholder input are essential to the Effective Health Care Program. Please visit the Web site (www.effectivehealthcare.ahrq.gov) to see draft research questions and reports or to join an email list to learn about new program products and opportunities for input.

We welcome comments on this systematic review. They may be sent by mail to the Task Order Officer named below at: Agency for Healthcare Research and Quality, 540 Gaither Road, Rockville, MD 20850, or by email to epc@ahrq.hhs.gov.

Richard G. Kronick, Ph.D.
Director
Agency for Healthcare Research and Quality

Yen-pin Chiang, Ph.D.
Acting Deputy Director
Center for Evidence and Practice Improvement
Agency for Healthcare Research and Quality

Stephanie Chang, M.D., M.P.H.
Director, EPC Program
Center for Evidence and Practice Improvement
Agency for Healthcare Research and Quality

Suchitra Iyer, Ph.D.
Task Order Officer
Center for Evidence and Practice Improvement
Agency for Healthcare Research and Quality

Acknowledgments

The authors gratefully acknowledge the following individuals for their contributions to this project: Suchitra Iyer, Ph.D., Task Order Officer; David Reuben, M.D., National Institutes of Health Working Group Chair; and the National Institutes of Health Working Group.

Key Informants

This topic was nominated to AHRQ from the National Institutes of Health. Therefore, in place of Key Informants, a National Institutes of Health Working Group Planning Meeting was conducted to provide input into the key questions and the scope of the report.

Technical Expert Panel

In designing the review questions and methodology at the outset of this report, the EPC consulted several technical and content experts, reflecting a variety of viewpoints relevant to this topic. Technical experts consulted are expected to have divergent and possibly conflicting opinions. This diversity is helpful in achieving a well-rounded report. The study questions, design, methodological approaches, and/or conclusions do not necessarily represent the views of individual technical and content experts.

Technical Experts must disclose any financial conflicts of interest greater than $10,000 and any other relevant business or professional conflicts of interest. Because of their unique clinical or content expertise, individuals with potential conflicts may be retained. The TOO and the EPC work to balance, manage, or mitigate any potential conflicts of interest identified.

The list of Technical Experts who participated in developing this report follows:

Matthew Bair, M.D., M.S.
Associate Professor of Medicine,
Indiana University School of Medicine
Research Scientist,
Indiana University Center for Health Services and Outcomes Research
Research Scientist,
Center for Health Services Research
Regenstrief Institute, Inc.
Core Investigator,
VA HSR&D Center for Health Information and Communication
Indianapolis, IN

Gilbert Fanciullo, M.D., M.S.
Director, Pain Management Center
Dartmouth-Hitchcock Medical Center
Lebanon, NH

Gary Franklin, M.D., M.P.H.
Research Professor
Environmental and Occupational Health Sciences
Adjunct Research Professor, Health Services
University of Washington
Seattle, WA

Charles Inturrisi, Ph.D.
Professor of Pharmacology
Weill Cornell Medical College
New York, NY

Robert Jamison, Ph.D.
Professor of Anaesthesia
Harvard Medical School
Psychologist
Brigham and Women's Hospital
Boston, MA

Erin E. Krebs, M.D., M.P.H.
Core Investigator, Center for Chronic Disease Outcomes Research
Minneapolis VA Health Care System
Associate Professor of Medicine,
University of Minnesota
Minneapolis, MN

Leonard Paulozzi, M.D., M.P.H.
Medical Epidemiologist
Division of Unintentional Injury Prevention
National Center for Injury Prevention and Control
Centers for Disease Control and Prevention
Atlanta, GA

Mark Wallace, M.D.
Chair, Division of Pain Management
University of California, San Diego
San Diego, CA

Lonnie Zeltzer, M.D.
Director, Children's Pain and Comfort Care Program
Mattel Children's Hospital UCLA
Distinguished Professor of Pediatrics,
Anesthesiology, Psychiatry and Biobehavioral Sciences
David Geffen School of Medicine
University of California, Los Angeles
Los Angeles, CA

Peer Reviewers

Prior to publication of the final evidence report, EPCs sought input from independent Peer Reviewers without financial conflicts of interest. However, the conclusions and synthesis of the scientific literature presented in this report does not necessarily represent the views of individual reviewers.

Peer Reviewers must disclose any financial conflicts of interest greater than $10,000 and any other relevant business or professional conflicts of interest. Because of their unique clinical or content expertise, individuals with potential non-financial conflicts may be retained. The TOO and the EPC work to balance, manage, or mitigate any potential non-financial conflicts of interest identified.

The list of Peer Reviewers follows:

Matthew Bair, M.D., M.S.
Associate Professor of Medicine,
Indiana University School of Medicine
Research Scientist,
Indiana University Center for Health Services and Outcomes Research
Research Scientist, Center for Health Services Research,
Regenstrief Institute, Inc.
Core Investigator,
VA HSR&D Center for Health Information and Communication
Indianapolis, IN

Daniel Carr, M.D., M.A.
Professor of Public Health and Community Medicine
Program Director, Pain, Research Education
& Policy
Tufts University School of Medicine
Boston, MA

Gary Franklin, M.D., M.P.H.
Research Professor, Environmental and Occupational Health Sciences
Adjunct Research Professor, Health Services
University of Washington
Seattle, WA

Aaron M. Gilson, M.S., M.S.S.W., Ph.D.
Research Program Manager/Senior Scientist
Pain & Policy Studies Group
Carbone Cancer Center
University of Wisconsin-Madison
Madison, WI

Douglas Gourlay M.D., M.Sc., FRCP(c), FASAM
Former Director, Pain and Chemical Dependency Division
Wasser Pain Center
Toronto, Ontario, Canada

Charles Inturrisi, Ph.D.
Professor of Pharmacology
Weill Cornell Medical College
New York, NY

Robert Jamison, Ph.D.
Professor of Anaesthesia, Harvard Medical School
Psychologist, Brigham and Women's Hospital
Boston, MA

Erin E. Krebs, M.D., M.P.H.
Core Investigator, Center for Chronic Disease Outcomes Research
Minneapolis VA Health Care System
Associate Professor of Medicine, University of Minnesota
Minneapolis, MN

Leonard Paulozzi, M.D., M.P.H.
Medical Epidemiologist
Division of Unintentional Injury Prevention
National Center for Injury Prevention and Control
Centers for Disease Control and Prevention
Atlanta, GA

Dennis Turk, Ph.D.
Professor, Department of Anesthesiology & Pain Medicine
University of Washington
Seattle, WA

Mark Wallace, M.D.
Chair, Division of Pain Management
University of California, San Diego
San Diego, CA

Lonnie Zeltzer, M.D.
Director, Children's Pain and Comfort Care Program
Mattel Children's Hospital UCLA
Distinguished Professor of Pediatrics, Anesthesiology,
Psychiatry and Biobehavioral Sciences
David Geffen School of Medicine
University of California, Los Angeles
Los Angeles, CA

The Effectiveness and Risks of Long-Term Opioid Treatment of Chronic Pain

Structured Abstract

Objectives. Chronic pain is common and use of long-term opioid therapy for chronic pain has increased dramatically. This report reviews the current evidence on effectiveness and harms of opioid therapy for chronic pain, focusing on long-term (≥ 1 year) outcomes.

Data sources. A prior systematic review (searches through October 2008), electronic databases (Ovid MEDLINE, Scopus, and the Cochrane Libraries January 2008 to August 2014), reference lists, and clinical trials registries.

Review methods. Using predefined criteria, we selected randomized trials and comparative observational studies of patients with cancer or noncancer chronic pain being considered for or prescribed long-term opioid therapy that addressed effectiveness or harms versus placebo, no opioid use, or nonopioid therapies; different opioid dosing methods; or risk mitigation strategies. We also included uncontrolled studies ≥ 1 year that reported rates of abuse, addiction, or misuse, and studies on the accuracy of risk prediction instruments for predicting subsequent opioid abuse or misuse. The quality of included studies was assessed, data were extracted, and results were summarized qualitatively.

Results. Of the 4,209 citations identified at the title and abstract level, a total of 39 studies were included. For a number of Key Questions, we identified no studies meeting inclusion criteria. Where studies were available, the strength of evidence was rated no higher than low, due to imprecision and methodological shortcomings, with the exception of buccal or intranasal fentanyl for pain relief outcomes within 2 hours after dosing (strength of evidence: moderate). No study evaluated effects of long-term opioid therapy versus no opioid therapy. In 10 uncontrolled studies, rates of opioid abuse were 0.6 percent to 8 percent and rates of dependence were 3.1 percent to 26 percent in primary care settings, but studies varied in methods used to define and ascertain outcomes. Rates of aberrant drug-related behaviors ranged from 5.7 percent to 37.1 percent. Compared with nonuse, long-term opioid therapy was associated with increased risk of abuse (one cohort study), overdose (one cohort study), fracture (two observational studies), myocardial infarction (two observational studies), and markers of sexual dysfunction (one cross-sectional study), with several studies showing a dose-dependent association. One randomized trial found no difference between a more liberal opioid dose escalation strategy and maintenance of current dose in pain or function, but differences between groups in daily opioid doses at the end of the trial were small. One cohort study found methadone associated with lower risk of mortality than long-acting morphine in a Veterans Affairs population in a propensity adjusted analysis (adjusted HR 0.56, 95 percent CI 0.51 to 0.62). Estimates of diagnostic accuracy for the Opioid Risk Tool were extremely inconsistent and other risk assessment instruments were evaluated in only one or two studies. No study evaluated the effectiveness of risk mitigation strategies on outcomes related to overdose, addiction, abuse, or misuse. Evidence was insufficient to evaluate benefits and harms of long-term opioid therapy in high-risk patients or in other subgroups.

Conclusions. Evidence on long-term opioid therapy for chronic pain is very limited but suggests an increased risk of serious harms that appears to be dose-dependent. More research is needed to understand long-term benefits, risk of abuse and related outcomes, and effectiveness of different opioid prescribing methods and risk mitigation strategies.

Contents

Introduction 1
   Background 1
   Scope of Review and Key Questions 2
      Key Question 1. Effectiveness and Comparative Effectiveness 2
      Key Question 2. Harms and Adverse Events 2
      Key Question 3. Dosing Strategies 3
   Key Question 4. Risk Assessment and Risk Mitigation Strategies 3

Methods 5
   Topic Refinement and Review Protocol 5
   Literature Search Strategy 5
   Study Selection 5
   Data Extraction 7
   Assessing Methodological Risk of Bias of Individual Studies 7
   Assessing Research Applicability 8
   Evidence Synthesis and Rating the Body of Evidence 9
   Peer Review and Public Commentary 9

Results 11
   Overview 12
   Key Question 1a. In patients with chronic pain, what is the effectiveness of long-term opioid therapy versus placebo or no opioid therapy for long-term (≥1 year) outcomes related to pain, function, and quality of life? 12
      Key Points 12
      Detailed Synthesis 12
   Key Question 1b. How does effectiveness vary depending on: (1) the specific type or cause of pain (e.g., neuropathic, musculoskeletal [including low back pain], fibromyalgia, sickle cell disease, inflammatory pain, and headache disorders); (2) patient demographics (e.g., age, race, ethnicity, gender); (3) patient comorbidities (including past or current alcohol or substance use disorders, mental health disorders, medical comorbidities and high risk for addiction)? 12
      Key Points 12
      Detailed Synthesis 12
   Key Question 1c. In patients with chronic pain, what is the comparative effectiveness of opioids versus nonopioid therapies (pharmacological or nonpharmacological) on outcomes related to pain, function, and quality of life? 13
      Key Points 13
      Detailed Synthesis 13
   Key Question 1d. In patients with chronic pain, what is the comparative effectiveness of opioids plus nonopioid interventions (pharmacological or nonpharmacological) versus opioids or nonopioid interventions alone on outcomes related to pain, function, quality of life, and doses of opioids used? 13
      Key Points 13
      Detailed Synthesis 13

Key Question 2a. In patients with chronic pain, what are the risks of opioids versus placebo or no opioid on: (1) opioid abuse, addiction, and related outcomes; (2) overdose; and (3) other harms, including gastrointestinal-related harms, falls, fractures, motor vehicle accidents, endocrinological harms, infections, cardiovascular events, cognitive harms, and psychological harms (e.g., depression)?..14
    Key Points 14
    Detailed Synthesis 15
Key Question 2b. How do harms vary depending on: (1) the specific type or cause of pain (e.g., neuropathic, musculoskeletal [including back pain], fibromyalgia, sickle cell disease, inflammatory pain, headache disorders); (2) patient demographics; (3) patient comorbidities (including past or current substance use disorder or at high risk for addiction); (4) the dose of opioids used?..24
    Key Points 25
    Detailed Synthesis 26
Key Question 3a. In patients with chronic pain, what is the comparative effectiveness of different methods for initiating and titrating opioids for outcomes related to pain, function, and quality of life; risk of overdose, addiction, abuse, or misuse; and doses of opioids used?.28
    Key Points 28
    Detailed Synthesis 28
Key Question 3b. In patients with chronic pain, what is the comparative effectiveness of short- versus long-acting opioids on outcomes related to pain, function, and quality of life;
    risk of overdose, addiction, abuse, or misuse; and doses of opioids used?.........................28
    Key Points 28
    Detailed Synthesis 28
Key Question 3c. In patients with chronic pain, what is the comparative effectiveness of different long-acting opioids on outcomes related to pain, function, and quality of life; and risk of overdose, addiction, abuse, or misuse?..30
    Key Points 30
    Detailed Synthesis 30
Key Question 3d. In patients with chronic pain, what is the comparative effectiveness of short- plus long-acting opioids versus long-acting opioids alone on outcomes related to pain, function, and quality of life; risk of overdose, addiction, abuse, or misuse; and doses of opioids used? 35
Key Question 3e. In patients with chronic pain, what is the comparative effectiveness of scheduled, continuous versus as-needed dosing of opioids on outcomes related to pain, function, and quality of life; risk of overdose, addiction, abuse, or misuse; and doses of opioids used? 35
    Key Points 35
    Detailed Synthesis 35
Key Question 3f. In patients with chronic pain on long-term opioid therapy, what is the comparative effectiveness of dose escalation versus dose maintenance or use of dose thresholds on outcomes related to pain, function, and quality of life?....................................35
    Key Points 35
    Detailed Synthesis 36

Key Question 3g. In patients on long-term opioid therapy, what is the comparative effectiveness of opioid rotation versus maintenance of current opioid therapy on outcomes related to pain, function, and quality of life; and doses of opioids used? 36
    Key Points 36
    Detailed Synthesis 37
Key Question 3h. In patients on long-term opioid therapy, what is the comparative effectiveness of different strategies for treating acute exacerbations of chronic pain on outcomes related to pain, function, and quality of life? 37
    Key Points 37
    Detailed Synthesis 37
Key Question 3i. In patients on long-term opioid therapy, what are the effects of decreasing opioid doses or of tapering off opioids versus continuation of opioids on outcomes related to pain, function, quality of life, and withdrawal? 40
    Key Points 40
    Detailed Synthesis 40
Key Question 3j. In patients on long-term opioid therapy, what is the comparative effectiveness of different tapering protocols and strategies on measures related to pain, function, quality of life, withdrawal symptoms, and likelihood of opioid cessation? 41
    Key Points 41
    Detailed Synthesis 41
Key Question 4a. In patients with chronic pain being considered for long-term opioid therapy, what is the accuracy of instruments for predicting risk of opioid overdose, addiction, abuse, or misuse? 41
    Key Points 41
    Detailed Synthesis 42
Key Question 4b. In patients with chronic pain, what is the effectiveness of use of risk prediction instruments on outcomes related to overdose, addiction, abuse, or misuse? 45
    Key Points 45
    Detailed Synthesis 46
Key Question 4c. In patients with chronic pain prescribed long-term opioid therapy, what is the effectiveness of risk mitigation strategies, including (1) opioid management plans, (2) patient education, (3) urine drug screening, (4) use of prescription drug monitoring program data, (5) use of monitoring instruments, (6) more frequent monitoring intervals, (7) pill counts, and (8) use of abuse-deterrent formulations on outcomes related to overdose, addiction, abuse, or misuse? 46
    Key Points 46
    Detailed Synthesis 46
Key Question 4d. What is the comparative effectiveness of treatment strategies for managing patients with addiction to prescription opioids on outcomes related to overdose, abuse, misuse, pain, function, and quality of life? 46
    Key Points 46
    Detailed Synthesis 46

Discussion 47
    Key Findings and Strength of Evidence 47
    Findings in Relationship to What is Already Known 54

    Applicability 55
    Implications for Clinical and Policy Decisionmaking 56
    Limitations of the Review Process 56
    Limitations of the Evidence Base 57
    Research Gaps 57
    Conclusions 58

References 59

Abbreviations and Acronyms 67

Figures
Figure A. Analytic framework ES-4
Figure B. Literature flow diagram ES-10
Figure 1. Analytic framework 4
Figure 2. Literature flow diagram 11

Tables
Table A. Summary of evidence ES-12
Table 1. Uncontrolled studies of long-term opioid use and abuse, misuse, and related
outcomes 17
Table 2. Head-to-head trials and observational studies of different long-acting opioids 32
Table 3. Trials of different strategies for treating acute exacerbations of chronic pain in
patients on long-term opioid therapy 38
Table 4. Studies of risk assessment instruments 44
Table 5. Predictive value of risk assessment instruments 45
Table 6. Summary of evidence 49

Appendixes
Appendix A. Search Strategy
Appendix B. PICOTS
Appendix C. Included Studies
Appendix D. Excluded Studies
Appendix E. Data Abstraction Tables
Appendix F. Quality Assessment Tables
Appendix G. Strength of Evidence Table

Executive Summary

Introduction

Background

Chronic pain, often defined as pain lasting longer than 3 months or past the time of normal tissue healing,[1] is extremely common. According to a recent Institute of Medicine report, up to one-third of U.S. adults report chronic pain.[2] Chronic pain is a major cause of decreased quality of life and disability and is often refractory to treatment.[3,4] There has been a dramatic increase over the past 10 to 20 years in the prescription of opioid medications for chronic pain,[5-7] despite limited evidence showing long-term beneficial effects.[8,9] In addition, accumulating evidence indicates that prescription opioids may be associated with important harms, including accidental overdose, abuse, addiction, diversion, and accidents involving injuries (such as falls and motor vehicle accidents).[10-20] Perhaps of most concern is the dramatic increase in overdose deaths associated with opioids. In 2011, there were 16,917 fatal overdoses involving prescription opioids.[21] Prescription opioid misuse and abuse resulted in almost 660,000 emergency department visits in 2010, over twice as many as in 2004.[13] Substance abuse treatment admissions for opiates other than heroin increased more than six-fold from 1999 to 2009.[12] Opioids are also associated with adverse effects such as constipation, nausea, and sedation.[22] Finally, data indicate potential associations between long-term opioid therapy and other harms, such as adverse endocrinological effects and hyperalgesia.[23-25]

These data underscore the complexity of clinical decisionmaking around long-term opioid therapy, which requires individualized assessments of the balance between benefits and harms; appropriate opioid selection, dose initiation, and titration strategies; integration of risk assessment and mitigation strategies; and consideration of the use of alternative, nonopioid therapies.[9] Risk mitigation strategies that have been suggested for patients prescribed long-term opioids include use of opioid medication agreements, application of dose thresholds that warrant increased caution, regular clinical followup and monitoring, urine drug screens, use of abuse- deterrent opioid formulations, and use of data from prescription drug monitoring programs.[9]

Understanding benefits and harms of long-term opioid therapy for chronic pain is a challenge because effects may vary depending on patient characteristics (e.g., age, sex, pain condition, psychosocial factors, comorbidities), opioid characteristics (e.g., specific opioid, short- versus long-acting opioid, mode of administration, dose), dosing strategies (e.g., round-the-clock versus as-needed dosing, application of dose thresholds), concomitant therapies (e.g., use of benzodiazepines or other drugs that may interact with opioids), and characteristics of the clinical setting. Other challenges in interpreting the literature include potential limitations in generalizability due to study design and other methodological shortcomings (e.g., duration of followup, exclusion of patients at higher risk for harms, under-representation of certain sociodemographic groups, and high dropout rates), and gaps in research on important scientific questions.[26] Although guidelines on use of opioids for chronic pain are available, most recommendations are based on weak or limited evidence.[9,27] The increase in use of long-term opioid therapy for chronic pain, new information concerning harms associated with long-term opioid therapy, continued wide variations in practice related to long-term opioid therapy, and the availability of new evidence underscore the need for a current systematic review in this area.

The purpose of this report is to systematically review the current evidence on long-term opioid therapy for chronic pain, which will be used by the National Institutes of Health (NIH) to inform a Pathways to Prevention Workshop on the role of opioids in the treatment of chronic pain. Although guidelines have been published from the American Pain Society (APS)/American Academy of Pain Medicine,[9] the Veterans Affairs (VA)/Department of Defense,[28] and other groups, the availability of new evidence warrants a new systematic review that could be used to inform updated or new guidelines, guide quality improvement efforts, and define and update priorities for further research in this area.[26] This review updates a prior systematic review on opioid therapy for chronic pain funded by the APS.[29] Differences between this review and the 2009 APS review are that it focuses specifically on benefits and harms associated with long-term use of opioid therapy and evaluates an additional Key Question on dose escalation versus maintenance of doses in patients on long-term opioid therapy, additional outcomes (e.g., cardiovascular events, infection, and psychological outcomes), and additional risk mitigation strategies (e.g., abuse-deterrent formulations and use of data from prescription drug monitoring programs).

Scope of Review and Key Questions

The Key Questions and analytic framework (Figure A) used to guide this report are shown below. The analytic framework shows the target populations, interventions, and outcomes that we examined.

Key Question 1. Effectiveness and Comparative Effectiveness

a. In patients with chronic pain, what is the effectiveness of long-term opioid therapy versus placebo or no opioid therapy for long-term (≥1 year) outcomes related to pain, function, and quality of life?
b. How does effectiveness vary depending on: (1) the specific type or cause of pain (e.g., neuropathic, musculoskeletal [including low back pain], fibromyalgia, sickle cell disease, inflammatory pain, and headache disorders); (2) patient demographics (e.g., age, race, ethnicity, gender); (3) patient comorbidities (including past or current alcohol or substance use disorders, mental health disorders, medical comorbidities and high risk for addiction)?
c. In patients with chronic pain, what is the comparative effectiveness of opioids versus nonopioid therapies (pharmacological or nonpharmacological) on outcomes related to pain, function, and quality of life?
d. In patients with chronic pain, what is the comparative effectiveness of opioids plus nonopioid interventions (pharmacological or nonpharmacological) versus opioids or nonopioid interventions alone on outcomes related to pain, function, quality of life, and doses of opioids used?

Key Question 2. Harms and Adverse Events

a. In patients with chronic pain, what are the risks of opioids versus placebo or no opioid on: (1) opioid abuse, addiction, and related outcomes; (2) overdose; and (3) other harms, including gastrointestinal-related harms, falls, fractures, motor vehicle accidents, endocrinological harms, infections, cardiovascular events, cognitive harms, and psychological harms (e.g., depression)?

b. How do harms vary depending on: (1) the specific type or cause of pain (e.g., neuropathic, musculoskeletal [including back pain], fibromyalgia, sickle cell disease, inflammatory pain, headache disorders); (2) patient demographics; (3) patient comorbidities (including past or current substance use disorder or at high risk for addiction); (4) the dose of opioids used?

Key Question 3. Dosing Strategies

a. In patients with chronic pain, what is the comparative effectiveness of different methods for initiating and titrating opioids for outcomes related to pain, function, and quality of life; risk of overdose, addiction, abuse, or misuse; and doses of opioids used?
b. In patients with chronic pain, what is the comparative effectiveness of short- versus long-acting opioids on outcomes related to pain, function, and quality of life; risk of overdose, addiction, abuse, or misuse; and doses of opioids used?
c. In patients with chronic pain, what is the comparative effectiveness of different long-acting opioids on outcomes related to pain, function, and quality of life; and risk of overdose, addiction, abuse, or misuse?
d. In patients with chronic pain, what is the comparative effectiveness of short- plus long-acting opioids versus long-acting opioids alone on outcomes related to pain, function, and quality of life; risk of overdose, addiction, abuse, or misuse; and doses of opioids used?
e. In patients with chronic pain, what is the comparative effectiveness of scheduled, continuous versus as-needed dosing of opioids on outcomes related to pain, function, and quality of life; risk of overdose, addiction, abuse, or misuse; and doses of opioids used?
f. In patients with chronic pain on long-term opioid therapy, what is the comparative effectiveness of dose escalation versus dose maintenance or use of dose thresholds on outcomes related to pain, function, and quality of life?
g. In patients on long-term opioid therapy, what is the comparative effectiveness of opioid rotation versus maintenance of current opioid therapy on outcomes related to pain, function, and quality of life; and doses of opioids used?
h. In patients on long-term opioid therapy, what is the comparative effectiveness of different strategies for treating acute exacerbations of chronic pain on outcomes related to pain, function, and quality of life?
i. In patients on long-term opioid therapy, what are the effects of decreasing opioid doses or of tapering off opioids versus continuation of opioids on outcomes related to pain, function, quality of life, and withdrawal?
j. In patients on long-term opioid therapy, what is the comparative effectiveness of different tapering protocols and strategies on measures related to pain, function, quality of life, withdrawal symptoms, and likelihood of opioid cessation?

Key Question 4. Risk Assessment and Risk Mitigation Strategies

a. In patients with chronic pain being considered for long-term opioid therapy, what is the accuracy of instruments for predicting risk of opioid overdose, addiction, abuse, or misuse?
b. In patients with chronic pain, what is the effectiveness of use of risk prediction instruments on outcomes related to overdose, addiction, abuse, or misuse?
c. In patients with chronic pain prescribed long-term opioid therapy, what is the effectiveness of risk mitigation strategies, including (1) opioid management plans, (2) patient education, (3) urine drug screening, (4) use of prescription drug monitoring

program data, (5) use of monitoring instruments, (6) more frequent monitoring intervals, (7) pill counts, and (8) use of abuse-deterrent formulations on outcomes related to overdose, addiction, abuse, or misuse?
d. What is the comparative effectiveness of treatment strategies for managing patients with addiction to prescription opioids on outcomes related to overdose, abuse, misuse, pain, function, and quality of life?

Figure A. Analytic framework

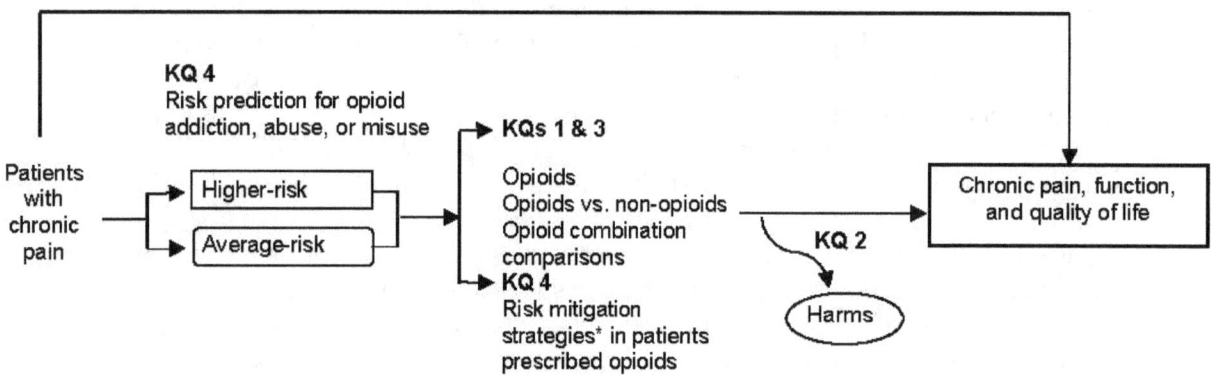

KQ, Key Question.

*Including opioid management plans, patient education, urine drug screening, use of prescription drug monitoring program data, use of monitoring instruments, more frequent monitoring intervals, pill counts, and use of abuse-deterrent formulations.

Methods

The methods for this Comparative Effectiveness Review (CER) follow the methods suggested in the Agency for Healthcare Research and Quality (AHRQ) Methods Guide for Effectiveness and Comparative Effectiveness Reviews.[30] All methods were determined a priori.

Topic Refinement and Review Protocol

This topic was selected for review based on a nomination from NIH. The initial Key Questions for this CER were developed with input from an NIH working group. The Key Questions and scope were further developed with input from a Technical Expert Panel (TEP) convened for this report. The TEP provided high-level content and methodological guidance to the review process and consisted of experts in health services research, internal medicine, psychology, pain medicine, pharmacology, neurology, occupational medicine, pediatrics, and epidemiology. TEP members disclosed all financial or other conflicts of interest prior to participation. The AHRQ Task Order Officer and the investigators reviewed the disclosures and determined that the TEP members had no conflicts of interest that precluded participation.

The protocol for this CER was developed prior to initiation of the review, and was posted on the AHRQ Web site on December 19, 2013 at: http://effectivehealthcare.ahrq.gov/ehc/products/557/1837/chronic-pain-opioid-treatment-protocol-131219.pdf. The protocol was also registered in the PROSPERO international database of prospectively registered systematic reviews.[31]

Literature Search Strategy

A research librarian conducted searches in Ovid MEDLINE, the Cochrane Central Register of Controlled Trials, the Cochrane Database of Systematic Reviews, PsychINFO, and CINAHL from 2008 to August 2014 (see Appendix A for full search strategies). We restricted search start dates to January 2008 because the searches in the prior APS review, which we used to identify potentially relevant studies, went through October 2008.[29] For outcomes (cardiovascular, infections, and psychological harms) and interventions (abuse-deterrent formulations, and use of prescription monitoring program data) not addressed in the APS review, we searched the same databases and did not apply any search date start restrictions.

We also hand-searched the reference lists of relevant studies and searched for unpublished studies in ClinicalTrials.gov. Scientific information packets (SIPs) with relevant published and unpublished studies were requested from 19 current application holders from the U.S. Food and Drug Administration (FDA) Risk Evaluation and Mitigation Strategy (REMS) Extended-Release and Long-Acting (ER/LA) Opioid Analgesics List.[32] We received five SIP submissions.

Study Selection

We developed criteria for inclusion and exclusion of articles based on the Key Questions and the populations, interventions, comparators, outcomes, timing, and setting (PICOTS) approach (Appendix B). Articles were selected for full-text review if they were about long-term opioid therapy for chronic pain, were relevant to a Key Question, and met the predefined inclusion criteria as shown below. We excluded studies published only as conference abstracts, restricted inclusion to English-language articles, and excluded studies of nonhuman subjects. Studies had to report original data to be included.

Each abstract was independently reviewed for potential inclusion and full-text review by two investigators. Two investigators independently reviewed all full-text articles for final inclusion. Discrepancies were resolved through discussion and consensus. A list of the included articles is available in Appendix C; excluded articles are shown Appendix D with primary reasons for exclusion.

We selected studies of adults (age ≥18 years) with chronic pain (defined as pain lasting >3 months) being considered for long-term opioid therapy (Key Questions 4a and 4b) or prescribed long-term opioid therapy (all other Key Questions). We defined long-term opioid therapy as use of opioids on most days for >3 months; this threshold was selected to differentiate ongoing opioid therapy (as often used for chronic pain) from short-term therapy. We included studies that did not explicitly report the duration of pain if the average duration of opioid therapy was >3 months. We included studies that did not explicitly report the duration of opioid therapy if patients were prescribed long-acting opioids, as these are not typically prescribed for short-term use. We included studies with patients with chronic pain related to current or previously treated cancer, but excluded studies with patients with pain at end of life (e.g., patients with cancer in hospice care). We excluded studies with patients with acute pain, pregnant or breastfeeding women, and patients treated with opioids for addiction.

We included studies of patients prescribed any long- or short-acting opioid used as long-term therapy, either alone or in combination with another agent (Key Question 1d). We included tapentadol, a dual mechanism medication with strong opioid mu-receptor affinity, but excluded tramadol, which is also a dual mechanism medication but with weak opioid mu-receptor affinity that has not been identified as a cause of unintentional prescription drug overdose deaths.[33] We also excluded studies of parenteral opioids.

We included studies that compared long-term opioid therapy versus placebo, no therapy, or another drug or nondrug therapy; studies that evaluated different dose initiation, titration, or rotation strategies; studies of different methods for tapering or discontinuing opioids; studies on methods for treating acute exacerbations of pain in people with chronic pain; and studies on various risk mitigation strategies for reducing harms associated with opioids. Risk mitigation strategies included opioid management plans, patient education, urine drug screening, use of prescription drug monitoring program data, use of monitoring instruments, more frequent monitoring intervals, pill counts, and use of abuse-deterrent formulations. We also included studies that compared the predictive accuracy of risk prediction instruments in people with chronic pain prior to initiation of opioids for predicting outcomes related to future misuse, abuse, or addiction, and studies on the effects of risk prediction instruments on clinical outcomes.

Outcomes were pain (intensity, severity, bothersomeness), function (physical disability, activity limitations, activity interference, work function), quality of life (including depression), and doses of opioids used. Evaluated harms included overdose, opioid use disorder, addiction, abuse, and misuse, as well as other opioid-related harms (including gastrointestinal harms, fractures, falls, motor vehicle accidents, endocrinological harms, infections, cardiovascular events, cognitive harms, and psychological harms [e.g., depression]). We focused on outcomes reported after at least 1 year of opioid therapy, with the exception of outcomes related to overdose and injuries (fractures, falls, and motor vehicle accidents), studies on treatment of acute exacerbations of chronic pain, studies on dose initiation and titration, and studies on discontinuation of opioid therapy, for which we included studies of any duration.

For all Key Questions, we included randomized trials and controlled observational studies (cohort studies, cross-sectional studies, and case-control studies) that performed adjustment on potential confounders. We included uncontrolled observational studies of patients with chronic pain prescribed opioid therapy for at least 1 year that reported abuse, misuse, or addiction as a primary outcome and described predefined methods to assess these outcomes. Otherwise, we excluded uncontrolled observational studies, case series, and case reports. We reviewed systematic reviews for potentially relevant references.

Data Extraction

We extracted the following information from included studies into evidence tables using Excel spreadsheets: study design, year, setting, inclusion and exclusion criteria, population characteristics (including sex, age, race, pain condition, and duration of pain), sample size, duration of followup, attrition, intervention characteristics (including specific opioid and formulation, dose, and duration of therapy), results, and funding sources.

For studies on the predictive accuracy of risk prediction instruments, we attempted to create two-by-two tables from information provided (sample size, prevalence, sensitivity, and specificity) and compared calculated measures of diagnostic accuracy based on the two-by-two tables with reported results. We noted discrepancies between calculated and reported results when present. When reported, we also recorded the area under the receiver operating characteristic curve (AUROC).[34,35]

For studies of interventions, we calculated relative risks (RR) and associated 95 percent confidence intervals (CI) based on the information provided (sample sizes and incidence of outcomes of interest in each intervention group). We noted discrepancies between calculated and reported results when present.

Data extraction for each study was performed by two investigators. The first investigator extracted the data, and the second investigator independently reviewed the extracted data for accuracy and completeness.

Assessing Methodological Risk of Bias of Individual Studies

We assessed risk of bias (quality) for each study using predefined criteria. We used the term "quality" rather than the alternate term "risk of bias;" both refer to internal validity. Randomized trials were evaluated with criteria and methods developed by the Cochrane Back Review Group.[36] Cohort studies, case-control studies, and cross-sectional studies were rated using criteria from the U.S. Preventive Services Task Force.[37] Risk prediction instrument studies were rated using criteria from various sources.[38-40] These criteria were applied in conjunction with the approach recommended in the chapter, Assessing the Risk of Bias of Individual Studies When Comparing Medical Interventions,[41] in the AHRQ Methods Guide. Studies of predictive accuracy of risk prediction instruments were assessed using an approach adapted from the AHRQ Methods Guide for Medical Test Reviews,[38] which is based on methods developed by the Quality Assessment of Diagnostic Accuracy Studies (QUADAS) group.[39] We reassessed the quality of studies included in the prior APS review to ensure consistency in quality assessment. Two investigators independently assessed the quality of each study. Discrepancies were resolved through discussion and consensus.

Individual studies were rated as having "poor," "fair," or "good" quality. We rated the quality of each randomized trial based on the methods used for randomization, allocation concealment, and blinding; the similarity of compared groups at baseline; whether attrition was adequately reported and acceptable; similarity in use of cointerventions; compliance to allocated treatments; the use of intent-to-treat analysis; and avoidance of selective outcomes reporting.[36,37]

We rated the quality of each cohort study based on whether it enrolled a consecutive or random sample of patients meeting inclusion criteria; whether it evaluated comparable groups; whether rates of loss to followup were reported and acceptable; whether it used accurate methods for ascertaining exposures, potential confounders, and outcomes; and whether it performed adjustment for important potential confounders.[37] For cross-sectional studies, we used criteria for cohort studies, but did not rate criteria related to loss to followup. For uncontrolled studies on risk of abuse or related outcomes, we evaluated whether it enrolled a consecutive or random sample, whether outcome assessors were blinded to patient characteristics, whether rates of loss to followup were reported (for longitudinal studies) and acceptable, and whether pre-specified outcomes were assessed in all patients.

We rated the quality of each case-control study based on whether it enrolled a consecutive or random sample of cases meeting predefined criteria; whether controls were derived from the same population as cases; whether cases and controls were comparable on key prognostic factors; whether it used accurate methods to ascertain outcomes, exposures, and potential confounders; and whether it performed adjustment for important potential confounders.[37]

We rated the quality of each study on the predictive value of risk prediction instruments based on whether it evaluated a consecutive or random sample of patients meeting pre-defined criteria, whether the patient population evaluated in the study was adequately described, whether the screening instrument included appropriate criteria, and whether outcomes were assessed in all patients independent of the results of the risk assessment instrument using adequately described methods.[38,39] We also evaluated whether the study was to develop a risk prediction instrument or to validate a previously developed instrument.[40]

Studies rated "good quality" were considered to have the least risk of bias and their results are likely to be valid. Studies rated "fair quality" have some methodological shortcomings, but no flaw or combination of flaws judged likely to cause major bias. In some cases, the article did not report important information, making it difficult to assess its methods or potential limitations. The moderate risk of bias category is broad and studies with this rating vary in their strengths and weaknesses; the results of some studies assessed to have moderate risk of bias are likely to be valid, while others may be only possibly valid. Studies rated "poor quality" have significant flaws that may invalidate the results. They have a serious or "fatal" flaw or combination of flaws in design, analysis, or reporting; large amounts of missing information; or serious discrepancies in reporting. The results of these studies are at least as likely to reflect flaws in the study design as the differences between the compared interventions. We did not exclude studies rated as having high risk of bias a priori, but they were considered the least reliable when synthesizing the evidence, particularly when discrepancies between studies were present.

Assessing Research Applicability

We recorded factors important for understanding the applicability of studies, such as whether the publication adequately described the study sample, the country in which the study was conducted, the characteristics of the patient sample (e.g., age, sex, race, pain condition, duration or severity of pain, medical comorbidities, and psychosocial factors), the characteristics of the interventions used (e.g., specific opioid, dose, mode of administration, or dosing strategy), the clinical setting (e.g., primary care or specialty setting), and the magnitude of effects on clinical outcomes.[42] We also recorded the funding source and role of the sponsor. We did not assign a rating of applicability (such as high or low) because applicability may differ based on the user of the report.

Evidence Synthesis and Rating the Body of Evidence

We constructed evidence tables summarizing study characteristics, results, and quality ratings for all included studies. We summarized evidence for each Key Question qualitatively used a hierarchy-of-evidence approach, where the best evidence was the focus of our synthesis for each Key Question. In the evidence tables, we included relevant studies from the prior APS review as well as new studies meeting inclusion criteria. Results were organized by Key Question. We did not attempt meta-analyses because of the small number of studies available for each Key Question; variability in study designs, patient samples, interventions, and measures; and methodological shortcomings in the available studies.

We assessed the overall strength of evidence (SOE) for each Key Question and outcome using the approach described in the AHRQ Methods Guide.[30] We synthesized the quality of the studies; the consistency of results within and between study designs; the directness of the evidence linking the intervention and health outcomes; and the precision of the estimate of effect (based on the number and size of studies and CIs for the estimates). We were not able to formally assess for publication bias due to small number of studies, methodological shortcomings, or differences across studies in designs, measured outcomes, and other factors. Rather, as described above, we searched for unpublished studies through searches of clinical trials registries and regulatory documents and by soliciting SIPs.

The SOE was based on the overall quality of each body of evidence, based on the risk of bias (graded low, moderate, or high); the consistency of results across studies (graded consistent, inconsistent, or unable to determine when only one study was available); the directness of the evidence linking the intervention and health outcomes (graded direct or indirect); and the precision of the estimate of effect, based on the number and size of studies and CIs for the estimates (graded precise or imprecise). We did not grade supplemental domains for cohort studies evaluating intermediate and clinical outcomes because too few studies were available for these factors to impact the SOE grades.

We graded the SOE for each Key Question using the four key categories recommended in the AHRQ Methods Guide.[30] A "high" grade indicates high confidence that the evidence reflects the true effect and that further research is very unlikely to change our confidence in the estimate of effect. A "moderate" grade indicates moderate confidence that the evidence reflects the true effect and further research may change our confidence in the estimate of effect and may change the estimate. A "low" grade indicates low confidence that the evidence reflects the true effect and further research is likely to change the confidence in the estimate of effect and is likely to change the estimate. An "insufficient" grade indicates evidence either is unavailable or is too limited to permit any conclusion, due to the availability of only poor-quality studies, extreme inconsistency, or extreme imprecision.

Peer Review and Public Commentary

Experts in chronic pain and opioid therapy, as well as individuals representing important stakeholder groups, were invited to provide external peer review of this CER. The AHRQ Task Order Officer and a designated EPC Associate Editor also provided comments and editorial review. To obtain public comment, the draft report was posted on the AHRQ Web site for 4 weeks. A disposition of comments report detailing the authors' responses to the peer and public review comments will be made available after AHRQ posts the final CER on the public Web site.

Results
Overview

The search and selection of articles are summarized in the study flow diagram (Figure B). Database searches resulted in 4,209 potentially relevant articles. After dual review of abstracts and titles, 667 articles were selected for full-text review, and 39 studies (in 40 publications) were determined by dual review at the full-text level to meet inclusion criteria and were included in this review. Data extraction and quality assessment tables for all included studies per Key Question are available in Appendixes E and F.

Figure B. Literature flow diagram

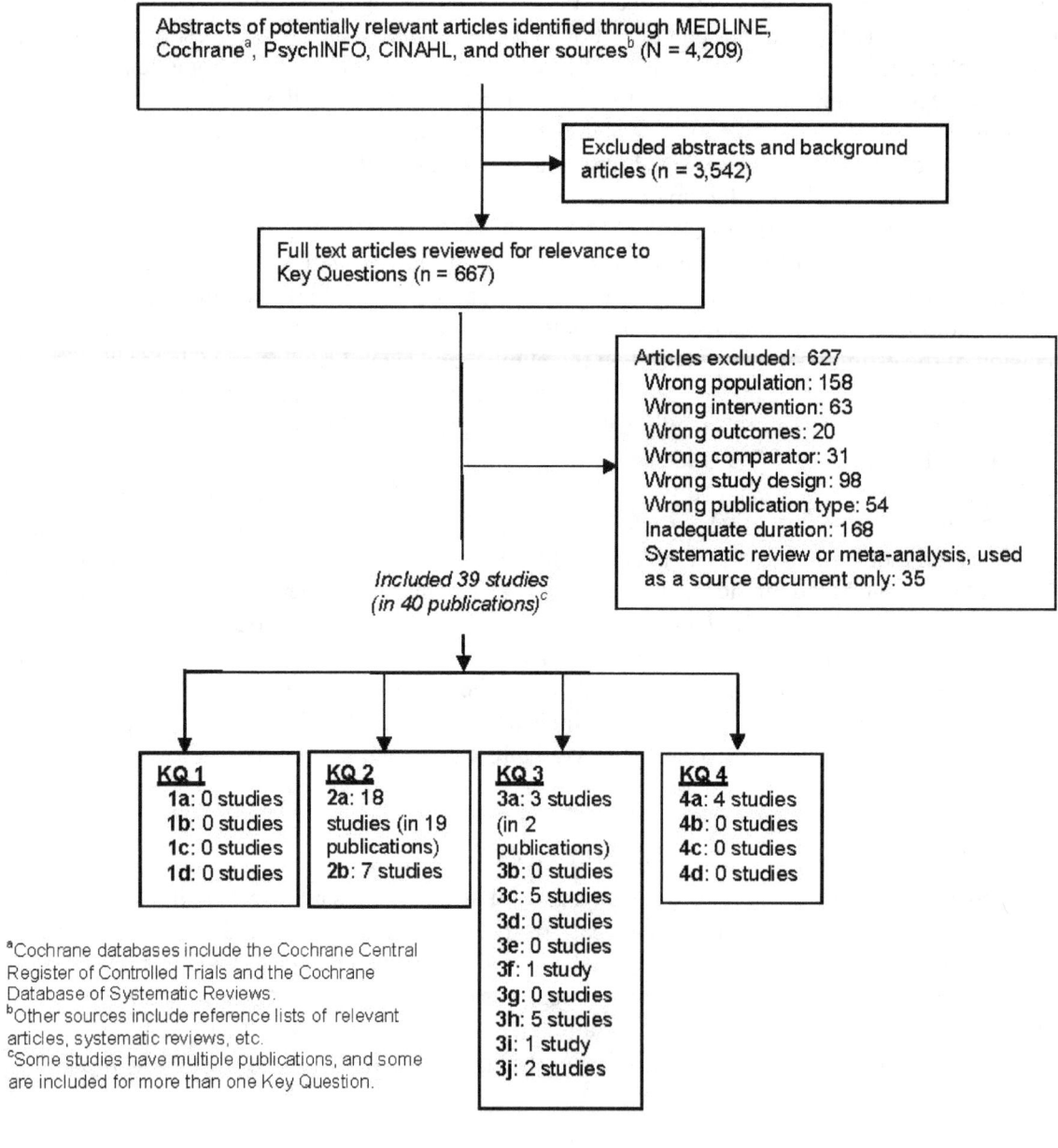

[a] Cochrane databases include the Cochrane Central Register of Controlled Trials and the Cochrane Database of Systematic Reviews.
[b] Other sources include reference lists of relevant articles, systematic reviews, etc.
[c] Some studies have multiple publications, and some are included for more than one Key Question.

Key Question 1. Effectiveness and Comparative Effectiveness

No study evaluated the effectiveness or comparative effectiveness of long-term opioid therapy versus placebo or no opioid therapy for long-term (≥1 year) outcomes related to pain, function, or quality of life in patients with chronic pain (SOE: insufficient).

Key Question 2. Harms and Adverse Events

In patients with chronic pain, 10 uncontrolled studies of patients on opioid therapy for at least 1 year that used predefined methods for ascertaining rates of abuse and related outcomes, rates of opioid abuse were 0.6 percent to 8 percent and rates of dependence were 3.1 percent to 26 percent in primary care settings, and rates of abuse were 14.4 percent, misuse 8 percent, and addiction 1.9 percent in pain clinic settings, but studies varied in methods used to define and ascertain outcomes. Rates of aberrant drug-related behaviors (e.g., positive urine drug tests, medication agreement violations) ranged from 5.7 percent to 37.1 percent (SOE: insufficient). In controlled observational studies, opioids were associated with increased risk of abuse (one study), overdose (one study), fracture (two studies), myocardial infarction (two studies), and use of testosterone replacement or medications for erectile dysfunction (one study) versus no opioid use (strength of evidence: low). No study evaluated effects of opioids versus placebo or no opioid on gastrointestinal harms, motor vehicle accidents, infections, and psychological or cognitive harms. In patients with chronic pain prescribed long-term opioid therapy, observational studies reported an association between higher doses of opioids and risk of abuse (one study), overdose (two studies), fracture (one study), myocardial infarction (one study), motor vehicle accidents (one study), and use or testosterone replacement or medications for erectile dysfunction (one study) (SOE: low). No study examined how harms vary depending on the specific type or cause of pain, patient demographics, or patient comorbidities (including past or current substance abuse disorder or being at high risk for addiction).

Key Question 3. Dosing Strategies

Three randomized, head-to-head trials of various long-acting opioids found no differences in long-term outcomes related to pain or function (SOE: low). One retrospective cohort study conducted in a Veterans Affairs setting that used a propensity-adjusted analysis found methadone associated with lower mortality risk than sustained-release morphine (SOE: low). One randomized trial found no difference between more liberal dose escalation versus maintenance of current doses on outcomes related to pain, function, or withdrawal due to opioid use, but doses of opioids at the end of the trial in the two groups were similar (52 versus 40 mg MED/day) (SOE: low). Five randomized trials found buccal or nasal fentanyl more effective than placebo or oral opioids for acute exacerbations of pain in patients with chronic pain, but focused on immediate (within 2 hours) outcomes (SOE: moderate). Studies on different methods for initiating and titrating opioids (three studies), decreasing doses or tapering off versus continuation (one study), and different tapering protocols and strategies (two studies), were limited in number, had methodological shortcomings, and showed no clear differences on outcomes related to pain and function (SOE: insufficient). No study examined effects of short- versus long-acting opioids, short- plus long-acting opioids versus long-acting opioids alone, scheduled, continuous versus as-needed dosing, or opioid rotation versus maintenance of current therapy in patients with chronic pain on long-term opioid therapy.

Key Question 4. Risk Assessment and Risk Mitigation Strategies

Four studies examined the accuracy of instruments for predicting risk of opioid overdose, addiction, abuse, or misuse in patients with chronic pain being considered for long-term opioid therapy. Three studies reported sensitivities for the Opioid Risk Tool that ranged from 0.20 to 0.99 (three studies) and specificities of 0.88 and 0.16 (two studies) (SOE: insufficient). Two studies found no clear differences between different risk assessment instruments in diagnostic accuracy. No study evaluated the effectiveness of the use of risk prediction instruments or other risk mitigation strategies, or the comparative effectiveness of treatment strategies for managing patients with a history of addiction on overdose, addiction, abuse, misuse, and related outcomes.

Key findings and SOE grades are summarized in the summary of evidence table (Table A). The factors used to determine the overall SOE grades are available in Appendix G.

Table A. Summary of evidence

Key Question Outcome	Strength of Evidence Grade	Conclusion
1. Effectiveness and comparative effectiveness		
a. In patients with chronic pain, what is the effectiveness of long-term opioid therapy versus placebo or no opioid therapy for long-term ($\geq$1 year) outcomes related to pain, function, and quality of life?		
Pain, function, quality of life	Insufficient	No study of opioid therapy versus placebo or no opioid therapy evaluated long-term ($\geq$1 year) outcomes related to pain, function, or quality of life
b. How does effectiveness vary depending on: 1) the specific type or cause of pain (e.g., neuropathic, musculoskeletal [including low back pain], fibromyalgia, sickle cell disease, inflammatory pain, and headache disorders); 2) patient demographics (e.g., age, race, ethnicity, gender); 3) patient comorbidities (including past or current alcohol or substance use disorders, mental health disorders, medical comorbidities and high risk for addiction)?		
Pain, function, quality of life	Insufficient	No studies
c. In patients with chronic pain, what is the comparative effectiveness of opioids versus nonopioid therapies (pharmacological or nonpharmacological) on outcomes related to pain, function, and quality of life?		
Pain, function, quality of life	Insufficient	No studies
d. In patients with chronic pain, what is the comparative effectiveness of opioids plus nonopioid interventions (pharmacological or nonpharmacological) versus opioids or nonopioid interventions alone on outcomes related to pain, function, quality of life, and doses of opioids used?		

Table A. Summary of evidence (continued)

Key Question Outcome	Strength of Evidence Grade	Conclusion
Pain, function, quality of life	Insufficient	No Studies
2. Harms and adverse events		
a. In patients with chronic pain, what are the risks of opioids versus placebo or no opioid on: 1) opioid abuse, addiction, and related outcomes; 2) overdose; and 3) other harms, including gastrointestinal-related harms, falls, fractures, motor vehicle accidents, endocrinological harms, infections, cardiovascular events, cognitive harms, and psychological harms (e.g., depression)?		
Abuse, addiction	Low	No randomized trial evaluated risk of opioid abuse, addiction, and related outcomes in patients with chronic pain prescribed opioid therapy. One retrospective cohort study found prescribed long-term opioid use associated with significantly increased risk of abuse or dependence versus no opioid use.
Abuse, addiction	Insufficient	In 10 uncontrolled studies, estimates of opioid abuse, addiction, and related outcomes varied substantially even after stratification by clinic setting
Overdose	Low	Current opioid use was associated with increased risk of any overdose events (adjusted HR 5.2, 95% CI 2.1 to 12) and serious overdose events (adjusted HR 8.4, 95% CI 2.5 to 28) versus current nonuse
Fractures	Low	Opioid use associated with increased risk of fracture in 1 cohort study (adjusted HR 1.28, 95% CI 0.99 to 1.64) and 1 case-control study (adjusted OR 1.27, 95% CI 1.21 to 1.33)
Myocardial infarction	Low	Current opioid use associated with increased risk of myocardial infarction versus nonuse (adjusted OR 1.28, 95% CI 1.19 to 1.37 and incidence rate ratio 2.66, 95% CI 2.30 to 3.08)
Endocrine	Low	Long-term opioid use associated with increased risk of use of medications for erectile dysfunction or testosterone replacement versus nonuse (adjusted OR 1.5, 95% CI 1.1 to 1.9)
Gastrointestinal harms, motor vehicle accidents, infections, psychological harms, cognitive harms	Insufficient	No studies
b. How do harms vary depending on: 1) the specific type or cause of pain (e.g., neuropathic, musculoskeletal [including back pain], fibromyalgia, sickle cell disease, inflammatory pain, headache disorders); 2) patient demographics; 3) patient comorbidities (including past or current substance use disorder or at high risk for addiction)?		

Table A. Summary of evidence (continued)

Key Question Outcome	Strength of Evidence Grade	Conclusion
Various harms	Insufficient	No studies
b. How do harms vary depending on the dose of opioids used?		
Abuse, addiction	Low	One retrospective cohort study found higher doses of long-term opioid therapy associated with increased risk of opioid abuse or dependence than lower doses. Compared to no opioid prescription, the adjusted odds ratios were 15 (95 percent CI 10 to 21) for 1-36 MED/day, 29 (95 percent CI 20 to 41) for 36-120 MED/day, and 122 (95 percent CI 73 to 205) for ≥120 MED/day.
Overdose	Low	Versus 1 to 19 mg MED/day, 1 cohort study found an adjusted HR for an overdose event of 1.44 (95% CI 0.57 to 3.62) for 20 to 49 mg MED/day that increased to 11.18 (95% CI 4.80 to 26.03) at >100 mg MED/day; 1 case-control study found an adjusted OR for an opioid-related death of 1.32 (95% CI 0.94 to 1.84) for 20 to 49 mg MED/day that increased to 2.88 (95% CI 1.79 to 4.63) at ≥200 mg MED/day
Fracture	Low	Risk of fracture increased from an adjusted HR of 1.20 (95% CI 0.92 to 1.56) at 1 to <20 mg MED/day to 2.00 (95% CI 1.24 to 3.24) at ≥50 mg MED/day; the trend was of borderline statistical significance
Myocardial infarction	Low	Relative to a cumulative dose of 0 to 1350 mg MED over 90 days, the incidence rate ratio for myocardial infarction for 1350 to <2700 mg was 1.21 (95% CI 1.02 to 1.45), for 2700 to <8100 mg was 1.42 (95% CI 1.21 to 1.67), for 8100 to <18,000 mg was 1.89 (95% CI 1.54 to 2.33), and for >18,000 mg was 1.73 (95% CI 1.32 to 2.26)
Motor vehicle accidents	Low	No association between opioid dose and risk of motor vehicle accidents.
Endocrine	Low	Relative to 0 to <20 mg MED/day, the adjusted OR for daily opioid dose of ≥120 mg MED/day for use of medications for erectile dysfunction or testosterone replacement was 1.6 (95% CI 1.0 to 2.4)

Table A. Summary of evidence (continued)

Key Question Outcome	Strength of Evidence Grade	Conclusion
3. Dosing strategies		
a. In patients with chronic pain, what is the comparative effectiveness of different methods for initiating and titrating opioids for outcomes related to pain, function, and quality of life; risks of overdose, addiction, abuse, or misuse; and doses of opioids used?		
Pain	Insufficient	Evidence from three trials on effects of titration with immediate-release versus sustained-release opioids reported inconsistent results on outcomes related to pain and are difficult to interpret due to additional differences between treatment arms in dosing protocols (titrated vs. fixed dosing) and doses of opioids used
Function, quality of life, outcomes related to abuse	Insufficient	No studies
b. In patients with chronic pain, what is the comparative effectiveness of short- versus long-acting opioids on outcomes related to pain, function, and quality of life; risk of overdose, addiction, abuse, or misuse; and doses of opioids used?		

Table A. Summary of evidence (continued)

Key Question Outcome	Strength of Evidence Grade	Conclusion
Pain, function, quality of life, outcomes related to abuse	Insufficient	No studies
c. In patients with chronic pain, what is the comparative effectiveness of different long-acting opioids on outcomes related to pain, function, and quality of life; and risk of overdose, addiction, abuse, or misuse?		
Pain and function	Low	No difference between various long-acting opioids
Assessment of risk of overdose, addiction, abuse, or misuse	Insufficient	No studies were designed to assess risk of overdose, addiction, abuse, or misuse
Overdose (as indicated by all-cause mortality)	Low	One cohort study found methadone to be associated with lower all-cause mortality risk than sustained-release morphine in a propensity adjusted analysis
Abuse and related outcomes	Insufficient	Another cohort study found some differences between long-acting opioids in rates of adverse outcomes related to abuse, but outcomes were nonspecific for opioid-related adverse events, precluding reliable conclusions
d. In patients with chronic pain, what is the comparative effectiveness of short- plus long-acting opioids vs. long-acting opioids alone on outcomes related to pain, function, and quality of life; risk of overdose, addiction, abuse, or misuse; and doses of opioids used?		
Pain, function, quality of life, outcomes related to abuse	Insufficient	No studies
e. In patients with chronic pain, what is the comparative effectiveness of scheduled, continuous versus as-needed dosing of opioids on outcomes related to pain, function, and quality of life; risk of overdose, addiction, abuse, or misuse; and doses of opioids used?		
Pain, function, quality of life, outcomes related to abuse	Insufficient	No studies
f. In patients with chronic pain on long-term opioid therapy, what is the comparative effectiveness of dose escalation versus dose maintenance or use of dose thresholds on outcomes related to pain, function, and quality of life?		
Pain, function, withdrawal due to opioid misuse	Low	No difference between more liberal dose escalation versus maintenance of current doses in pain, function, or risk of withdrawal due to opioid misuse, but there was limited separation in opioid doses between groups (52 vs. 40 mg MED/day at the end of the trial)
g. In patients on long-term opioid therapy, what is the comparative effectiveness of opioid rotation versus maintenance of current opioid therapy on outcomes related to pain, function, and quality of life; and doses of opioids used?		
Pain, function, quality of life, outcomes related to abuse	Insufficient	No studies

Table A. Summary of evidence (continued)

Key Question Outcome	Strength of Evidence Grade	Conclusion
h. In patients on long-term opioid therapy, what is the comparative effectiveness of different strategies for treating acute exacerbations of chronic pain on outcomes related to pain, function, and quality of life?		
Pain	Moderate	Two randomized trials found buccal fentanyl more effective than placebo for treating acute exacerbations of pain and three randomized trials found buccal fentanyl or intranasal fentanyl more effective than oral opioids for treating acute exacerbations of pain in patients on long-term opioid therapy, based on outcomes measured up to 2 hours after dosing
Abuse and related outcomes	Insufficient	No studies
i. In patients on long-term opioid therapy, what are the effects of decreasing opioid doses or of tapering off opioids versus continuation of opioids on outcomes related to pain, function, quality of life, and withdrawal?		
Pain, function	Insufficient	Abrupt cessation of morphine was associated with increased pain and decreased function compared to continuation of morphine
j. In patients on long-term opioid therapy, what is the comparative effectiveness of different tapering protocols and strategies on measures related to pain, function, quality of life, withdrawal symptoms, and likelihood of opioid cessation?		
Opioid abstinence	Insufficient	No clear differences between different methods for opioid discontinuation or tapering in likelihood of opioid abstinence after 3 to 6 months
4. Risk assessment and risk mitigation strategies		
a. In patients with chronic pain being considered for long-term opioid therapy, what is the accuracy of instruments for predicting risk of opioid overdose, addiction, abuse, or misuse?		
Diagnostic accuracy: Opioid Risk Tool	Insufficient	Based on a cutoff of >4, three studies (one poor-quality, two poor-quality) reported very inconsistent estimates of diagnostic accuracy, precluding reliable conclusions
Diagnostic accuracy: Screening and Opioid Assessment for Patients with Pain (SOAPP) version 1	Low	Based on a cutoff score of ≥ 8, sensitivity was 0.68 and specificity of 0.38 in 1 study, for a PLR of 1.11 and NLR of 0.83. Based on a cutoff score of >6, sensitivity was 0.73 in 1 study
b. In patients with chronic pain, what is the effectiveness of use of risk prediction instruments on outcomes related to overdose, addiction, abuse, or misuse?		
Outcomes related to abuse	Insufficient	No study evaluated the effectiveness of risk prediction instruments for reducing outcomes related to overdose, addiction, abuse, or misuse

Table A. Summary of evidence (continued)

Key Question Outcome	Strength of Evidence Grade	Conclusion
c. In patients with chronic pain prescribed long-term opioid therapy, what is the effectiveness of risk mitigation strategies, including 1) opioid management plans, 2) patient education, 3) urine drug screening, 4) use of prescription drug monitoring program data, 5) use of monitoring instruments, 6) more frequent monitoring intervals, 7) pill counts, and 8) use of abuse-deterrent formulations on outcomes related to overdose, addiction, abuse, or misuse?		
Outcomes related to abuse	Insufficient	No studies
d. What is the comparative effectiveness of treatment strategies for managing patients with addiction to prescription opioids on outcomes related to overdose, abuse, misuse, pain, function, and quality of life?		
Outcomes related to abuse	Insufficient	No studies

Abbreviations: CI=confidence interval, HR=hazard ratio, MED= morphine equivalent dose, mg=milligrams, NLR=negative likelihood ratio, OR=odds ratio, PLR=positive likelihood ratio, SOAPP= Screening and Opioid Assessment for Patients with Pain.

Discussion

Key Findings and Strength of Evidence

The key findings of this review are summarized in the summary of evidence table (Table A) and the factors used to determine the overall SOE grades are summarized in Appendix G. For a number of Key Questions, we identified no studies meeting inclusion criteria. For Key Questions where studies were available, the SOE was rated no higher than low, due to small numbers of studies and methodological shortcomings, with the exception of buccal or intranasal fentanyl for pain relief outcomes within 2 hours after dosing, for which the SOE was rated moderate.

For effectiveness and comparative effectiveness, we identified no studies of long-term opioid therapy in patients with chronic pain versus no opioid therapy or nonopioid alternative therapies that evaluated outcomes at 1 year or longer. No studies examined how effectiveness varies based on various factors, including type of pain and patient characteristics. Most placebo-controlled randomized trials were shorter than 6 weeks in duration[43] and no cohort studies on the effects of long-term opioid therapy versus no opioid therapy on outcomes related to pain, function, or quality of life were found. Although uncontrolled studies of patients prescribed opioids are available,[8] findings are difficult to interpret due to the lack of a nonopioid comparison group.

Regarding harms, new evidence (published since the APS review) from observational studies suggests that being prescribed long-term opioids for chronic pain is associated with increased risk of abuse,[44] overdose,[45] fractures,[18,46] and myocardial infarction,[47] versus not currently being prescribed opioids. In addition, several recent studies suggest that the risk is dose-dependent, with higher opioid doses associated with increased risk.[11,18,44,45,48,49] Although two studies found an association between opioid dose and increased risk of overdose starting at relatively low doses (20 to 49 mg MED/day), estimates at higher doses were variable (adjusted HR 11.18 at >100 mg MED/day versus adjusted OR 2.88 for ≥200 mg MED/day).[45,49] However, few studies evaluated each outcome and the population evaluated and duration of opioid therapy were not always well characterized. In addition, as in all observational studies, findings are susceptible to residual confounding despite use of statistical adjustment and other techniques such as matching. A study also found long-term opioid therapy associated with increased likelihood of receiving prescriptions for erectile dysfunction or testosterone, which may be markers for sexual dysfunction due to presumed endocrinological effects of opioids.[11] However, it did not directly measure sexual dysfunction, and patients may seek or receive these medications for other reasons.

No study assessed the risk of abuse, addiction, or related outcomes associated with long-term opioid therapy use versus placebo or no opioid therapy. In uncontrolled studies, rates of abuse and related outcomes varied substantially, even after restricting inclusion to studies that evaluated patients on opioid therapy for at least one year and used pre-defined methods for ascertaining these outcomes, and stratifying studies according to whether they evaluated primary care populations or patients evaluated in pain clinic settings.[50-60] An important reason for the variability in estimates is differences in patient samples and in how terms such as addiction, abuse, misuse, and dependence were defined in the studies, and in methods used to identify these outcomes (e.g., formal diagnostic interview with patients versus chart review or informal assessment). In one study, estimates of opioid misuse were lower based on independent review than based on assessments by the treating physician.[59] No study evaluated patients with "opioid use disorder" as recently defined in the new DSM-V.[61]

Evidence on the effectiveness of different opioid dosing strategies is also extremely limited. One new trial of a more liberal dose escalation strategy versus maintenance of current doses found no differences in outcomes related to pain, function, or risk of withdrawal from the study due to opioid misuse, but the difference in opioid doses between groups at the end of the trial was small (52 versus 40 mg MED/day).[62] One study from Washington State reported a decrease in the number of opioid-associated overdose deaths after implementing a dose threshold,[63] but did not meet inclusion criteria for this review because it was an ecological, before-after study, and it is not possible to reliably determine whether changes in the number of opioid overdose deaths were related to other factors that could have impacted opioid prescribing practices. Evidence on benefits and harms of different methods for initiating and titrating opioids, short- versus long-acting opioids, scheduled and continuous versus as-needed dosing of opioids, use of opioid rotation, and methods for titrating or discontinuing patients off opioids was not available or too limited to reach reliable conclusions.

We also found limited evidence on the comparative benefits and harms of specific opioids. Three head-to-head trials found few differences in pain relief between various long-acting opioids at 1 year followup,[64-66] but the usefulness of these studies for evaluating comparative effectiveness may be limited because patients in each arm had doses titrated to achieve adequate pain control. None of the trials was designed to evaluate abuse, addiction, or related outcomes.

Methadone has been an opioid of particular interest because it is disproportionately represented in case series and epidemiological studies of opioid-associated deaths.[67] Characteristics of methadone that may be associated with increased risk of serious harms are its long and variable half-life, which could increase the risk for accidental overdose, and its association with electrocardiographic QTc interval prolongation, which could increase the risk of potentially life-threatening ventricular arrhythmia.[68] However, the highest-quality observational study, which was conducted in VA patients with chronic pain and controlled well for confounders using a propensity-adjusted analysis, found methadone to be associated with lower risk of mortality as compared with sustained-release morphine.[69] These results suggest that in some settings, methadone may not be associated with increased mortality risk, though research is needed to understand the factors that contribute to safer prescribing in different clinical settings.

Although five randomized trials found buccal or intranasal fentanyl more effective than placebo or oral opioids for treating acute exacerbations of chronic pain, all focused on short-term treatment and immediate outcomes in the minutes or hours after administration.[70-74] No study was designed to assess long-term benefits or harms, including accidental overdose, abuse, or addiction. In 2007, the U.S. FDA released a public health advisory due to case reports of deaths and other life-threatening adverse effects in patients prescribed buccal fentanyl.[75]

Evidence also remains limited on the utility of opioid risk assessment instruments, used prior to initiation of opioid therapy, for predicting likelihood of subsequent opioid abuse or misuse. In three studies of the ORT, estimates were extremely inconsistent (sensitivity ranged from 0.20 to 0.99).[76-78] A study that directly compared the accuracy of the ORT and two other risk assessment instruments reported weak likelihood ratios for predicting future abuse or misuse (PLR 1.27 to 1.65 and NLR 0.86 to 0.91).[76] Risk prediction instruments other than the ORT (such as the SOAPP version 1, revised SOAPP, or DIRE) were only evaluated in one or two studies, and require further validation. Studies on the accuracy of risk instruments for identifying aberrant behavior in patients already prescribed opioids are available,[53,56,76,79-85] but were outside the scope of this review.

No study evaluated the effectiveness of risk mitigation strategies, such as use of risk assessment instruments, opioid management plans, patient education, urine drug screening, prescription drug monitoring program data, monitoring instruments, more frequent monitoring intervals, pill counts, or abuse-deterrent formulations on outcomes related to overdose, addiction, abuse or misuse. Studies on effects of risk mitigation strategies were primarily focused on ability to detect misuse (e.g., urine drug testing and prescription monitoring program data) or on effects on markers of risky prescribing practices or medication-taking behaviors,[86] and did not meet inclusion criteria for this review, which focused on effects on clinical outcomes. One study found that rates of poison center treatment incidents and opioid-related treatment admissions increased at a lower rate in States with a prescription drug monitoring program than in States without one, but used an ecological design, did not evaluate a cohort of patients prescribed opioids for chronic pain, and was not designed to account for other factors that could have impacted opioid prescribing practices.[86]

Although evidence indicates that patients with a history of substance abuse or at higher risk for abuse or misuse due to other risk factors are more likely to be prescribed opioids than patients without these risk factors,[87-90] we identified no study on the effectiveness of methods for mitigating potential harms associated with long-term opioid therapy in high-risk patients.

Findings in Relationship to What is Already Known

Our findings are generally consistent with prior systematic reviews of opioid therapy for chronic pain that also found no long-term, placebo-controlled randomized trials.[8,43] One systematic review of outcomes associated with long-term opioid therapy concluded that many patients discontinue treatment due to adverse events or insufficient pain relief, though patients who continue opioid therapy experience clinically significant pain relief.[8] However, results of the studies included in this review are difficult to interpret because the studies had no nonopioid therapy control group, reported substantial between-study heterogeneity, and were susceptible to potential attrition and selection bias. Our findings are also consistent with a systematic review on comparative benefits and harms of various long-acting opioids and short- versus long-acting opioids, which found no clear differences, primarily based on short-term randomized trials.[91]

Our review reported rates of abuse and related outcomes that are higher than a previously published systematic review of long-term opioid therapy that reported a very low rate of opioid addiction (0.27 percent).[8] Factors that may explain this discrepancy are that the prior review included studies that did not report predefined methods for ascertaining opioid addiction, potentially resulting in underreporting, and primarily included studies that excluded high-risk patients. Like a previous systematic review, we found variability in estimates of abuse and related outcomes, with some potential differences in estimates based on clinical setting (primary care versus pain clinic) and patient characteristics (e.g., exclusion of high-risk patients).[92]

Regarding risk mitigation strategies, our findings were similar to a previously published systematic review that found weak evidence with which to evaluate risk prediction instruments.[93] Unlike our review, which found no evidence on effects of risk mitigation strategies on risk of abuse, addiction, or related outcomes, a previously published review found use of opioid management plans and urine drug screens to be associated with decreased risk of misuse behaviors.[14] However, this conclusion was based on four studies that did not meet inclusion criteria for our review because effects of opioid management plans and urine drug screens could not be separated from other concurrent opioid prescribing interventions,[94,95] use of a historical control group,[96,97] or before-after study design.[94]

Applicability

A number of issues could impact the applicability of our findings. One challenge was difficulty in determining whether studies focused on patients with chronic pain. Although a number of large observational studies reported harms based on analyses of administrative databases, they were frequently limited in their ability to assess important clinical factors such as the duration or severity of pain. For some of these studies, we inferred the presence of chronic pain from prescribing data, such as the number of prescriptions over a defined period or the use of long-acting opioid preparations. Some potentially relevant studies were excluded because it was not possible to determine whether the sample evaluated had chronic pain or received long-term therapy.[16,98-103]

Another issue that could impact applicability is the type of opioid used in the studies. Both long-acting and short-acting opioids are often prescribed for chronic pain. In some studies, use of short-acting opioids predominated.[11,18,49] Results of studies of short-acting opioids may not generalize to patients prescribed long-acting opioids.

Selection of patients could also impact applicability. The few randomized trials that met inclusion criteria typically excluded patients at high risk of abuse or misuse and frequently used run-in periods prior to allocating treatments. The use of a run-in period preselects patients who respond to and tolerate initial exposure to the studied treatment. Therefore, benefits observed in the trials might be greater and harms lower than seen in actual clinical practice.[104]

Another factor impacting applicability is that most trials were not designed or powered to assess risk of abuse, addiction, or related outcomes. For example, trials of buccal fentanyl for acute exacerbations of chronic pain focused exclusively on immediate (episode-based) outcomes and were not designed to assess long-term outcomes, including outcomes related to the potential for abuse.[70-74] Long-term head-to-head trials of long-acting opioids excluded patients at high risk for these outcomes and reported no events.[64-66]

The setting in which studies were conducted could also impact applicability. As noted in other sections of this report, rates of overdose, abuse, addiction, and related outcomes are likely to vary based on the clinical setting. Therefore, we stratified studies reporting rates of abuse according to whether they were performed in primary care or pain clinic settings. The highest-quality comparative study of methadone versus another opioid (long-acting morphine) found decreased mortality risk but was conducted in a VA setting,[69] which could limit applicability to other settings, due to factors such as how clinicians were trained in methadone use, policies on opioid prescribing, availability of resources to manage opioid prescribing, or other factors.

Implications for Clinical and Policy Decisionmaking

Our review has important implications for clinical and policy decisionmaking. Based on our review, most clinical and policy decisions regarding use of long-term opioid therapy must necessarily still be made on the basis of weak or insufficient evidence. This is in accordance with findings from a 2009 U.S. guideline on use of opioids for chronic pain, which found 21 of 25 recommendations supported by only low-quality evidence,[105] and a 2010 Canadian guideline,[106] which classified 3 of 24 recommendations as based on (short-term) randomized trials and 19 recommendations as based solely or partially on consensus opinion. Although randomized trials show short-term, moderate improvements in pain in highly selected, low-risk populations with chronic pain, such efficacy-based evidence is of limited usefulness for informing long-term opioid prescribing decisions in clinical practice.

Given the marked increase in numbers of overdose deaths and other serious adverse events that have occurred following the marked increase in opioid prescribing for chronic pain, recent policy efforts have focused on safer prescribing of opioids. A recent review of opioid guidelines found broad agreement regarding a number of risk mitigation strategies despite weak evidence, such as risk-assessment guided patient assessment for opioid therapy, urine drug testing, use of prescription monitoring program data, abuse-deterrent formulations, and opioid management plans.[107] Based on low-quality evidence regarding harms associated with long-term opioid therapy, our review provides some limited support for clinical policy efforts aimed at reducing harms. One area in which there has been less agreement across guidelines is whether dose thresholds that warrant more intense monitoring or used to define maximum ceiling doses should be implemented, and if so, what is the appropriate threshold. Some evidence is now available on dose-dependent harms associated with opioids,[45,49] which could help inform policies related to dose thresholds. However, research on the effects of implementing dose thresholds on clinical outcomes is limited to a single ecological study.[63] In addition, although two observational studies were consistent in reporting a relationship between higher opioid dose and risk of overdose, estimates were highly variable at similar doses.[45,49] This makes it difficult to determine an optimal maximum dose threshold based on an objective parameter, such as a dose inflection point where risk rises markedly. Other studies have begun to characterize cardiovascular, endocrinological, and injury-related harms associated with long-term opioid therapy and could be used to inform clinical decisions, though using such information in balanced assessments to inform clinical and policy decisionmaking remains a challenge given the lack of evidence regarding long-term benefits.

Limitations of the Review Process

We excluded non-English language articles and did not search for studies published only as abstracts. We did not attempt meta-analysis or assess for publication bias using graphical or statistical methods to detect small sample effects due to the paucity of evidence. Although we found no evidence of unpublished studies through searches on clinical trial registries and regulatory documents and solicitation of unpublished studies through SIP requests, the usefulness of such methods for identifying unpublished observational studies may be limited, as such studies are often not registered. We identified no unpublished randomized trials meeting inclusion criteria. We focused on studies that reported outcomes after at least one year of opioid therapy, though applying a shorter duration threshold for inclusion could have provided additional evidence. However, we identified no placebo-controlled trials of opioid therapy for at least 6 months.

Limitations of the Evidence Base

As noted previously, the critical limitation of our review is the lack of evidence in the target population (patients with chronic pain) and intervention (long-term opioid therapy), despite broadening of inclusion criteria to incorporate studies in which we assumed that patients were being treated for chronic pain due to the type of opioid prescribed (long-acting opioid) or number of prescriptions. We were also unable to determine how benefits and harms vary in subgroups, such as those defined by demographic characteristics, characteristics of the pain condition, and other patient characteristics (e.g., medical or psychological comorbidities). Due to the lack of evidence and methodological shortcomings in the available studies, no body of evidence (with the exception of buccal or intranasal fentanyl for immediate pain relief) was rated higher than low, meaning that conclusions are highly uncertain.

Research Gaps

Many research gaps limit the full understanding of the effectiveness, comparative effectiveness, and harms of long-term opioid therapy, as well as of the effectiveness of different dosing methods and risk mitigation strategies, and effectiveness in special populations. Longer-term studies of patients clearly with chronic pain comparing those who are prescribed long-term opioid therapy with those receiving other pharmacological and non-pharmacological therapies are needed. Studies that include higher-risk patients, commonly treated with opioids in clinical practice, and that measure multiple important outcomes, including pain, physical and psychological functioning, as well as misuse and abuse, would be more helpful than efficacy studies focused solely on pain intensity. Greater standardization of methods for defining and identifying abuse-related outcomes in studies that report these outcomes are needed. The Initiative on Methods, Measurement, and Pain Assessment in Clinical Trials (IMMPACT) group recently issued recommendations on measuring abuse liability in analgesic clinical trials.[108]

Additional research is also needed to develop and validate risk prediction instruments, and to determine how using them impacts treatment decisions and, ultimately, patient outcomes. More research is needed on the comparative benefits and harms of different opioids or formulations and different prescribing methods. Studies comparing effectiveness and harms of methadone versus other long-acting opioids, to determine if findings from a study[69] conducted in a VA setting are reproducible in other settings, and to better understand factors associated with safer methadone prescribing.

Research is also needed to understand the effects of risk mitigation strategies such as urine drug screening, use of prescription drug monitoring program data, and abuse-deterrent formulations on clinical outcomes such as rates of overdose, abuse, addiction, and misuse. In one before-after study, the introduction of an abuse-deterrent opioid was followed by patients switching to other prescription opioids or illicit opioids,[109] underscoring the need for research to understand both the positive and negative clinical effects of risk mitigation strategies.

Long-term randomized trials of opioid therapy are difficult to implement due to attrition, challenges in recruitment, or ethical factors (e.g., long-term allocation of patients with pain to placebo or allocation to non-use of risk mitigation strategies recommended in clinical practice guidelines). Nonetheless, pragmatic and other non-traditional randomized trial approaches could be used to address these challenges.[110] Observational studies could also help address a number of these research questions, but should be specifically designed to evaluate patients with chronic pain prescribed long-term opioid therapy and appropriately measure and address potential confounders. Well-designed clinical registries that enroll patients with chronic pain prescribed and not prescribed chronic opioids could help address the limitations of studies based solely or primarily on administrative databases, which are often unable to fully characterize the pain condition (e.g., duration, type, and severity) or other clinical characteristics and frequently do not have information regarding outcomes related to pain, function, and quality of life. Such registry studies could be designed to extend the observations from randomized trials of opioids versus placebo or other treatments, but would differ from currently available studies by following patients who discontinue or do not start opioids, in addition to those who continue on or start opioid therapy.

Conclusions

Evidence on long-term opioid therapy for chronic pain is very limited, but suggests an increased risk of serious harms that appears to be dose-dependent. Based on our review, most clinical and policy decisions regarding use of long-term opioid therapy must necessarily still be made on the basis of weak or insufficient evidence. More research is needed to understand long-term benefits, risk of abuse and related outcomes, and effectiveness of different opioid prescribing methods and risk mitigation strategies.

References

1. International Association for the Study of Pain. Classification of chronic pain: Descriptions of chronic pain syndromes and definitions of pain terms. Pain. 1986;3:S1-226. PMID 3461421.
2. Institute of Medicine (U.S.) Committee on Advancing Pain Research Care and Education. Relieving Pain in America: A Blueprint for Transforming Prevention, Care, Education, and Research. Washington, DC: National Academies Press; 2011.
3. Ballantyne JC, Shin NS. Efficacy of opioids for chronic pain: A review of the evidence. Clinical J Pain. 2008;24(6):469-478. PMID 18574357.
4. Eriksen J, Sjogren P, Bruera E, Ekholm O, Rasmussen NK. Critical issues on opioids in chronic non-cancer pain: an epidemiological study. Pain. 2006;125(1-2):172-179. PMID 16842922.
5. Sullivan MD, Edlund MJ, Fan M-Y, DeVries A, Brennan Braden J, Martin BC. Trends in use of opioids for non-cancer pain conditions 2000–2005 in Commercial and Medicaid insurance plans: The TROUP study. Pain. 2008;138(2):440-449. PMID 18547726.
6. Boudreau D, Von Korff M, Rutter CM, et al. Trends in long-term opioid therapy for chronic non-cancer pain. Pharmacoepidemiol Drug Saf. 2009;18(12):1166-1175. PMID 19718704.
7. Olsen Y, Daumit GL, Ford DE. Opioid prescriptions by U.S. primary care physicians from 1992 to 2001. J Pain. 2006;7(4):225-235. PMID 16618466.
8. Noble M, Treadwell JR, Tregear SJ, et al. Long-term opioid management for chronic noncancer pain. Cochrane Database Syst Rev. 2010(11):CD006605. doi: 10.1002/14651858.CD006605.pub2. PMID 20091598.
9. Chou R, Fanciullo GJ, Fine PG, et al. Clinical guidelines for the use of chronic opioid therapy in chronic noncancer pain. J Pain. 2009;10(2):113-130. PMID 19187889.
10. Starrels JL, Becker WC, Weiner MG, Li X, Heo M, Turner BJ. Low use of opioid risk reduction strategies in primary care even for high-risk patients with chronic pain. J Gen Intern Med. 2011;26(9):958-964. PMID 21347877.
11. Deyo RA, Smith DH, Johnson ES, et al. Prescription opioids for back pain and use of medications for erectile dysfunction. Spine. 2013;38(11):909-915. PMID 23459134.
12. Substance Abuse and Mental Health Services Administration. Treatment Episode Data Set (TEDS). 1999 - 2009. National Admissions to Substance Abuse Treatment Services, DASIS Series: S-56. Rockville, MD: Substance Abuse and Mental Health Services Administration; 2011.
13. Substance Abuse and Mental Health Services Administration. The DAWN Report: Highlights of the 2010 Drug Abuse Warning Network (DAWN) Findings on Drug-Related Emergency Department Visits. Rockville, MD: Center for Behavioral Health Statistics and Quality; 2012.
14. Starrels JL, Becker WC, Alford DP, Kapoor A, Williams A, Turner BJ. Systematic review: treatment agreements and urine drug testing to reduce opioid misuse in patients with chronic pain. Ann Intern Med. 2010;152:712-720. PMID 20513829.
15. Warner M, Chen LH, Makuc DM, Anderson RN, Minino AM. Drug poisoning deaths in the United States, 1980-2008. NCHS Data Brief. 2011;81:1-8. PMID 22617462.
16. Bohnert ASB, Valenstein M, Bair MJ, et al. Association between opioid prescribing patterns and opioid overdose-related deaths. JAMA. 2011;305(13):1315-1321. PMID 21467284.
17. Volkow ND, McLellan TA. Curtailing diversion and abuse of opioid analgesics without jeopardizing pain treatment. JAMA. 2011;305(13):1346-1347. PMID 21467287.
18. Saunders KW, Dunn KM, Merrill JO, et al. Relationship of opioid use and dosage levels to fractures in older chronic pain patients. J Gen Intern Med. 2010;25(4):310-315. PMID 20049546.
19. Rolita L, Spegman A, Tang X, Cronstein BN. Greater number of narcotic analgesic prescriptions for osteoarthritis is associated with falls and fractures in elderly adults. J Am Geriatr Soc. 2013;61(3):335-340. PMID 23452054.
20. Gomes T, Redelmeier DA, Juurlink DN, Dhalla IA, Camacho X, Mamdani MM. Opioid dose and risk of road trauma in Canada: a population-based study. JAMA

21. Intern Med. 2013;173(3):196-201. PMID 23318919.
22. Centers for Disease Control and Prevention. Prescription Drug Overdose in the United States: Fact Sheet. 2014. Available at: http://www.cdc.gov/homeandrecreationalsafety/overdose/facts.html. Accessed July 17, 2014.
22. Furlan AD, Sandoval JA, Mailis-Gagnon A, Tunks E. Opioids for chronic noncancer pain: a meta-analysis of effectiveness and side effects. CMAJ. 2006;174(11):1589-1594. PMID 16717269.
23. Daniell HW. Hypogonadism in men consuming sustained-action oral opioids. J Pain. 2002;3:377-384. PMID 14622741.
24. Daniell HW. Opioid endocrinopathy in women consuming prescribed sustained-action opioids for control of nonmalignant pain. J Pain. 2008;9:28-36. PMID 14622741.
25. Angst MS, Clark JD. Opioid-induced hyperalgesia: a qualitative systematic review. Anesthesiology. 2006;104(3):570-587. PMID 16508405.
26. Chou R, Ballantyne JC, Fanciullo GJ, Fine PG, Miaskowski C. Research gaps on use of opioids for chronic noncancer pain: findings from a review of the evidence for an American Pain Society and American Academy of Pain Medicine clinical practice guideline. J Pain. 2009;10(2):147-159. PMID 19187891.
27. Furlan AD, Reardon R, Weppler C, National Opioid Use Guideline Group (NOUGG). Opioids for chronic noncancer pain: a new Canadian practice guideline. CMAJ. 2011;182(9):923-930. PMID 20439443.
28. United States Department of Veterans Affairs, The Management of Opioid Therapy for Chronic Pain Working Group. VA/DoD Clinical Practice Guideline for Management of Opioid Therapy for Chronic Pain' 2010. Available at http://www.healthquality.va.gov/Chronic_Opioid_Therapy_COT.asp. Accessed on September 19, 2014.
29. American Pain Society-American Academy of Pain Medicine Opioids Guidelines Panel. Guideline for the Use of Chronic Opioid Therapy in Chronic Noncancer Pain: Evidence Review. Available at: http://www.americanpainsociety.org/uploads/pdfs/Opioid_Final_Evidence_Report.pdf 2009. Accessed on September 19, 2014.
30. Owens D, Lohr KN, Atkins D, et al. Methods Guide for Effectiveness and Comparative Effectiveness Reviews. Rockville, MD: Agency for Healthcare Research and Quality. 2011.
31. Chou R. The effectiveness and risks of long-term opioid treatment of chronic pain. PROSPERO 2014:CRD42014007016; 2013. Available at: http://www.crd.york.ac.uk/PROSPERO/display_record.asp?ID=CRD42014007016. Accessed September 19, 2014.
32. U.S. Food and Drug Administration. Extended-Release and Long-Acting (ER/LA) Opioid Analgesics Risk Evaluation and Mitigation Strategy (REMS) a single shared system - Current Application Holders. Available at: http://www.fda.gov/downloads/Drugs/DrugSafety/InformationbyDrugClass/UCM348818.pdf. Accessed September 19, 2014
33. Hall AJ, Logan JE, Toblin RL, et al. Patterns of abuse among unintentional pharmaceutical overdose fatalities. JAMA. 2008;300(22):2613-2620. PMID 19066381.
34. Altman DG, Bland JM. Diagnostic tests 3: receiver operating characteristic plots. BMJ. 1994;309(6948):188. PMID 8044101.
35. Zweig MH, Campbell G. Receiver-operating characteristic (ROC) plots: a fundamental evaluation tool in clinical medicine. Clin Chem. 1993;39(4):561-577. PMID 8472349.
36. Furlan AD, Pennick V, Bombardier C, van Tulder M. 2009 updated methods guidelines for systematic reviews in the Cochrane Back Review Group. Spine. 2009;24:1929-1941. PMID 19680101.
37. U.S. Preventive Services Task Force. U.S. Preventive Services Task Force Procedure Manual. AHRQ Publication No. 08-05118-EF, July 2008. Available at: http://www.uspreventiveservicestaskforce.org/uspstf08/methods/procmanual.htm. 2008. Accessed September 19, 2014.
38. Agency for Healthcare Research and Quality. Methods Guide for Medical Test Reviews. Agency for Healthcare Research and Quality: Rockville, MD; 2010. Available at: http://effectivehealthcare.ahrq.gov/index.cfm/search-for-guides-reviews-and-reports/?pageaction=displayproduct&productid=558 Accessed September 19, 2014.
39. Whiting PF, Rutjes AWS, Westwood ME, et al. QUADAS-2: A revised tool for the Quality Assessment of Diagnostic Accuracy

Studies. Ann Intern Med. 2011;155(8):529-536. PMID 22007046.
40. McGinn TG, Guyatt GH, Wyer PC, et al. Users' guides to the medical literature: XXII: how to use articles about clinical decision rules. JAMA. 2000;284(1):79-84. PMID 10872017.
41. Agency for Healthcare Research and Quality. Methods guide for Effectiveness and Comparative Effectiveness Reviews. AHRQ Publication No. 10(13)-EHC063-EF. Rockville, MD: Agency for Healthcare Research and Quality. November 2013. Chapters available at: www.effectivehealthcare.ahrq.gov. Accessed September 19, 2014.
42. Atkins D, Chang SM, Gartlehner G, et al. Assessing applicability when comparing medical interventions: AHRQ and the Effective Health Care Program. J Clin Epidemiol. 2011;64(11):1198-1207. PMID 21463926.
43. Furlan A, Chaparro LE, Irvin E, Mailis-Gagnon A. A comparison between enriched and nonenriched enrollment randomized withdrawal trials of opioids for chronic noncancer pain. Pain Res Manag. 2011;16(5):337-351. PMID 22059206.
44. Edlund MJ, Martin BC, Russo JE, Devries A, Braden JB, Sullivan M, D. The role of opioid prescription in incident opioid abuse and dependence among individuals with chronic noncancer pain. Clin J Pain. 2014;30(7):557-564. PMID 24281273.
45. Dunn KM, Saunders KW, Rutter CM, et al. Opioid prescriptions for chronic pain and overdose: a cohort study. Ann Intern Med. 2010;152(2):85-92. PMID 20083827.
46. Li L, Setoguchi S, Cabral H, Jick S. Opioid use for noncancer pain and risk of fracture in adults: a nested case-control study using the general practice research database. Am J Epidemiol. 2013;178(4):559-569. PMID 23639937.
47. Li L, Setoguchi S, Cabral H, Jick S. Opioid use for noncancer pain and risk of myocardial infarction amongst adults. J Intern Med. 2013;273(5):511-526. PMID 23331508.
48. Carman WJ, Su S, Cook SF, Wurzelmann JI, McAfee A. Coronary heart disease outcomes among chronic opioid and cyclooxygenase-2 users compared with a general population cohort. Pharmacoepidemiol Drug Saf. 2011;20(7):754-762. PMID 21567652.
49. Gomes T, Mamdani MM, Dhalla IA, Paterson JM, Juurlink DN. Opioid dose and drug-related mortality in patients with nonmalignant pain. Arch Intern Med. 2011;171(7):686-691. PMID 21482846.
50. Martell BA, O'Connor PG, Kerns RD, et al. Systematic review: opioid treatment for chronic back pain: prevalence, efficacy, and association with addiction. Ann Intern Med. 2007;146(2):116-127. PMID 17227935.
51. Banta-Green CJ, Merrill JO, Doyle SR, Boudreau DM, Calsyn DA. Opioid use behaviors, mental health and pain--development of a typology of chronic pain patients. Drug Alcohol Depend. 2009;104(1-2):34-42. PMID 19473786.
52. Boscarino JA, Rukstalis M, Hoffman SN, et al. Risk factors for drug dependence among out-patients on opioid therapy in a large U.S. health-care system. Addiction. 2010;105(10):1776-1782. PMID 20712819.
53. Compton PA, Wu SM, Schieffer B, Pham Q, Naliboff BD. Introduction of a self-report version of the Prescription Drug Use Questionnaire and relationship to medication agreement noncompliance. J Pain Symptom Manag. 2008;36(4):383-395. PMID 18508231.
54. Cowan DT, Wilson-Barnett J, Griffiths P, Allan LG. A survey of chronic noncancer pain patients prescribed opioid analgesics. Pain Medicine. 2003;4(4):340-351. PMID 14750910.
55. Fleming MF, Balousek SL, Klessig CL, Mundt MP, Brown DD. Substance use disorders in a primary care sample receiving daily opioid therapy. J Pain. 2007;8(7):573-582. PMID 17499555.
56. Hojsted J, Nielsen PR, Guldstrand SK, Frich L, Sjogren P. Classification and identification of opioid addiction in chronic pain patients. Eur J Pain. 2010;14(10):1014-1020. PMID 20494598.
57. Portenoy RK, Farrar JT, Backonja MM, et al. Long-term use of controlled-release oxycodone for noncancer pain: results of a 3-year registry study. Clin J Pain. 2007;23(4):287-299. PMID 17449988.
58. Saffier K, Colombo C, Brown D, Mundt MP, Fleming MF. Addiction Severity Index in a chronic pain sample receiving opioid therapy. J Subst Abuse Treat. 2007;33(3):303-311. PMID 17376639.
59. Schneider JP, Kirsh KL. Defining clinical issues around tolerance, hyperalgesia, and addiction: a quantitative and qualitative

59. outcome study of long-term opioid dosing in a chronic pain practice. J Opioid Manag. 2010;6(6):385-395. PMID 21268999.
60. Wasan AD, Butler SF, Budman SH, et al. Does report of craving opioid medication predict aberrant drug behavior among chronic pain patients? Clin J Pain. 2009;25(3):193-198. PMID 19333168.
61. American Psychiatric Association. Diagnostic and statistical manual of mental disorders, Fifth Edition. Arlington, VA: Amerian Psychiatric Association; 2013.
62. Naliboff BD, Wu SM, Schieffer B, et al. A randomized trial of 2 prescription strategies for opioid treatment of chronic nonmalignant pain. J Pain. 2011;12(2):288-296. PMID 21111684.
63. Franklin GM, Mai J, Turner J, Sullivan M, Wickizer T, Fulton-Kehoe D. Bending the prescription opioid dosing and mortality curves: impact of the Washington State opioid dosing guideline. Am J Ind Med. 2012;55(4):325-331. PMID 22213274.
64. Allan L, Richarz U, Simpson K, Slappendel R. Transdermal fentanyl versus sustained release oral morphine in strong-opioid naive patients with chronic low back pain. Spine (Phila Pa 1976). 2005;30(22):2484-2490. PMID 16284584.
65. Mitra F, Chowdhury S, Shelley M, Williams G. A feasibility study of transdermal buprenorphine versus transdermal fentanyl in the long-term management of persistent non-cancer pain. Pain Med. 2013;14(1):75-83. PMID 23320402.
66. Wild JE, Grond S, Kuperwasser B, et al. Long-term safety and tolerability of tapentadol extended release for the management of chronic low back pain or osteoarthritis pain. Pain Pract. 2010;10(5):416-427. PMID 20602712.
67. Chou R, Cruciani RA, Fiellin DA, et al. Methadone safety: a clinical practice guideline from the American Pain Society and College on Problems of Drug Dependence, in collaboration with the Heart Rhythm Society. J Pain. 2014;15(4):321-337. PMID 24685458.
68. Chou R, Weimer MB, Dana T. Methadone overdose and cardiac arrhythmia potential: findings from a review of the evidence for an American Pain Society and College on Problems of Drug Dependence clinical practice guideline. J Pain. 2014;15(4):338-365. PMID 24685459.
69. Krebs EE, Becker WC, Zerzan J, Bair MJ, McCoy K, Hui S. Comparative mortality among Department of Veterans Affairs patients prescribed methadone or long-acting morphine for chronic pain. Pain. Aug;152(8):1789-1795. PMID 21524850.
70. Ashburn MA, Slevin KA, Messina J, Xie F. The efficacy and safety of fentanyl buccal tablet compared with immediate-release oxycodone for the management of breakthrough pain in opioid-tolerant patients with chronic pain. Anesth Analg. 2011;112(3):693-702. PMID 21304148.
71. Davies A, Sitte T, Elsner F, et al. Consistency of efficacy, patient acceptability, and nasal tolerability of fentanyl pectin nasal spray compared with immediate-release morphine sulfate in breakthrough cancer pain. J Pain Symptom Manag. 2011;41(2):358-366. PMID 21334555.
72. Portenoy RK, Messina J, Xie F, Peppin J. Fentanyl buccal tablet (FBT) for relief of breakthrough pain in opioid-treated patients with chronic low back pain: a randomized, placebo-controlled study. Curr Med Res Opin. 2007;23(1):223-233. PMID 17207304.
73. Simpson DM, Messina J, Xie F, Hale M. Fentanyl buccal tablet for the relief of breakthrough pain in opioid-tolerant adult patients with chronic neuropathic pain: a multicenter, randomized, double-blind, placebo-controlled study. Clin Ther. 2007;29(4):588-601. PMID 17617282.
74. Webster LR, Slevin KA, Narayana A, Earl CQ, Yang R. Fentanyl buccal tablet compared with immediate-release oxycodone for the management of breakthrough pain in opioid-tolerant patients with chronic cancer and noncancer pain: a randomized, double-blind, crossover study followed by a 12-week open-label phase to evaluate patient outcomes. Pain Med. 2013;14(9):1332-1345. PMID 23855816.
75. U.S. Food and Drug Administration. Public Health Advisory: Important Information for the Safe Use of Fentora (fentanyl buccal tablets). 2013. Available at:http://www.fda.gov/Drugs/DrugSafety/PostmarketDrugSafetyInformationforPatientsandProviders/DrugSafetyInformationforHeathcareProfessionals/PublicHealthAdvisories/ucm051273.htm. Accessed on May 22, 2014.

76. Jones T, Moore T. Preliminary data on a new opioid risk assessment measure: the Brief Risk Interview. J Opioid Manag. 2013;9(1):19-27. PMID 23709300.
77. Moore TM, Jones T, Browder JH, Daffron S, Passik SD. A comparison of common screening methods for predicting aberrant drug-related behavior among patients receiving opioids for chronic pain management. Pain Med. 2009;10(8):1426-1433. PMID 20021601.
78. Webster LR, Webster RM. Predicting aberrant behaviors in opioid-treated patients: preliminary validation of the Opioid Risk Tool. Pain Med. 2005;6(6):432-442. PMID 16336480.
79. Butler SF, Budman SH, Fanciullo GJ, Jamison RN. Cross validation of the current opioid misuse measure to monitor chronic pain patients on opioid therapy. Clin J Pain. 2010;26(9):770-776. PMID 20842012.
80. Butler SF, Budman SH, Fernandez KC, Fanciullo GJ, Jamison RN. Cross-validation of a screener to predict opioid misuse in chronic pain patients (SOAPP-R). J Addict Med. 2009;3(2):66-73. PMID 20161199.
81. Fleming MF, Davis J, Passik SD. Reported lifetime aberrant drug-taking behaviors are predictive of current substance use and mental health problems in primary care patients. Pain Med. 2008;9(8):1098-1106. PMID 18721174.
82. Meltzer EC, Rybin D, Saitz R, et al. Identifying prescription opioid use disorder in primary care: diagnostic characteristics of the Current Opioid Misuse Measure (COMM). Pain. 2011;152(2):397-402. PMID 21177035.
83. Butler SF, Budman SH, Fernandez KC, et al. Development and validation of the Current Opioid Misuse Measure. Pain. 2007;130(1-2):144-156. PMID 17493754.
84. Holmes CP, Gatchel RJ, Adams LL, et al. An opioid screening instrument: long-term evaluation of the utility of the Pain Medication Questionnaire. Pain Pract. 2006;6(2):74-88. PMID 17309714.
85. Butler SF, Fernandez K, Benoit C, Budman SH, Jamison RN. Validation of the revised Screener and Opioid Assessment for Patients with Pain (SOAPP-R). J Pain. 2008;9(4):360-372. PMID 18203666.
86. Reifler LM, Droz D, Bailey JE, et al. Do prescription monitoring programsi mpact State trends in opioid abuse/misuse? Pain Med. 2012;13(3):434-442. PMID 22299725.
87. Deyo RA, Smith DH, Johnson ES, et al. Opioids for back pain patients: primary care prescribing patterns and use of services. J Am Board Fam Med. 2011;24(6):717-727. PMID 22086815.
88. Seal KH, Shi Y, Cohen G, et al. Association of mental health disorders with prescription opioids and high-risk opioid use in us veterans of Iraq and Afghanistan. JAMA. 2012;307(9):940-947. PMID 22396516.
89. Sullivan MD, Edlund MJ, Zhang L, Unutzer J, Wells KB. Association between mental health disorders, problem drug use, and regular prescription opioid use. Arch Intern Med. 2006;166(19):2087-2093. PMID 17060538.
90. Morasco BJ, Duckart JP, Carr TP, Deyo RA, Dobscha SK. Clinical characteristics of veterans prescribed high doses of opioid medications for chronic non-cancer pain. Pain. 2010;151(3):625-632. PMID 20801580.
91. Carson S, Thakurta S, Low A, Smith B, Chou R. Drug Class Review: Long-Acting Opioid Analgesics: Final Update 6 Report. Portland, OR: Oregon Health & Science University; 2011. PMID: 21977550.
92. Fishbain DA, Cole B, Lewis J, Rosomoff HL, Rosomoff RS. What percentage of chronic nonmalignant pain patients exposed to chronic opioid analgesic therapy develop abuse/addiction and/or aberrant drug-related behaviors? A structured evidence-based review. Pain Med. 2008;9(4):444-459. PMID 18489635.
93. Turk DC, Swanson KS, Gatchel RJ. Predicting opioid misuse by chronic pain patients: a systematic review and literature synthesis. Clin J Pain. 2008;24(6):497-508. PMID 18574359.
94. Wiedemer NL, Harden PS, Arndt IO, Gallagher RM. The opioid renewal clinic: a primary care, managed approach to opioid therapy in chronic pain patients at risk for substance abuse. Pain Med. 2007;8(7):573-584. PMID 17883742.
95. Goldberg KC, Simel DL, Oddone EZ. Effect of an opioid management system on opioid prescribing and unscheduled visits in a large primary care clinic. JCOM. 2005;12(12): 621-628.
96. Manchikanti L, Manchukonda R, Damron KS, Brandon D, McManus CD, Cash K. Does adherence monitoring reduce controlled substance abuse in chronic pain

97. patients? Pain Physician. 2006;9(1):57-60. PMID 16700282.
97. Manchikanti L, Manchukonda R, Pampati V, et al. Does random urine drug testing reduce illicit drug use in chronic pain patients receiving opioids? Pain Physician. 2006;9(2):123-129. PMID 16703972.
98. Paulozzi LJ, Kilbourne EM, Shah NG, et al. A history of being prescribed controlled substances and risk of drug overdose death. Pain Med. 2012;13(1):87-95. PMID 22026451.
99. Byas-Smith MG, Chapman SL, Reed B, Cotsonis G. The effect of opioids on driving and psychomotor performance in patients with chronic pain. Clin J Pain. 2005;21(4):345-352. PMID 15951653.
100. Gaertner J, Frank M, Bosse B, et al. [Oral controlled-release oxycodone for the treatment of chronic pain. Data from 4196 patients]. Schmerz. 2006;20(1):61-68. PMID 15926076.
101. Galski T, Williams JB, Ehle HT. Effects of opioids on driving ability. J Pain Symptom Manage. 2000;19(3):200-208. PMID 10760625.
102. Sabatowski R, Schwalen S, Rettig K, Herberg KW, Kasper SM, Radbruch L. Driving ability under long-term treatment with transdermal fentanyl. J Pain Symptom Manage. 2003;25(1):38-47. PMID 12565187.
103. Menefee LA, Frank ED, Crerand C, et al. The effects of transdermal fentanyl on driving, cognitive performance, and balance in patients with chronic nonmalignant pain conditions. Pain Med. 2004;5(1):42-49. PMID 14996236.
104. Pablos-Mendez A, Barr RG, Shea S. Run-in periods in randomized trials: implications for hte application of results in clinical practice. JAMA. 1998;279(3):222-225. PMID 9438743.
105. Chou R, Fanciullo GJ, Fine PG, Miaskowski C, Passik SD, Portenoy RK. Opioids for chronic noncancer pain: prediction and identification of aberrant drug-related behaviors: a review of the evidence for an American Pain Society and American Academy of Pain Medicine clinical practice guideline. J Pain. 2009;10(2):131-146. PMID 19187890.
106. Furlan AD, Reardon R, Weppler C. Opioids for chronic noncancer pain: a new Canadian practice guideline. CMAJ. 2010;182(9):923-930. PMID 20439443.
107. Nuckols TK, Anderson L, Popescu I, et al. Opioid prescribing: a systematic review and critical appraisal of guidelines for chronic pain. Annals Intern Med. 2014;160(1):38-47. PMID 24217469.
108. O'Connor AB, Turk DC, Dworkin RH, et al. Abuse liability measures for use in analgesic clinical trials in patients with pain: IMMPACT Recommendations. Pain. 2013;154(11):2324-2334. PMID 24148704.
109. Cicero TJ, Ellis MS, Surratt HL. Effect of abuse-deterrent formulation of OxyContin. N Engl J Med. 2012;367(2):187-189. PMID 22784140.
110. Roland M, Torgerson DJ. Understanding controlled trials: What are pragmatic trials? BMJ. 1998;316:285. PMID 947251

Introduction

Background

Chronic pain, often defined as pain lasting longer than 3 months or past the time of normal tissue healing,[1] is extremely common. According to a recent Institute of Medicine report, up to one-third of U.S. adults report chronic pain.[2] Chronic pain is a major cause of decreased quality of life and disability and is often refractory to treatment.[3,4] There has been a dramatic increase over the past 10 to 20 years in the prescription of opioid medications for chronic pain,[5-7] despite limited evidence showing long-term beneficial effects.[8,9] In addition, accumulating evidence indicates that prescription opioids may be associated with important harms, including accidental overdose, abuse, addiction, diversion, and accidents involving injuries (such as falls and motor vehicle accidents).[10-20] Perhaps of most concern is the dramatic increase in overdose deaths associated with opioids. In 2011, there were 16,917 fatal overdoses involving prescription opioids.[21] Prescription opioid misuse and abuse resulted in almost 660,000 emergency department visits in 2010, over twice as many as in 2004.[13] Substance abuse treatment admissions for opiates other than heroin increased more than six-fold from 1999 to 2009.[12] Opioids are also associated with adverse effects such as constipation, nausea, and sedation.[22] Finally, data indicate potential associations between long-term opioid therapy and other harms, such as adverse endocrinological effects and hyperalgesia.[23-25]

These data underscore the complexity of clinical decisionmaking around long-term opioid therapy, which requires individualized assessments of the balance between benefits and harms; appropriate opioid selection, dose initiation, and titration strategies; integration of risk assessment and mitigation strategies; and consideration of the use of alternative, nonopioid therapies.[9] Risk mitigation strategies that have been suggested for patients prescribed long-term opioids include use of opioid medication agreements, application of dose thresholds that warrant increased caution, regular clinical followup and monitoring, urine drug screens, use of abuse-deterrent opioid formulations, and use of data from prescription drug monitoring programs.[9]

Understanding benefits and harms of long-term opioid therapy for chronic pain is a challenge because effects may vary depending on patient characteristics (e.g., age, sex, pain condition, psychosocial factors, comorbidities), opioid characteristics (e.g., specific opioid, short- versus long-acting opioid, mode of administration, dose), dosing strategies (e.g., round-the-clock versus as-needed dosing, application of dose thresholds), concomitant therapies (e.g., use of benzodiazepines or other drugs that may interact with opioids), and characteristics of the clinical setting. Other challenges in interpreting the literature include potential limitations in generalizability due to study design and other methodological shortcomings (e.g., duration of followup, exclusion of patients at higher risk for harms, under-representation of certain sociodemographic groups, and high dropout rates), and gaps in research on important scientific questions.[26] Although guidelines on use of opioids for chronic pain are available, most recommendations are based on weak or limited evidence.[9,27] The increase in use of long-term opioid therapy for chronic pain, new information concerning harms associated with long-term opioid therapy, continued wide variations in practice related to long-term opioid therapy, and the availability of new evidence underscore the need for a current systematic review in this area.

The purpose of this report is to systematically review the current evidence on long-term opioid therapy for chronic pain, which will be used by the National Institutes of Health (NIH) to inform a Pathways to Prevention Workshop on the role of opioids in the treatment of chronic pain. Although guidelines have been published from the American Pain Society (APS)/

American Academy of Pain Medicine,[9] the Veterans Affairs (VA)/Department of Defense,[28] and other groups, the availability of new evidence warrants a new systematic review that could be used to inform updated or new guidelines, guide quality improvement efforts, and define and update priorities for further research in this area.[26] This review updates a prior systematic review on opioid therapy for chronic pain funded by the APS.[29] Differences between this review and the 2009 APS review are that it focuses specifically on benefits and harms associated with long-term use of opioid therapy and evaluates an additional Key Question on dose escalation versus maintenance of doses in patients on long-term opioid therapy, additional outcomes (e.g., cardiovascular events, infection, and psychological outcomes), and additional risk mitigation strategies (e.g., abuse-deterrent formulations and use of data from prescription drug monitoring programs).

Scope of Review and Key Questions

The Key Questions and analytic framework (Figure 1) used to guide this report are shown below. The analytic framework shows the target populations, interventions, and outcomes that we examined.

Key Question 1. Effectiveness and Comparative Effectiveness

a. In patients with chronic pain, what is the effectiveness of long-term opioid therapy versus placebo or no opioid therapy for long-term (≥1 year) outcomes related to pain, function, and quality of life?
b. How does effectiveness vary depending on: (1) the specific type or cause of pain (e.g., neuropathic, musculoskeletal [including low back pain], fibromyalgia, sickle cell disease, inflammatory pain, and headache disorders); (2) patient demographics (e.g., age, race, ethnicity, gender); (3) patient comorbidities (including past or current alcohol or substance use disorders, mental health disorders, medical comorbidities and high risk for addiction)?
c. In patients with chronic pain, what is the comparative effectiveness of opioids versus nonopioid therapies (pharmacological or nonpharmacological) on outcomes related to pain, function, and quality of life?
d. In patients with chronic pain, what is the comparative effectiveness of opioids plus nonopioid interventions (pharmacological or nonpharmacological) versus opioids or nonopioid interventions alone on outcomes related to pain, function, quality of life, and doses of opioids used?

Key Question 2. Harms and Adverse Events

a. In patients with chronic pain, what are the risks of opioids versus placebo or no opioid on: (1) opioid abuse, addiction, and related outcomes; (2) overdose; and (3) other harms, including gastrointestinal-related harms, falls, fractures, motor vehicle accidents, endocrinological harms, infections, cardiovascular events, cognitive harms, and psychological harms (e.g., depression)?
b. How do harms vary depending on: (1) the specific type or cause of pain (e.g., neuropathic, musculoskeletal [including back pain], fibromyalgia, sickle cell disease, inflammatory pain, headache disorders); (2) patient demographics; (3) patient comorbidities (including past or current substance use disorder or at high risk for addiction); 4) the dose of opioids used?

Key Question 3. Dosing Strategies

a. In patients with chronic pain, what is the comparative effectiveness of different methods for initiating and titrating opioids for outcomes related to pain, function, and quality of life; risk of overdose, addiction, abuse, or misuse; and doses of opioids used?
b. In patients with chronic pain, what is the comparative effectiveness of short- versus long-acting opioids on outcomes related to pain, function, and quality of life; risk of overdose, addiction, abuse, or misuse; and doses of opioids used?
c. In patients with chronic pain, what is the comparative effectiveness of different long-acting opioids on outcomes related to pain, function, and quality of life; and risk of overdose, addiction, abuse, or misuse?
d. In patients with chronic pain, what is the comparative effectiveness of short- plus long-acting opioids versus long-acting opioids alone on outcomes related to pain, function, and quality of life; risk of overdose, addiction, abuse, or misuse; and doses of opioids used?
e. In patients with chronic pain, what is the comparative effectiveness of scheduled, continuous versus as-needed dosing of opioids on outcomes related to pain, function, and quality of life; risk of overdose, addiction, abuse, or misuse; and doses of opioids used?
f. In patients with chronic pain on long-term opioid therapy, what is the comparative effectiveness of dose escalation versus dose maintenance or use of dose thresholds on outcomes related to pain, function, and quality of life?
g. In patients on long-term opioid therapy, what is the comparative effectiveness of opioid rotation versus maintenance of current opioid therapy on outcomes related to pain, function, and quality of life; and doses of opioids used?
h. In patients on long-term opioid therapy, what is the comparative effectiveness of different strategies for treating acute exacerbations of chronic pain on outcomes related to pain, function, and quality of life?
i. In patients on long-term opioid therapy, what are the effects of decreasing opioid doses or of tapering off opioids versus continuation of opioids on outcomes related to pain, function, quality of life, and withdrawal?
j. In patients on long-term opioid therapy, what is the comparative effectiveness of different tapering protocols and strategies on measures related to pain, function, quality of life, withdrawal symptoms, and likelihood of opioid cessation?

Key Question 4. Risk Assessment and Risk Mitigation Strategies

a. In patients with chronic pain being considered for long-term opioid therapy, what is the accuracy of instruments for predicting risk of opioid overdose, addiction, abuse, or misuse?
b. In patients with chronic pain, what is the effectiveness of use of risk prediction instruments on outcomes related to overdose, addiction, abuse, or misuse?
c. In patients with chronic pain prescribed long-term opioid therapy, what is the effectiveness of risk mitigation strategies, including (1) opioid management plans, (2) patient education, (3) urine drug screening, (4) use of prescription drug monitoring program data, (5) use of monitoring instruments, (6) more frequent monitoring intervals, (7) pill counts, and (8) use of abuse-deterrent formulations on outcomes related to overdose, addiction, abuse, or misuse?
d. What is the comparative effectiveness of treatment strategies for managing patients with addiction to prescription opioids on outcomes related to overdose, abuse, misuse, pain, function, and quality of life?

Figure 1. Analytic framework

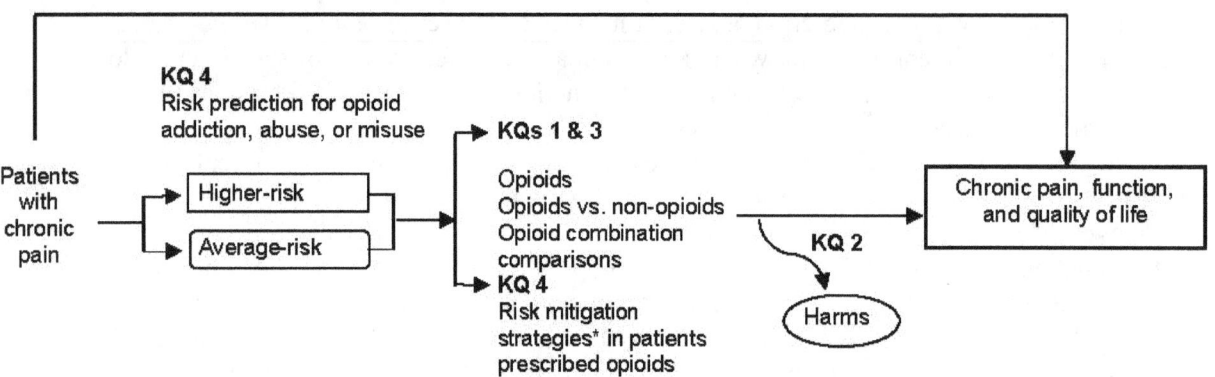

KQ, Key Question.

*Including opioid management plans, patient education, urine drug screening, use of prescription drug monitoring program data, use of monitoring instruments, more frequent monitoring intervals, pill counts, and use of abuse-deterrent formulations.

Methods

The methods for this Comparative Effectiveness Review (CER) follows the methods suggested in the Agency for Healthcare Research and Quality (AHRQ) Methods Guide for Effectiveness and Comparative Effectiveness Reviews.[30] All methods were determined a priori.

Topic Refinement and Review Protocol

This topic was selected for review based on a nomination from NIH. The initial Key Questions for this CER were developed with input from an NIH working group. The Key Questions and scope were further developed with input from a Technical Expert Panel (TEP) convened for this report. The TEP provided high-level content and methodological guidance to the review process and consisted of experts in health services research, internal medicine, psychology, pain medicine, pharmacology, neurology, occupational medicine, pediatrics, and epidemiology. TEP members disclosed all financial or other conflicts of interest prior to participation. The AHRQ Task Order Officer and the investigators reviewed the disclosures and determined that the TEP members had no conflicts of interest that precluded participation.

The protocol for this CER was developed prior to initiation of the review, and was posted on the AHRQ Web site on December 19, 2013 at: http://effectivehealthcare.ahrq.gov/ehc/products/557/1837/chronic-pain-opioid-treatment-protocol-131219.pdf. The protocol was also registered in the PROSPERO international database of prospectively registered systematic reviews.[31]

Literature Search Strategy

A research librarian conducted searches in Ovid MEDLINE, the Cochrane Central Register of Controlled Trials, the Cochrane Database of Systematic Reviews, PsychINFO, and CINAHL from 2008 to August 2014 (see Appendix A for full search strategies). We restricted search start dates to January 2008 because the searches in the prior APS review, which we used to identify potentially relevant studies, went through October 2008.[29] For outcomes (cardiovascular, infections, and psychological harms) and interventions (abuse-deterrent formulations, and use of prescription monitoring program data) not addressed in the APS review, we searched the same databases and did not apply any search date start restrictions.

We also hand-searched the reference lists of relevant studies and searched for unpublished studies in ClinicalTrials.gov. Scientific information packets (SIPs) with relevant published and unpublished studies were requested from nineteen current application holders from the U.S. Food and Drug Administration (FDA) Risk Evaluation and Mitigation Strategy (REMS) Extended-Release and Long-Acting (ER/LA) Opioid Analgesics List.[32] We received five SIP submissions.

Study Selection

We developed criteria for inclusion and exclusion of articles based on the Key Questions and the populations, interventions, comparators, outcomes, timing, and setting (PICOTS) approach (Appendix B). Articles were selected for full-text review if they were about long-term opioid therapy for chronic pain, were relevant to a Key Question, and met the predefined inclusion criteria as shown below. We excluded studies published only as conference abstracts, restricted inclusion to English-language articles, and excluded studies of nonhuman subjects. Studies had to report original data to be included.

Each abstract was independently reviewed for potential inclusion and full-text review by two investigators. Two investigators independently reviewed all full-text articles for final inclusion. Discrepancies were resolved through discussion and consensus. A list of the included articles is available in Appendix C; excluded articles are shown Appendix D with primary reasons for exclusion.

We selected studies of adults (age ≥18 years) with chronic pain (defined as pain lasting >3 months) being considered for long-term opioid therapy (Key Questions 4a and 4b) or prescribed long-term opioid therapy (all other Key Questions). We defined long-term opioid therapy as use of opioids on most days for >3 months; this threshold was selected to differentiate ongoing opioid therapy (as often used for chronic pain) from short-term therapy. We included studies that did not explicitly report the duration of pain if the average duration of opioid therapy was >3 months. We included studies that did not explicitly report the duration of opioid therapy if patients were prescribed long-acting opioids, as these are not typically prescribed for short-term use. We included studies with patients with chronic pain related to current or previously treated cancer, but excluded studies with patients with pain at end of life (e.g., patients with cancer in hospice care). We excluded studies with patients with acute pain, pregnant or breastfeeding women, and patients treated with opioids for addiction.

We included studies of patients prescribed any long- or short-acting opioid used as long-term therapy, either alone or in combination with another agent (Key Question 1d). We included tapentadol, a dual mechanism medication with strong opioid mu-receptor affinity, but excluded tramadol, which is also a dual mechanism medication but with weak opioid mu-receptor affinity that has not been identified as a cause of unintentional prescription drug overdose deaths.[33] We also excluded studies of parenteral opioids.

We included studies that compared long-term opioid therapy versus placebo, no therapy, or another drug or nondrug therapy; studies that evaluated different dose initiation, titration, or rotation strategies; studies of different methods for tapering or discontinuing opioids; studies on methods for treating acute exacerbations of pain in people with chronic pain; and studies on various risk mitigation strategies for reducing harms associated with opioids. Risk mitigation strategies included opioid management plans, patient education, urine drug screening, use of prescription drug monitoring program data, use of monitoring instruments, more frequent monitoring intervals, pill counts, and use of abuse-deterrent formulations. We also included studies that compared the predictive accuracy of risk prediction instruments in people with chronic pain prior to initiation of opioids for predicting outcomes related to future misuse, abuse, or addiction, and studies on the effects of risk prediction instruments on clinical outcomes.

Outcomes were pain (intensity, severity, bothersomeness), function (physical disability, activity limitations, activity interference, work function), quality of life (including depression), and doses of opioids used. Evaluated harms included overdose, opioid use disorder, addiction, abuse, and misuse, as well as other opioid-related harms (including gastrointestinal, fractures, falls, motor vehicle accidents, endocrinological harms, infections, cardiovascular events, cognitive harms, and psychological harms [e.g., depression]). We focused on outcomes reported after at least 1 year of opioid therapy, with the exception of outcomes related to overdose and injuries (fractures, falls, and motor vehicle accidents), studies on treatment of acute exacerbations of chronic pain, studies on dose initiation and titration, and studies on discontinuation of opioid therapy, for which we included studies of any duration.

For all Key Questions, we included randomized trials and controlled observational studies (cohort studies, cross-sectional studies, and case-control studies) that performed adjustment on potential confounders. We included uncontrolled observational studies of patients with chronic pain prescribed opioid therapy for at least 1 year that reported abuse, misuse, or addiction as a primary outcome and described predefined methods to assess these outcomes. Otherwise, we excluded uncontrolled observational studies, case series, and case reports. We reviewed systematic reviews for potentially relevant references.

Data Extraction

We extracted the following information from included studies into evidence tables using Excel spreadsheets: study design, year, setting, inclusion and exclusion criteria, population characteristics (including sex, age, race, pain condition, and duration of pain), sample size, duration of followup, attrition, intervention characteristics (including specific opioid and formulation, dose, and duration of therapy), results, and funding sources.

For studies on the predictive accuracy of risk prediction instruments, we attempted to create two-by-two tables from information provided (sample size, prevalence, sensitivity, and specificity) and compared calculated measures of diagnostic accuracy based on the two-by-two tables with reported results. We noted discrepancies between calculated and reported results when present. When reported, we also recorded the area under the receiver operating characteristic curve (AUROC).[34, 35]

For studies of interventions, we calculated relative risks (RR) and associated 95 percent confidence intervals (CI) based on the information provided (sample sizes and incidence of outcomes of interest in each intervention group). We noted discrepancies between calculated and reported results when present.

Data extraction for each study was performed by two investigators. The first investigator extracted the data, and the second investigator independently reviewed the extracted data for accuracy and completeness.

Assessing Methodological Risk of Bias of Individual Studies

We assessed risk of bias (quality) for each study using predefined criteria. We used the term "quality" rather than the alternate term "risk of bias;" both refer to internal validity. Randomized trials were evaluated with criteria and methods developed by the Cochrane Back Review Group.[36] Cohort studies, case-control studies, and cross-sectional studies were rated using criteria from the U.S. Preventive Services Task Force.[37] Risk prediction instrument studies were rated using criteria from various sources.[38-40] These criteria were applied in conjunction with the approach recommended in the chapter, Assessing the Risk of Bias of Individual Studies When Comparing Medical Interventions,[41] in the AHRQ Methods Guide. Studies of predictive accuracy of risk prediction instruments were assessed using an approach adapted from the AHRQ Methods Guide for Medical Test Reviews,[38] which is based on methods developed by the Quality Assessment of Diagnostic Accuracy Studies (QUADAS) group.[39] We reassessed the quality of studies included in the prior APS review to ensure consistency in quality assessment. Two investigators independently assessed the quality of each study. Discrepancies were resolved through discussion and consensus.

Individual studies were rated as having "poor," "fair," or "good" quality. We rated the quality of each randomized trial based on the methods used for randomization, allocation concealment, and blinding; the similarity of compared groups at baseline; whether attrition was adequately reported and acceptable; similarity in use of cointerventions; compliance to allocated treatments; the use of intent-to-treat analysis; and avoidance of selective outcomes reporting.[36,37]

We rated the quality of each cohort study based on whether it enrolled a consecutive or random sample of patients meeting inclusion criteria; whether it evaluated comparable groups; whether rates of loss to followup were reported and acceptable; whether it used accurate methods for ascertaining exposures, potential confounders, and outcomes; and whether it performed adjustment for important potential confounders.[37] For cross-sectional studies, we used criteria for cohort studies, but did not rate criteria related to loss to followup. For uncontrolled studies on risk of abuse or related outcomes, we evaluated whether it enrolled a consecutive or random sample, whether outcome assessors were blinded to patient characteristics, whether rates of loss to followup were reported (for longitudinal studies) and acceptable, and whether pre-specified outcomes were assessed in all patients.

We rated the quality of each case-control study based on whether it enrolled a consecutive or random sample of cases meeting predefined criteria; whether controls were derived from the same population as cases; whether cases and controls were comparable on key prognostic factors; whether it used accurate methods to ascertain outcomes, exposures, and potential confounders; and whether it performed adjustment for important potential confounders.[37]

We rated the quality of each study on the predictive value of risk prediction instruments based on whether it evaluated a consecutive or random sample of patients meeting pre-defined criteria, whether the patient population evaluated in the study was adequately described, whether the screening instrument included appropriate criteria, and whether outcomes were assessed in all patients independent of the results of the risk assessment instrument using adequately described methods.[38,39] We also evaluated whether the study was to develop a risk prediction instrument or to validate a previously developed instrument.[40]

Studies rated "good quality" were considered to have the least risk of bias and their results are likely to be valid. Studies rated "fair quality" have some methodological shortcomings, but no flaw or combination of flaws judged likely to cause major bias. In some cases, the article did not report important information, making it difficult to assess its methods or potential limitations. The moderate risk of bias category is broad and studies with this rating vary in their strengths and weaknesses; the results of some studies assessed to have moderate risk of bias are likely to be valid, while others may be only possibly valid. Studies rated "poor quality" have significant flaws that may invalidate the results. They have a serious or "fatal" flaw or combination of flaws in design, analysis, or reporting; large amounts of missing information; or serious discrepancies in reporting. The results of these studies are at least as likely to reflect flaws in the study design as the differences between the compared interventions. We did not exclude studies rated as having high risk of bias a priori, but they were considered the least reliable when synthesizing the evidence, particularly when discrepancies between studies were present.

Assessing Research Applicability

We recorded factors important for understanding the applicability of studies, such as whether the publication adequately described the study sample, the country in which the study was conducted, the characteristics of the patient sample (e.g., age, sex, race, pain condition, duration or severity of pain, medical comorbidities, and psychosocial factors), the characteristics of the interventions used (e.g., specific opioid, dose, mode of administration, or dosing strategy), the clinical setting (e.g., primary care or specialty setting), and the magnitude of effects on clinical outcomes.[42] We also recorded the funding source and role of the sponsor. We did not assign a rating of applicability (such as high or low) because applicability may differ based on the user of the report.

Evidence Synthesis and Rating the Body of Evidence

We constructed evidence tables summarizing study characteristics, results, and quality ratings for all included studies. We summarized evidence for each Key Question qualitatively used a hierarchy-of-evidence approach, where the best evidence was the focus of our synthesis for each Key Question. In the evidence tables, we included relevant studies from the prior APS review as well as new studies meeting inclusion criteria. Results were organized by Key Question. We did not attempt meta-analyses because of the small number of studies available for each Key Question; variability in study designs, patient samples, interventions, and measures; and methodological shortcomings in the available studies.

We assessed the overall strength of evidence (SOE) for each Key Question and outcome using the approach described in the AHRQ Methods Guide.[30] We synthesized the quality of the studies; the consistency of results within and between study designs; the directness of the evidence linking the intervention and health outcomes; and the precision of the estimate of effect (based on the number and size of studies and CIs for the estimates). We were not able to formally assess for publication bias due to small number of studies, methodological shortcomings, or differences across studies in designs, measured outcomes, and other factors. Rather, as described above, we searched for unpublished studies through searches of clinical trials registries and regulatory documents and by soliciting SIPs.

The SOE was based on the overall quality of each body of evidence, based on the risk of bias (graded low, moderate, or high); the consistency of results across studies (graded consistent, inconsistent, or unable to determine when only one study was available); the directness of the evidence linking the intervention and health outcomes (graded direct or indirect); and the precision of the estimate of effect, based on the number and size of studies and CIs for the estimates (graded precise or imprecise). We did not grade supplemental domains for cohort studies evaluating intermediate and clinical outcomes because too few studies were available for these factors to impact the SOE grades.

We graded the SOE for each Key Question using the four key categories recommended in the AHRQ Methods Guide.[30] A "high" grade indicates high confidence that the evidence reflects the true effect and that further research is very unlikely to change our confidence in the estimate of effect. A "moderate" grade indicates moderate confidence that the evidence reflects the true effect and further research may change our confidence in the estimate of effect and may change the estimate. A "low" grade indicates low confidence that the evidence reflects the true effect and further research is likely to change the confidence in the estimate of effect and is likely to change the estimate. An "insufficient" grade indicates evidence either is unavailable or is too limited to permit any conclusion, due to the availability of only poor-quality studies, extreme inconsistency, or extreme imprecision.

Peer Review and Public Commentary

Experts in chronic pain and opioid therapy, as well as individuals representing important stakeholder groups, were invited to provide external peer review of this CER. The AHRQ Task Order Officer and a designated EPC Associate Editor also provided comments and editorial review. To obtain public comment, the draft report was posted on the AHRQ Web site for 4 weeks. A disposition of comments report detailing the authors' responses to the peer and public review comments will be made available after AHRQ posts the final CER on the public Web site.

Results

Overview

The search and selection of articles are summarized in the study flow diagram (Figure 2). Database searches resulted in 4,209 potentially relevant articles. After dual review of abstracts and titles, 667 articles were selected for full-text review, and 39 studies (in 40 publications) were determined by dual review at the full-text level to meet inclusion criteria and were included in this review. Data extraction and quality assessment tables for all included studies per Key Question are available in Appendixes E and F.

Figure 2. Literature flow diagram

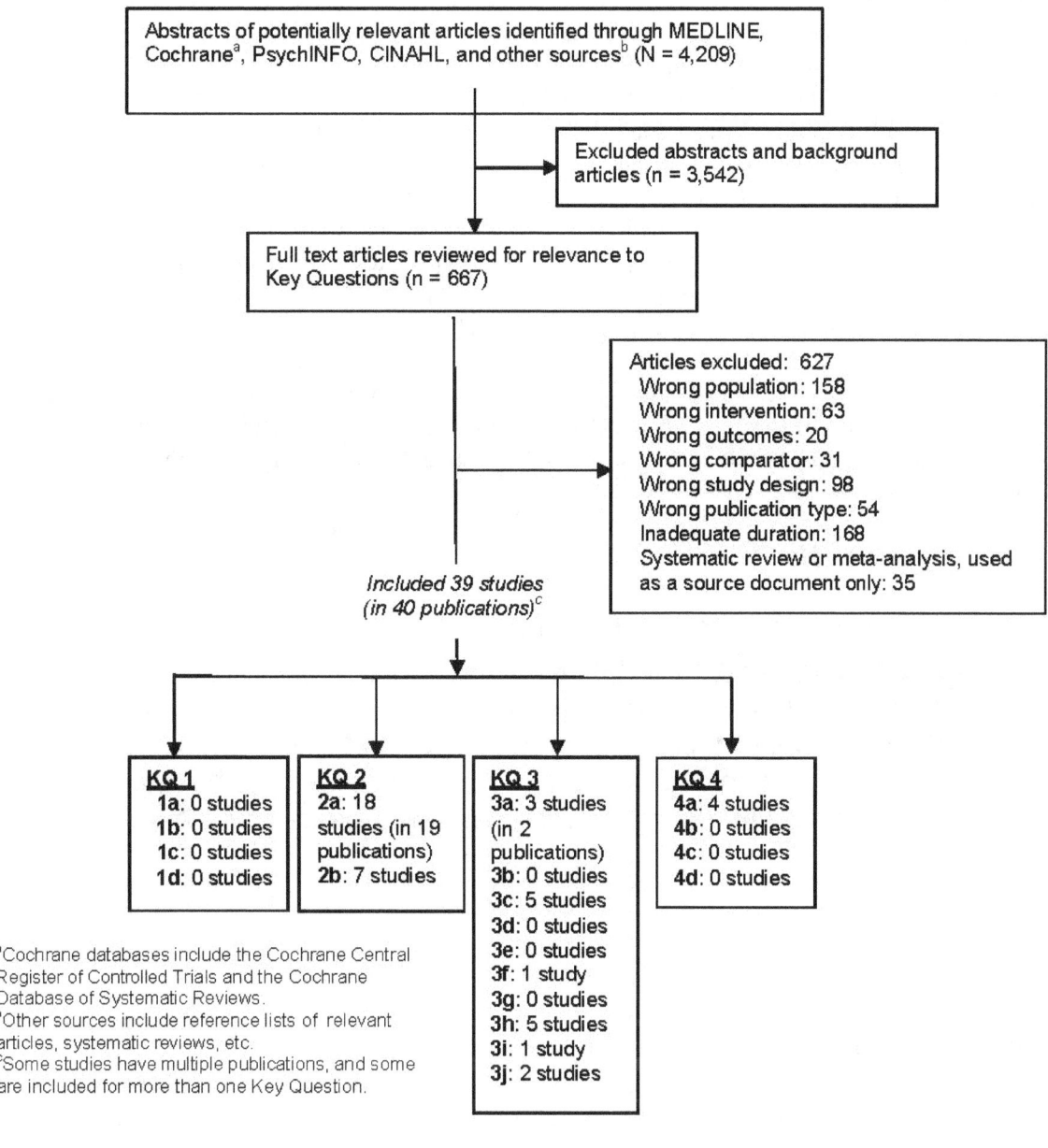

[a] Cochrane databases include the Cochrane Central Register of Controlled Trials and the Cochrane Database of Systematic Reviews.
[b] Other sources include reference lists of relevant articles, systematic reviews, etc.
[c] Some studies have multiple publications, and some are included for more than one Key Question.

Key Question 1a

In patients with chronic pain, what is the effectiveness of long-term opioid therapy versus placebo or no opioid therapy for long-term (≥1 year) outcomes related to pain, function, and quality of life?

Key Points

- No study of opioid therapy versus placebo or no opioid therapy evaluated long-term (≥1 year) outcomes related to pain, function, or quality of life (SOE: Insufficient).

Detailed Synthesis

All studies in the 2009 APS review evaluated outcomes related to pain, function, and quality of life at less than 1 year (typically at ≤12 weeks) and did not meet inclusion criteria for the current review. We also identified no studies published since the 2009 APS review that met inclusion criteria. Although a systematic review[8] of long-term opioid therapy included 10 studies of oral opioids and five studies of transdermal opioids that evaluated outcomes after at least 6 months, all were case series or uncontrolled long-term continuations of patients enrolled in clinical trials, with the exception of one head-to-head randomized trial that compared two long-acting opioids (see Key Question 3c).[43] In the systematic review, the pooled estimate for discontinuation due to insufficient pain relief was 10.3 percent (95 percent CI 7.6 to 13.9 percent) with oral opioids and 5.8 percent (95 percent CI 4.2 to 7.9) with transdermal opioids. Among patients who remained on oral opioids for at least 6 months, pain scores were generally reduced, but estimates varied substantially. Effects on quality of life and functional status were inconclusive. Findings of this review are difficult to interpret due to the lack of a nonopioid comparison group in the included studies, marked statistical heterogeneity, and other methodological shortcomings of the studies.

Key Question 1b

How does effectiveness vary depending on: (1) the specific type or cause of pain (e.g., neuropathic, musculoskeletal [including low back pain], fibromyalgia, sickle cell disease, inflammatory pain, and headache disorders); (2) patient demographics (e.g., age, race, ethnicity, gender); (3) patient comorbidities (including past or current alcohol or substance use disorders, mental health disorders, medical comorbidities and high risk for addiction)?

Key Points

- No study met inclusion criteria (see Key Question 1a) (SOE: Insufficient).

Detailed Synthesis

No study met inclusion criteria (see Key Question 1a). Although one systematic review[44] reported similar short-term effects of opioids versus placebo on improvement in pain scores for nociceptive (31 studies) and neuropathic (13 studies) pain, the studies included in the review did not meet inclusion criteria due to the short duration of followup. In the review, 61 of 62 included randomized trials were 16 weeks or shorter in duration, and the other trial was 24 weeks. There were too few trials of fibromyalgia (two studies) or mixed pain conditions (one study) to reliably estimate effects of opioids for these pain conditions.

Key Question 1c

In patients with chronic pain, what is the comparative effectiveness of opioids versus nonopioid therapies (pharmacological or nonpharmacological) on outcomes related to pain, function, and quality of life?

Key Points
- No study met inclusion criteria (SOE: Insufficient).

Detailed Synthesis

We identified no study on the comparative effectiveness of long-term opioid therapy versus nonopioid therapies on long-term outcomes related to pain, function, and quality of life.

Key Question 1d

In patients with chronic pain, what is the comparative effectiveness of opioids plus nonopioid interventions (pharmacological or nonpharmacological) versus opioids or nonopioid interventions alone on outcomes related to pain, function, quality of life, and doses of opioids used?

Key Points
- No study met inclusion criteria (SOE: Insufficient).

Detailed Synthesis

We identified no study on the comparative effectiveness of long-term opioid therapy plus nonopioid interventions versus opioids or nonopioid interventions alone on long-term outcomes related to pain, function, and quality of life.

Key Question 2a

In patients with chronic pain, what are the risks of opioids versus placebo or no opioid on: (1) opioid abuse, addiction, and related outcomes; (2) overdose; and (3) other harms, including gastrointestinal-related harms, falls, fractures, motor vehicle accidents, endocrinological harms, infections, cardiovascular events, cognitive harms, and psychological harms (e.g., depression)?

Key Points

- One fair-quality retrospective review of a large database of claims from commercial health plans found long-term (≥91 days supply) prescribed opioid use associated with significantly increased risk of opioid abuse or dependence diagnosis versus no opioid use (1-36 MED/day: OR 15, 95 percent CI 10 to 21; 36-120 MED/day: OR 29, 95 percent CI 20 to 41; ≥120 MED/day: OR 122, 95 percent CI 73 to 206) (SOE: Low).
- In 10 uncontrolled studies, estimates of opioid abuse, addiction, and related outcomes varied substantially even after stratification by clinic setting. Rates of diagnosed opioid abuse were 0.6 percent to 8 percent and rates of dependence were 3 percent to 26 percent in primary care settings. In pain clinic settings, rates of misuse were 8 to 16 percent and addiction 2 to 14 percent, but studies varied in methods used to define and ascertain outcomes. Rates of (variably-defined) aberrant drug-related behaviors (e.g., positive urine drug tests, medication agreement violations) ranged from 5.7 percent to 37.1 percent (SOE: Insufficient).
- One fair-quality retrospective cohort study found recent opioid use to be associated with increased risk of any overdose events (adjusted hazard ratio [HR] 5.2, 95 percent CI 2.1 to 12) and serious overdose events (adjusted HR 8.4, 95 percent CI 2.5 to 28) versus current nonuse in chronic pain patients who had received opioids at some point (SOE: Low).
- One fair-quality cohort study and one good-quality case-control study found use of opioids to be associated with increased risk of fracture (adjusted HR 1.28, 95 percent CI 0.99 to 1.64 and adjusted OR 1.27, 95 percent CI 1.21 to 1.33) though the estimate was not statistically significant in the cohort study and the risk was no longer present with more than 20 cumulative prescriptions in the other (SOE: Low).
- One good-quality case-control study found current opioid use versus nonuse to be associated with increased risk of myocardial infarction (adjusted OR 1.28, 95 percent CI 1.19 to 1.37). The risk was highest with 11 to 50 cumulative prescriptions (OR 1.38, 95 percent CI 1.28 to 1.49). A fair-quality cohort study found chronic opioid therapy, compared to the general population, to be associated with increased risk of myocardial infarction (adjusted incidence rate ratio [IRR] 2.66, 95 percent CI 2.30 to 3.08) and of myocardial infarction or revascularization (adjusted IRR 2.38, 95 percent CI 2.15 to 2.63) (SOE: Low).
- One fair-quality cross-sectional study of men with back pain (n=11,327) found long-term opioid use versus nonuse of opioids to be associated with increased risk for use of

medications for erectile dysfunction or testosterone replacement (adjusted OR 1.5, 95 percent CI 1.1 to 1.9) (SOE: Low)
- No study evaluated the association between long-term opioid therapy for chronic pain versus no opioid therapy and risk of motor vehicle accidents, infections, psychological harms, or cognitive harms.

Detailed Synthesis

Opioid Abuse, Addiction, and Related Outcomes

The 2009 APS review included two systematic reviews on use of opioids for chronic pain and rates of opioid abuse, addiction, or related outcomes.[45, 46] One systematic review that restricted inclusion to studies with at least 1 year of followup reported signs of opioid addiction in 0.27 percent of patients prescribed opioids in studies that reported this outcome.[45] However, none of the studies met inclusion criteria for the current review because addiction was not the primary outcome and they did not describe pre-specified methods for defining or ascertaining these outcomes. The other systematic review focused on patients with low back pain and reported rates of aberrant medication-taking behaviors that ranged from 5 to 24 percent.[46] The studies did not meet inclusion criteria for the current review because they did not include patients with at least 1 year of followup, did not clearly separate abuse and addiction related to opioid use versus other substances, or did not report pre-specified methods for the outcomes, with the exception of one retrospective cohort study.[47] It reported rates of opioid abuse behaviors in patients with chronic pain in primary care settings, based on chart review findings of one or more reports of lost or stolen opioid medications, documented use of other sources to obtain opioid medications, or requests for two or more early refills. Rates of opioid abuse behaviors were 24 percent (12/50) in a VA primary care setting and 31 percent (15/48) in a non-VA, urban hospital-based primary care setting. Factors associated with decreased risk of opioid abuse behaviors were no history of substance use disorder (adjusted OR 0.72, 95 percent CI 0.45 to 1.1) and older age (adjusted OR 0.94, 95 percent CI 0.94 to 0.99).

We identified no randomized trial published since the APS review on risk of opioid abuse, addiction, and related outcomes in patients with chronic pain prescribed long-term opioid therapy. One fair-quality retrospective study of patients in a large administrative database newly diagnosed with chronic (non-cancer) pain and followed for 18 months found prescribed long-term opioid use (receipt of ≥91 days' supply of opioids within a 12-month period), versus no prescribed opioids, associated with increased risk of opioid use disorder (defined as opioid abuse and dependence based on ICD-9 codes) (Appendix E1 and F1).[48] Rates of opioid abuse or dependence were 0.72, 1.28 and 6.1 percent in those prescribed low (1-36 mg MED/day), medium (36-120 mg MED/day) and high (≥120 mg MED/day) opioid doses, respectively, during the 12 months after the new chronic pain diagnosis, versus 0.004 percent in those with no opioid prescription. Compared to no opioid prescription and after adjustment for age, sex, history of substance abuse/dependence diagnosis and other comorbidities, chronic opioid use was associated with significantly increased risk of abuse or dependence for all doses of opioids (low dose: OR 15, 95 percent CI 10 to 21; medium dose: OR 29, 95 percent CI 20 to 41; high dose: OR 122, 95 percent CI 73 to 206).

Ten additional uncontrolled studies (in 11 publications) of patients with chronic pain, the majority of whom were prescribed opioids for at least 1 year, evaluated abuse and related outcomes as a primary outcome using explicit, predefined criteria (Table 1 below; Appendix E1 and F2).[49-58] All were rated fair-quality; none of the studies reported blinding of outcome assessors to patient characteristics, such as risk factors for substance abuse or psychological comorbidities. Another shortcoming in some studies was failure to assess the predefined outcomes in all patients.

Four of the new studies were performed exclusively or primarily in U.S. primary care settings.[47, 49, 50, 53] One study[53] found that 0.6 percent of primary care clinic patients receiving daily prescription opioids (96 percent for more than a year; total n=801) met the Diagnostic and Statistical Manual of Mental Disorders Fourth Edition (DSM-IV) criteria for opioid abuse disorder and 3.1 percent for opioid dependence, based on formal diagnostic interviews.

Behaviors indicative of opioid misuse were more common. Thirty-seven percent reported increasing doses on their own, 33 percent feeling intoxicated from pain medication, 24 percent purposeful over-sedation, 16 percent using opioids for purposes other than pain management, and 20 percent drinking alcohol to relieve pain. Twenty-four percent of patients had urine drug screens positive for illicit drugs (mostly cannabinoids).[53] A retrospective study of chronic pain patients receiving long-term opioid therapy in an integrated managed care health system (n=704) found that 13 percent met DSM-IV criteria for opioid dependence and 8 percent met criteria for opioid abuse without dependence, based on structured phone interviews.[49] Another study, which performed diagnostic interviews in 9 primary care and 3 specialty clinics with patients who received 4 or more opioid prescriptions over a year (n=705), found that 26 percent met DSM-IV criteria for current opioid dependence.[50] In multivariate logistic regression models, factors associated with current opioid dependence were age less than 65 years (OR 2.3, 95 percent CI 1.6 to 3.5), history of opioid abuse (OR 3.8, 95 percent CI 2.6 to 5.7), higher lifetime opioid dependence severity (OR 1.9, 95 percent CI 1.4 to 2.5), history of major depression (OR 1.3, 95 percent CI 1.1 to 1.6), and current use of psychotropic medications (OR 1.7, 95 percent CI 1.2 to 2.5). Rates of opioid abuse or misuse behaviors were not reported.

Six other studies were performed in pain clinic settings. Pain clinics may have a higher proportion of patients with opioid abuse and related problems because of referral patterns. Despite initial screening to exclude current substance abuse on entry, one study from a VA pain clinic found that after 1 year of followup, 28 percent of patients prescribed opioids (n=135) were discontinued from the clinic because of medication agreement violations.[51] Among these were 8 percent with specific opioid misuse behaviors such as unsanctioned dose increases or use of opioids other than those prescribed. In a cross-sectional study of Danish pain clinic patients with cancer and noncancer pain (mean duration of opioid use among those taking opioids = 6.8 years), 14.4 percent of those using opioids (n=187) met International Classification of Diseases (ICD-10) criteria for "addiction to opioids," which correspond most closely to the DSM-IV criteria for opioid abuse.[54] A cross-sectional study of UK NHS hospital pain clinic patients who had been prescribed opioids (n=104) found that 1.9 percent of the patients self-reported addiction using the Substance Use Questionnaire, 2.9 percent reported that they had craved opioids and 0.9 percent reported that they used alcohol to enhance the effects of opioids.[52] A prospective registry study of patients who had participated in five clinical trials of CR oxycodone and who continued to take this medication (n=227) found that 5.7 percent of the patients were identified by their physicians as exhibiting problematic drug-related behaviors, based on a brief physician-completed questionnaire.[55] However, verification by an independent panel resulted in a lower rate of 2.2 percent. A chart review conducted in a single pain clinic (n=197) reported that 15.7 percent of patients had aberrant drug-related behaviors noted in their charts and 8.7 percent had positive urine drug tests.[57] Finally, a cross-sectional study of patients attending five pain clinics (n=622) 0 found that 37.1 percent had positive urine drug tests (defined as presence of an illicit substance or unprescribed opioid), while 24 percent had positive scores ≥2 (the cutoff for "high risk") on the Prescription Opioid Therapy

Questionnaire and 29.1 percent had scores ≥11 (the cutoff for "at risk") on the Prescription Drug Use Questionnaire.[58]

A challenge in interpreting the evidence on rates of opioid abuse, addiction, and related outcomes is inconsistency in how these outcomes were defined, as well as variability in methods used to ascertain these outcomes. In addition, definitions and usage of these terms have changed over time. The studies described above were all conducted prior to the American Psychiatric Association's new DSM-V[59] diagnostic criteria for current opioid use disorder.

Overall, because of methodological limitations in the available studies and because estimates for opioid abuse, addiction, and related outcomes were highly variable even after stratifying by clinical setting, the SOE was rated Insufficient.

Table 1. Uncontrolled studies of long-term opioid use and abuse, misuse, and related outcomes

Author, Year Duration, If Applicable	Sample Characteristics Opioid Dose, Opioid Duration, and Pain Type	Method of Ascertaining and Defining Abuse/Misuse	Main Results
Banta-Green, 2009[49] Cross-sectional	n=704 Integrated group practice patients in a nonprofit healthcare system in Washington State Mean age: 55 years Female sex: 62% Race: 89% non-Hispanic White Dose: mean 50 mg/day MED, past year Duration: NR Pain type: NR	Composite International Diagnostic Interview (CIDI) for DSM-IV opioid diagnoses	Opioid dependence: 13% (91/704) Opioid abuse without dependence: 8% (56/704)
Boscarino, 2010[50] Cross-sectional	n=705 Primary and specialty care patients in integrated healthcare system in Pennsylvania who received 4+ opioid prescriptions in past 12 months Age: 18-64 years: 79% 65+ years: 21% Female sex: 61% White race: 98% Dose: NR Duration: mean of 10.7 opioid prescriptions over 1 year Pain type: non-cancer, otherwise not described	Composite International Diagnostic Interview (CIDI) for DSM-IV criteria for opioid dependence UDT: not examined	25.8% (95% CI: 22.0-29.9) met criteria for current opioid dependence; 35.5% (95% CI: 31.1-40.2) met criteria for lifetime dependence Factors associated with current dependence: Age <65 years (OR 2.3, 95% CI 1.6 to 3.5) History of opioid abuse (OR 3.8, 95% CI 2.6 to 5.7) History of high dependence severity (OR 1.9, 95% CI 1.4 to 2.5) History of major depression (OR 1.3, 95% CI 1.1 to 1.6) Current use of psychotropic medications (OR 1.7, 95% CI 1.2 to 2.5)

Table 1. Uncontrolled studies of long-term opioid use and abuse, misuse, and related outcomes (continued)

Author, Year Duration, If Applicable	Sample Characteristics Opioid Dose, Opioid Duration, and Pain Type	Method of Ascertaining and Defining Abuse/Misuse	Main Results
Carrington Reid, 2002[47] Retrospective cohort	n=98 (50 at VA and 48 at urban primary care clinic) patients with 6+ months of opioid prescriptions during 1 year VA primary care clinic vs. urban hospital primary care clinic Median age: 54 vs. 55 years Female sex: 8% vs. 67% Race: 88% White, 12% Black vs. 52% White, 36% Black, 10% Hispanic Median duration of pain: 10 vs. 13 years Dose: NR Duration: 6+ months of opioid prescriptions during past year Pain type: Non-cancer, Various (low back 44% vs 25%)	Chart review for reports of lost or stolen opioids, documented use of other sources to obtain opioids, and requests for ≥2 early refills UDT: not examined	VA site vs. urban primary care site Opioid abuse behaviors: 24% (12/50) vs. 31% (15/48) Median time to onset of abuse behaviors: 24 months Factors associated with odds of opioid abuse behaviors: History of substance use disorder (adjusted OR 3.8, 95% CI 1.4 to 10.8) Age (adjusted OR 0.4, 95% CI 0.9 to 1.0) Number of medical diseases (adjusted OR 0.7, 95% CI 0.5-1.1)
Compton, 2008[51] 1 year	n=135 veterans at a VA pain clinic Mean age: 53 years Female sex: 6% Race: NR Baseline mean usual pain VAS (0-10) rating: 6.75 Dose: NR Duration: NR Pain type: 77% musculoskeletal, 19% neuropathic, 4% multi-category	Chart review for opioid discontinuation due to medication agreement violation (including for opioid misuse or abuse) UDT: not examined	Discontinuation due to medication agreement violation: 28% (38/135) Discontinuation due to specific problematic opioid misuse behaviors: 8% (11/135)
Cowan, 2003[52] Cross-sectional	n=104 patients who had been prescribed opioids at a pain clinic in a UK NHS hospital Mean age: 55.4 years Female sex: 39% Race: NR Mean duration of pain: 10.5 years Dose: NR Duration: mean 14.1 months; 57% of the 104 patients had permanently stopped opioid therapy Pain type: 34% degenerative disease other than OA, 24% failed back/neck surgery syndrome, 10% complex regional pain syndrome, 10% osteoarthritis	SUQ UDT: not examined	Self-reported addiction: 1.9% (2/104) Craving opioids: 2.9% (3/104) Has taken drugs to enhance the effect of opioids: 0.9% (1/104) Has used alcohol to enhance the effect of opioids: 0.9% (1/104)

Table 1. Uncontrolled studies of long-term opioid use and abuse, misuse, and related outcomes (continued)

Author, Year Duration, If Applicable	Sample Characteristics Opioid Dose, Opioid Duration, and Pain Type	Method of Ascertaining and Defining Abuse/Misuse	Main Results
Fleming, 2007[53] See also: Saffier, 2007[56] Cross-sectional	n=801 primary care patients on daily opioid therapy Mean age: 48.6 years Female sex: 68% Race: 75.6% White; 23.1% African American; 1% other Disability income: 48% Mean daily dose: 92 mg MED Duration: 96% prescribed COT for ≥12 mos. Pain type: Degenerative aarthritis: 24%; low back pain: 21%; migraine headache 8%; neuropathy 5.5%	In-person interviews with Addiction Severity Index (ASI); Substance Dependence Severity Scale (SDSS); Aberrant Behavior 12-item List UDT: sample collected at end of interview	Met DSM-IV criteria for opioid dependence: 3.1% Met DSM-IV criteria for opioid abuse: 0.6% Any illicit drug on UDT: 24% (mostly marijuana) Purposely over-sedated: 24% (186/785) Felt intoxicated from pain medication: 33% (260/785) Requested early refills: 45% (359/785) Increased dose on own: 37% (288/785) Medications lost or stolen: 30% (236/785) Used opioid for purpose other than pain: 16% (125/785) Drank alcohol to relieve pain: 20% (154/785)
Hojsted, 2010[54] Cross-sectional	n=253 patients at a pain clinic (236 non-cancer and 17 cancer pain) Mean age: 52 years Female sex: 64% Race: NR Receiving opioids: 74% (187/253) Dose: Median daily dose = 90 mg MED among those taking opioids Duration: mean 6.8 years among those taking opioids who returned a questionnaire Pain type: 28% nociceptive pain, 33% neuropathic pain, 39% mixed nociceptive and neuropathic	Addiction screening by physician and nurse (blinded to each other) using the ICD-10 and Portenoy's Criteria; a positive screen by either provider was considered positive UDT: not examined	Addiction to opioids or hypnotics, ICD-10: total sample 11% (28/253); among those taking addictive drugs 13%; among those taking opioids 14% Addiction to opioids, ICD-10, among those taking opioids: 14.4% (27/187) Addiction to opioids or hypnotics, Portenoy's Criteria. among those taking opioids: 19% (36/187) Addiction to opioids, Portenoy's Criteria: 19% (36/187)

Table 1. Uncontrolled studies of long-term opioid use and abuse, misuse, and related outcomes (continued)

Author, Year Duration, If Applicable	Sample Characteristics Opioid Dose, Opioid Duration, and Pain Type	Method of Ascertaining and Defining Abuse/Misuse	Main Results
Portenoy, 2007[55] 3 years	n=227 patients enrolled in a registry study of patients who had participated in a previous controlled clinical trial of CR oxycodone for noncancer pain and who continued to take CR oxycodone Mean age: 56 years Female sex: 57% Race: 90% White BPI average pain score: 6.4 Dose: mean 52.5 mg MED/day Duration: mean 541 days Pain type: 38% osteoarthritis pain, 31% diabetic neuropathy, 31% low back pain	Physician-completed brief questionnaire assessing problematic drug-related behavior with verification by an independent panel of experts UDT: not examined	Problematic drug-related behavior identified by physicians: 5.7% (13/227) Problematic drug-related behavior adjudicated by expert panel as meeting DSM-IV criteria for drug abuse or dependence: 0 Problematic drug-related behavior adjudicated by expert panel as positive: 2.2% (5/227) Problematic drug-related behavior adjudicated by expert panel as possible: 0.4% (1/227) Problematic drug-related behavior adjudicated by expert panel as withdrawal but no indication of abuse: 0.4% (1/227) Problematic drug-related behavior adjudicated by expert panel as suspected abuse/dependence but insufficient information to draw definitive conclusion: 2.2% (5/227) Problematic drug-related behavior adjudicated by expert panel as no evidence of abuse, dependence, or euphoria: 0.4% (1/227) Overdose deaths: 1 (phenylpropanolamine, oxycodone, and alcohol)

Table 1. Uncontrolled studies of long-term opioid use and abuse, misuse, and related outcomes (continued)

Author, Year Duration, If Applicable	Sample Characteristics Opioid Dose, Opioid Duration, and Pain Type	Method of Ascertaining and Defining Abuse/Misuse	Main Results
Schneider, 2010[57] Retrospective chart review	n=197 patients treated by a pain specialist for at least one year Mean age: 49 years Female sex: 67% Race: NR Dose: mean 180 mg/day MED (long-acting), 49 mg/day MED (short-acting) Duration: mean 4.7 years Pain type: 51% back pain, 10% neck pain, 9% fibromyalgia, 8% other myofascial pain	UDT: immunoassay followed by confirmatory GC/MS	Positive UDT: 8.7% (14/161) Aberrant drug-related behaviors noted in chart: 15.7% (31/197)
Wasan, 2009[58] Cross-sectional	n=622 chronic noncancer pain patients from pain management centers on long-term opioid therapy Mean age: 50.4 years Female sex: 55% Race: 80% White Mean pain rating (0-10): 5.96 Dose: NR Duration: mean 6.2 years Pain type: 61% low back pain	POTQ, PDUQ, and UDT (immunoassay and confirmatory GCMS)	Positive scores of ≥2 on POTQ: 24% (115/480) Score ≥11 on PDUQ: 29.1% (130/447) Positive UDT: 37.1% (134/356)

Abbreviations: ASI= Addiction Severity Index, CI=confidence interval, CIDI=Composite International Diagnostic Interview, DSM-IV= Diagnostic and Statistical Manual Fifth Edition, GC/MS=gas chromatography mass spectrometry, ICD-10=International Statistical Classification of Diseases and Related Health Problems Version 10, MED=morphine-equivalent dose, NA=not applicable, NR= not reported, OR=odds ratio, PDUQ=Prescription Drug Use Questionnaire, POTQ=Prescription Opioid Therapy Questionnaire, SDSS=Dependence Severity Scale, SUQ=Self-report Substance Use Questionnaire, UDT=urine drug test, VA=Veterans Affairs.

Overdose

The 2009 APS review identified no studies on the risk of overdose in patients with chronic pain prescribed long-term opioid therapy versus placebo or no opioid. Epidemiological studies that reported opioid-related deaths did not have a nonopioid control group, did not have denominators for the numbers of people prescribed opioids, were not designed to distinguish deaths related to prescribed opioids from deaths related to illicit use of opioids, or did not focus on patients on long-term opioid therapy.[60]

We identified one fair-quality retrospective cohort study published since the APS review that reported risk of overdose with opioid use versus nonuse in patients (n=9,940) in a U.S. integrated health care system with a new episode of opioid use (defined as no opioid prescription in the past 6 months), a chronic noncancer pain diagnosis within 2 weeks before the initial opioid prescription, and at least 3 opioid prescriptions in the first 90 days of the episode (Appendix E2 and F1).[61] The mean duration of followup was 42 months, and short-acting opioids were the most frequently prescribed type; only 10 percent of the patients received predominantly long- acting opioids. Overdoses were identified through ICD-9 codes and a State mortality registry, with verification through medical record review. Risk estimates were based on recently dispensed opioids at the time of the overdose event. Therefore, results may be interpreted as risk of overdose with current use versus nonuse in people previously prescribed opioid therapy for several months.

The annual overdose rate was 256 per 100,000 person-years in patients who recently received prescribed opioids versus 36 per 100,000 person-years in people who did not. After adjustment for smoking, depression, substance abuse, comorbid conditions, pain site, age, sex, recent sedative-hypnotic prescription, and recent initiation of opioid use, recent receipt of any prescribed opioids, compared to no opioid receipt, was associated with increased risk of any overdose events (HR 5.2, 95 percent CI 2.1 to 12.5) and serious overdose events (HR 8.4, 95 percent CI 2.5 to 28) (SOE: Low).

Gastrointestinal Harms

The APS review identified no studies on risk of gastrointestinal harms with long-term opioid therapy versus placebo or nonuse, and we identified no studies published since the APS review meeting inclusion criteria. Systematic reviews included in the APS review were based on short-term trials that reported frequent nausea, constipation, and vomiting in patients prescribed opioids.[22, 62, 63]

Fractures

The APS review included a systematic review of six observational studies of the association between opioid use and fracture. All six studies reported a statistically significant association, with a pooled RR of 1.38 (95 percent CI 1.15 to 1.66).[64] The APS review also included a case-control study not in the systematic review that also found use of various opioids to be associated with increased risk of fracture (OR estimates ranged from 1.1 to 2.2).[65] However, none of these studies meet inclusion criteria for the current review, because they did not specifically evaluate patients with chronic pain or on long-term opioid therapy. In addition, the studies had important methodological limitations, including failure to adjust for important confounders. Other studies published since the 2009 APS review also evaluated the association between opioid use and fractures, but did not meet inclusion criteria for similar reasons.[66-70]

We identified one cohort study[18] and one case-control study[71] published since the APS review on the association between opioid use and fracture in patients with chronic pain or on long-term opioid therapy (Appendix E3, F1, and F3). The cohort study identified patients 60 years and older with a diagnosis of noncancer pain initiating a new episode of opioid use (no opioid prescription fills in the prior 6 months) who had at least three opioid prescriptions in the first 90 days of the episode.[18] Patients were followed for a mean of 33 months. The overall annual confirmed nonvertebral fracture rate was 5 percent (6 percent among current opioid users and 4 percent among people not currently using opioids; HR 1.28, 95 percent CI 0.99 to 1.64, adjusted for demographic factors, prior fractures, comorbidities, and concomitant medication use). The most commonly prescribed opioids were hydrocodone (42 percent), oxycodone (24 percent), and codeine combinations (14 percent). The study was rated fair-quality due to failure to report loss to followup and unclear blinding of outcomes assessors.

One good-quality case-control study evaluated 21,739 people with hip, humerus, or wrist fractures from the UK General Practice Research Database and 85,326 nonfracture controls matched on age, sex, date of fracture diagnosis, and practice site.[71] Although the study did not specifically focus on patients with chronic pain, the analysis was stratified by duration of opioid use, based on the cumulative number of opioid prescriptions before the index date. After adjustment for a number of factors, including smoking status, comorbidities, concomitant medications, type of pain, and recent or past opioid use, current opioid therapy was associated with increased risk of fracture versus nonuse (OR 1.27, 95 percent CI 1.21 to 1.33). The risk was highest with one prescription (OR 2.70, 95 percent CI 2.34 to 3.13) and decreased with higher numbers of prescriptions, with no increased risk for patients with more than 20 cumulative prescriptions, suggesting that increased risk of fracture may be associated with more recent initiation of opioid therapy.

The SOE for the association between opioid use versus non-use and risk of fractures was rated Low.

Motor Vehicle Accidents

The APS review included two systematic reviews[72, 73] (25 and 48 observational studies) and five other observational studies[74-78] on the association between opioid use and driving safety, but none of the studies met inclusion criteria for the current review because they did not report duration of opioid use, included individuals treated for opioid addiction or using opioids illicitly, focused on surrogate markers of driving safety such as simulated driving tests or measures of cognitive performance rather than actual motor vehicle accidents, or did not include a comparison arm of chronic pain patients not prescribed opioids. We identified no studies published since the APS review on risk of motor vehicle accidents in patients with chronic pain on long-term opioid therapy versus no opioid therapy.

Cardiovascular Events

The APS review did not evaluate the association between opioid therapy for chronic pain and risk of cardiovascular events. We identified one cohort study[79] and one case-control study[80] on the association between long-term opioid use for chronic pain and risk of myocardial infarction (Appendix E4, F2, and F3). The cohort study included individuals with claims for opioids or a nonselective cyclo-oxygenase-2 (COX-2) inhibitor over a cumulative period of $\geq$180 days over a 3.5 year period.[79] Individuals were excluded if they had cancer pain or a history of myocardial infarction or cancer and were matched on age, sex and cohort entry date to people in the general population who did not receive $\geq$180 days of opioids or COX-2 selective non-steroidal anti-inflammatory drugs (NSAIDs). Compared to the general population, chronic opioid therapy was associated with increased risk of myocardial infarction (adjusted IRR 2.66, 95 percent CI 2.30 to 3.08) and of myocardial infarction or revascularization (adjusted IRR 2.38, 95 percent CI 2.15 to 2.63), after controlling for age, sex, cardiovascular and other comorbidities, and concomitant medication use. The study was rated fair quality because there was no attempt to match patients on pain condition or severity of pain, or to adjust for these factors.

A good-quality case-control study compared 11,693 people with myocardial infarction from the UK General Practice Research Database to 44,897 controls with no myocardial infarction matched on age, sex, index date, and practice site.[80] The most commonly prescribed opioids were codeine, propoxyphene, and dihydrocodeine. Although it did not specifically enroll patients with chronic pain, the study included an analysis stratified by duration of opioid use, based on the number of cumulative opioid prescriptions at the time of myocardial infarction. After adjustment for a number of factors, including smoking status, comorbidities, concomitant medications, type of pain, and recent or past opioid use, it found current opioid therapy use associated with increased risk of myocardial infarction versus nonuse (adjusted OR 1.28, 95 percent CI 1.19 to 1.37). Recent (within 31 to 365 days) use was also associated with increased risk (OR 1.17, 95 percent CI 1.10 to 1.24). The risk was highest with 11 to 50 cumulative prescriptions (OR 1.38, 95 percent CI 1.28 to 1.49) but was statistically significant with 1-2, 3-10, or >50 cumulative prescriptions (OR range 1.09 to 1.25).

The SOE for the association between opioid use versus non-use and risk of myocardial infarction was rated Low.

We identified no study on the association between long-term opioid therapy for chronic pain versus no opioid therapy and risk of arrhythmia or sudden death.

Endocrinological Harms

The APS review included four studies on the effects of oral opioid use on endocrinological effects. One cross-sectional study of women with chronic pain (n=37, mean duration of opioid use 31 months) found no association between opioid use versus nonuse and growth hormone, corticotrophin, cortisol, thyroxine, thyrotropin, prolactin, estradiol, follicle stimulating hormone, luteinizing hormone, or testosterone levels, but did not meet inclusion criteria because it did not adjust for potential confounders.[81] Three other cross-sectional studies found opioid use to be associated with decreased levels of gonadal hormone or dehydroepiandrosterone sulfate in men and women, but it was unclear in two of the studies whether patients had chronic pain, the duration of opioid use was not reported, none of the studies adjusted for potential confounders, and it was unclear how patients were selected, making it difficult to determine whether patients on opioids with signs of sexual or endocrinological dysfunction were preferentially enrolled.[23, 24, 82]

We identified one study published since the APS review on the association between opioid use versus nonuse and endocrinological harms (Appendix E5 and F2).[11] In a cross-sectional analysis of men with back pain (n=11,327) in an integrated health care system, long-term opioid use (defined as ≥120 days or >90 days with 10 or more fills), compared with no opioid use, was associated with increased likelihood of use of medications for erectile dysfunction or testosterone replacement (adjusted OR 1.5, 95 percent CI 1.1 to 1.9), after adjustment for age, co-morbidities, hospitalizations, use of sedative-hypnotics, dose of opioids, type of opioid, depression, and smoking status. Median opioid dose in men on chronic opioids was 30 mg morphine equivalent dose (MED)/day (19 percent received ≥120 mg) and 42 percent received long-acting opioids. A limitation of this study is that the patient sample was a mix of acute, subacute, and chronic back pain, and the study could not control for duration of pain. In all studies, the cross-sectional design makes it impossible to determine whether endocrinological problems preceded opioid use or resulted from opioid use. One other cross-sectional study published since the prior APS review reported an association between long-term opioid use and laboratory markers of endocrinological dysfunction, but did not meet inclusion criteria because it did not perform adjustment for potential confounders.[83]

The SOE for the association between opioid use versus non-use and risk of endocrinological harms was rated Low.

Other Harms

We identified no studies on the association between long-term opioid therapy for chronic pain versus no opioid use and risk of falls, infections, cognitive harms, or psychological harms. These outcomes were not evaluated in the APS review.

Key Question 2b

How do harms vary depending on: (1) the specific type or cause of pain (e.g., neuropathic, musculoskeletal [including back pain], fibromyalgia, sickle cell disease, inflammatory pain, headache disorders); (2) patient demographics; (3) patient comorbidities (including past or current substance abuse disorder or at high risk for addiction); (4) the dose of opioids used?

Key Points

- No study evaluated how harms associated with long-term opioid therapy vary depending on the specific type or cause of pain, patient demographics, or patient comorbidities (SOE: Insufficient).
- One fair-quality retrospective database study found higher doses of long-term opioid therapy associated with increased risk of opioid abuse or dependence than lower doses. Compared to no opioid prescription, the adjusted odds ratios were 15 (95 percent CI 10 to 21) for 1-36 mg MED/day, 29 (95 percent CI 20 to 41) for 36-120 mg MED/day, and 122 (95 percent CI 73 to 206) for ≥120 mg MED/day (SOE: Low).
- One fair-quality retrospective cohort study and one good-quality nested case-control study found an association between higher doses of long-term opioid therapy and risk of overdose. In the cohort study, versus 1 to 19 mg MED/day, the adjusted HR for an overdose event was 1.44 (95 percent CI 0.57 to 3.62) with 20 to 49 mg MED/day and increased with higher doses to 8.87 (95 percent CI 3.99 to 19.72) for ≥100 mg MED/day. The risk for serious overdose showed a similar pattern, with HRs of 1.19 (95 percent CI 0.4 to 3.6) for 20 to <50 mg MED/day, 3.11 (95 percent CI 1.01 to 9.51) for 50 to 99 mg/day, and 11.18 (95 percent CI 4.80 to 26.03) for ≥100 mg/day (all relative to 1-19 mg/day). In the case-control study, versus 1 to 19 mg MED/day, the adjusted OR for an opioid-related death was 1.32 (95 percent CI 0.94 to 1.84) for 20 to 49 mg MED/day and increased to 2.88 (95 percent CI 1.79 to 4.63) for ≥200 mg MED/day (SOE: Low).
- One fair-quality cohort study found that risk of fracture increased from an adjusted HR of 1.20 (95 percent CI 0.92 to 1.56) at 1 to <20 mg MED/day to 2.00 (95 percent CI 1.24 to 3.24) at ≥50 mg MED/day; the overall test for dose response did not reach statistical significance (P = 0.06) (SOE: Low).
- One fair-quality cohort study found that relative to a cumulative dose of 0 to <1350 mg MED over 90 days, the adjusted IRR for myocardial infarction for 1350 to <2700 mg was 1.21 (95 percent CI 1.02 to 1.45), for 2700 to <8100 mg was 1.42 (95 percent CI 1.21 to 1.67), for 8100 to <18,000 mg was 1.89 (95 percent CI 1.54 to 2.33), and for ≥18,000 mg was 1.73 (95 percent CI 1.32 to 2.26) (SOE: Low).
- One good-quality case-control study found no association between opioid dose and odds of road trauma injury among drivers and passengers.

Doses of opioids >20 mg MED/day were associated with increased odds of road trauma injury when the analysis was restricted to drivers. There was no dose-dependent association at doses higher than 20 mg MED/day. Relative to 1 to <20 mg MED/day, the adjusted odds of road trauma injury among drivers were 1.21 (1.02 to 1.42) for 20 to 49 (1.02 to 1.49) for >200 mg. (SOE: Low).

One fair-quality cross-sectional study of men found a daily opioid dose of ≥120 mg MED/day to be associated with increased odds of use of medications for erectile dysfunction or testosterone replacement versus 0 to <20 mg MED/day (adjusted OR 1.6, 95 percent CI 1.03 to 2.4). Odds were not increased at doses of 20 to <120 mg MED/day (SOE: Low).

Detailed Synthesis

We identified no study on how harms associated with long-term opioid therapy vary depending on the specific type or cause of pain, patient demographics, or patient comorbidities, including those with a history of or at high risk for addiction.

The APS review identified no studies on the association between opioid dose and risk of harms in patients with chronic pain on long-term opioid therapy. We identified six studies published since the APS review on the association between opioid dose and risk of opioid-related deaths or overdose,[61,84] fractures,[18] myocardial infarction,[79] motor vehicle accidents,[20] and endocrinological effects.[11]

Opioid Abuse, Addiction, and Related Outcomes

A previously described (see KQ 2a) fair-quality retrospective database study found a dose-dependent association between dose of long-term opioid therapy for chronic pain and risk of abuse or dependence.[48] Based on ICD-9 diagnosis codes, rates of abuse or dependence were 0.7 percent with low-dose opioids (1-36 mg MED/day), 1.3 percent with medium-dose (36-120 mg MED/day), and 6.1 percent with high-dose (≥120 mg MED/day). Compared to no opioid prescription, the odds ratio for abuse or dependence after adjustment for age, sex, history of substance abuse and other comorbidities was 15 (95 percent CI 10 to 21) for low-dose, 29 (95 percent CI 20 to 41) for medium-dose, and 122 (95 percent CI 73 to 205) for high-dose opioids (Appendix E1) (SOE: Low).

Overdose

Two studies found an association between opioid dose and risk of overdose (Appendix E2, F1, and F3).[61,84] A previously described (see KQ 2a), fair-quality retrospective cohort study of patients (n=9,940) with recently diagnosed noncancer pain and prescribed opioid therapy followed patients for a mean duration of 42 months.[61] Fifty-one patients experienced overdose events (148 per 100,000 person-years); 40 were serious overdose events (116 per 100,000 person-years) and 6 were fatal overdose events (17 per 100,000 person-years). After adjusting for smoking, depression, substance abuse, comorbid conditions, pain site, age, sex, recent sedative-hypnotic prescription, and recent initiation of opioid use, higher opioid dose was associated with increased risk of any overdose event. Relative to 1 to 19 mg MED/day, 20 to 49 mg/day was associated with a HR of 1.44 (0.57-3.62), 50-99 mg/day with a HR of 3.73 (1.47-9.5), and ≥100 mg/day with a HR of 8.87 (3.99-19.72). The risk for serious overdose showed a similar pattern, with HRs of 1.19 (95 percent CI 0.4 to 3.6) for 20 to 49 mg MED/day, 3.11 (95 percent CI 1.01 to 9.51) for 50 to 99 mg/day, and 11.18 (95 percent CI 4.80 to 26.03) for ≥100 mg/day (all relative to 1-19 mg/day).

A good-quality, population-based, nested case-control study of Canadian patients eligible for publicly funded prescription drug coverage who had received an opioid for noncancer pain identified 498 cases of opioid-associated deaths.[84] Cases were matched on age, sex, index year, the Charlson comorbidity index, and a disease risk index based on comorbidities to 1714 controls. Opioid-associated deaths were identified using coroner records and defined as deaths in which the coroner identified a combination of drugs including at least one opioid or in which forensic toxicology testing showed an opioid concentration sufficiently high to cause death.

Mean duration of opioid use was 5 years in cases and 4 years in controls. Long-acting opioids were dispensed at some point in the exposure period to 46 percent of cases and 30 percent of controls. After adjusting for previous drugs used, number of drugs, duration of opioid treatment, the number of physicians prescribing opioids, the number of pharmacies dispensing opioids, and prescribing of long-acting opioids, higher doses of opioids were associated with increased odds of opioid-associated mortality. Relative to 1 to 19 mg MED/day, the adjusted OR for opioid-associated mortality was 1.32 (95 percent CI 0.94 to 1.84) for 20 to 49 mg/day, 1.92 (95 percent CI 1.30 to 2.85) for 50 to 99 mg/day, 2.04 (95 percent CI 1.28 to 3.24) for 100 to 199 mg/day, and 2.88 (95 percent CI 1.79 to 4.63) for ≥200 mg/day (SOE: Low).

Three other observational studies also found an association between higher opioid doses and risk of opioid overdose-related deaths, but did not meet inclusion criteria because duration of opioid use was not reported,[16,85] emergency room visits for opioid-related overdose events were combined with emergency room visits for alcohol,[86] or it did not evaluate patients with chronic pain prescribed long-term opioid therapy.[85]

Fractures

A previously described, fair-quality cohort study (see Key Question 2a) on the association between current use of opioids and risk of fractures in people aged 60 and older found that risk of fracture increased from an adjusted hazard ratio of 1.20 (95 percent CI 0.92 to 1.56) at 1 to <20 mg MED/day to 2.00 (95 percent CI 1.24 to 3.24) at ≥50 mg MED/day, although the overall test for dose response did not reach statistical significance (p = 0.06) (Appendix E3 and F2) (SOE: Low).[18]

Cardiovascular Events

A previously described fair-quality cohort study (see Key Question 2a) on the association between current use of opioids and risk of myocardial infarction in patients using long-term opioid therapy found a trend towards increased risk of myocardial infarction with higher cumulative opioid exposure (Appendix E4 and F1).[79] Compared to a cumulative dose of 0 to <1350 mg MED over 90 days, the adjusted IRR for myocardial infarction for 1350 to <2700 mg was 1.21 (95 percent CI 1.02 to 1.45), for 2700 to <8100 mg was 1.42 (95 percent CI 1.21 to 1.67), for 8100 to <18,000 mg was 1.89 (95 percent CI 1.54 to 2.33), and for ≥18,000 mg was 1.73 (95 percent CI 1.32 to 2.26) (SOE: Low).

Motor Vehicle Accidents

We identified one good-quality case-control study (n=10,600) on the association of opioid dose with risk of motor vehicle accidents in Ontario, Canada among individuals eligible for provincial prescription drug coverage who received at least one opioid prescription (Appendix E6 and F3).[20] It identified 5,300 cases who visited an emergency department with an injury related to road trauma. Cases were matched on sex, age, index year, and disease risk index to

5300 controls who did not visit the emergency department for road trauma. Although it did not specifically identify chronic pain patients on long-term opioid therapy, the average duration of opioid use was 7.1 years in cases and 6.8 years in controls. Individuals prescribed methadone were excluded because methadone is typically used to treat addiction in this area. Although there was no association between opioid dose and risk of road trauma in drivers or passengers at the time of the accident, doses of opioids >20 mg MED/day were associated with increased odds of road trauma when the analysis was restricted to drivers. There was no dose-dependent association at doses higher than 20 mg MED/day. Relative to 1 to <20 mg MED/day, the odds of road trauma among drivers after adjustment for age, alcoholism history, concomitant medication use, total number of drugs, and number of physician and emergency department visits was 1.21 (95 percent CI 1.02 to 1.42) for 20 to 49 mg, 1.29 (95 percent CI 1.06 to 1.57) for 50-99 mg, 1.42 (95 percent CI 1.15 to 1.76) for 100 to 199 mg, and 1.23 (95 percent CI 1.02 to 1.49) for ≥200 mg (SOE: Low).

Endocrinological Harms

One previously described fair-quality study cross-sectional analysis of men with back pain (n=11,327) found a daily opioid dose of ≥120 mg MED/day associated with increased risk of use of medications for erectile dysfunction or testosterone replacement versus 0 to <20 mg MED/day (OR 1.6, 95 percent CI 1.03 to 2.4), after adjustment for duration of opioid use, age, co-morbidities, hospitalizations, use of sedative-/hypnotics, type of opioid, depression, and smoking status (Appendix E5 and F2) (SOE: Low).[11] There was no increased risk at doses of 20 to <120 mg MED/day.

Key Question 3a

In patients with chronic pain, what is the comparative effectiveness of different methods for initiating and titrating opioids for outcomes related to pain, function, and quality of life; risk of overdose, addiction, abuse, or misuse; and doses of opioids used?

Key Points

- Evidence from three trials on effects of titration with immediate-release versus sustained-release opioids reported inconsistent results on outcomes related to pain and are difficult to interpret due to additional differences between treatment arms in dosing protocols (titrated versus fixed dosing) and doses of opioids used (SOE: Insufficient).
- No trial was designed to assess risk of addiction, abuse, or misuse (SOE: Insufficient).

Detailed Synthesis

The APS review included three fair-quality, open-label trials of sustained-release versus immediate release opioids for titrating patients to stable pain control (Appendix E7 and F4).[87, 88] Two trials comparing controlled-release (CR) versus immediate-release (IR) oxycodone were reported in one publication.[87] The first involved a sample of 48 patients with cancer pain and dose titration for a period up to 21 days.[87] The second trial titrated 57 patients with low back pain for a period of up to 10 days.[87] Most patients in both trials were converted to oxycodone from other opioids. Results of both trials showed no difference between CR and IR oxycodone with respect to the percentage of patients achieving stable pain control, the time to achieve stable pain control, and the degree of pain control achieved. Another trial found titrated doses of sustained-release morphine plus immediate-release oxycodone slightly superior to fixed-dose, immediate-release oxycodone for pain intensity, but no differences on measures of function, sleep, and psychological distress.[88] Results of this trial are difficult to interpret because maximum doses of opioids varied in the two arms (up to 200 mg MED/day in titrated dose arm, versus up to 20 mg/day in the fixed-dose oxycodone arm), and average doses of opioids were not reported. None of the three trials was designed to assess outcomes related to risk of overdose, addiction, abuse, or misuse. Due to study limitations, inconsistent results, and differences between study arms other than use of sustained-release versus immediate-release opioids, the SOE was rated Insufficient.

We identified no study published since the APS review on the comparative effectiveness of different methods for initiating and titrating opioids.

Key Question 3b

In patients with chronic pain, what is the comparative effectiveness of short- versus long-acting opioids on outcomes related to pain, function, and quality of life; risk of overdose, addiction, abuse, or misuse; and doses of opioids used?

Key Points

- No study compared effectiveness of short- versus long-acting opioids on long-term outcomes in patients with chronic pain (SOE: Insufficient).

Detailed Synthesis

The APS review included a systematic review[89] of seven trials[87, 88, 90-94] of short- versus long-acting opioid formulations, but none of the trials met inclusion criteria for the current review. Six trials[87, 90-94] were 30 days or shorter in duration and the other[88] was 16 weeks in duration. Five of the trials found no difference between sustained-release and immediate-release opioid formulations in pain control.[87, 90, 91, 93, 94] Although two trials found regimens including sustained-release preparations more effective for pain control than regimens restricted to immediate-release preparations, results are difficult to interpret because the regimens were not given at therapeutically equivalent doses.[88, 92] No trial was designed to evaluate risk of overdose, addiction, abuse, or misuse.

We identified no trials of short- versus long-acting opioids published since the APS review that met inclusion criteria.

Key Question 3c

In patients with chronic pain, what is the comparative effectiveness of different long-acting opioids on outcomes related to pain, function, and quality of life; and risk of overdose, addiction, abuse, or misuse?

Key Points

- Three randomized, head-to-head trials of various long-acting opioids found no differences in long-term outcomes related to pain or function (SOE: Low).
- No trial was designed to assess risk of overdose, addiction, abuse, or misuse (SOE: Insufficient).
- One cohort study found sustained-release methadone to be associated with lower mortality risk (presumably related to accidental overdose) as compared to morphine in a propensity-adjusted analysis (SOE: Low).
- Another cohort study found some differences between long-acting opioids in rates of adverse outcomes related to abuse, but outcomes were nonspecific for opioid-related adverse events, precluding reliable conclusions (SOE: Insufficient).

Detailed Synthesis

The APS review included one fair-quality, open-label randomized trial (n=680) of transdermal fentanyl versus sustained-release morphine in patients with chronic low back pain that evaluated outcomes through 13 months[43] (Table 2 below; Appendix E8a, E8b, and F4). The study found no differences between these long-acting opioids in pain relief, pain intensity, use of supplemental analgesic medications, work loss, and quality of life. The study was not designed to assess overdose and addiction or related outcomes, and no cases of these outcomes were reported. The APS review also included a fair-quality retrospective cohort study based on Oregon Medicaid administrative data (n=5,684) that evaluated abuse and other related outcomes in patients with cancer or noncancer pain and at least one new 28-day prescription of methadone, sustained-release oxycodone, sustained-release morphine, or transdermal fentanyl over a 4-year timeframe.[95] Adverse events were based on clinical encounters and ICD-9 codes and defined as emergency department (ED) visits or hospitalization for opioid-related events, all-cause ED visits or hospitalizations, opioid poisoning, overdose symptoms, and death. After adjusting for opioid dose, co-morbidities, concomitant medications, and other potential confounders, sustained-release oxycodone was associated with lower risk than sustained-release morphine of an ED encounter or hospitalization involving an opioid-related adverse event (HR 0.45, 95 percent CI 0.26 to 0.77) or death (HR 0.71, 95 percent CI 0.54 to 0.94). Among patients with noncancer pain, compared with sustained-release morphine, fentanyl was associated with higher risk of ED encounters (HR 1.27, 95 percent CI 1.02 to 1.59) and methadone was associated with greater risk of overdose symptoms (HR 1.57, 95 percent CI 1.03 to 2.40). There were no significant differences between methadone and long-acting morphine in risk of death (adjusted HR 0.71, 95 percent CI 0.46 to 1.08) or overdose symptoms. Some limitations of this study include large, statistically significant differences in baseline characteristics between patients prescribed different long-acting opioids and analysis of outcomes not specific for opioid-related adverse events. For example, overdose symptoms were defined as alteration of consciousness, malaise, fatigue, lethargy, or respiratory failure.

We identified two randomized trials[96, 97] and one retrospective cohort study[98] published since the APS review that compared different long-acting opioids in patients receiving long-term opioid therapy. One large (n=1,117) fair-quality trial of patients with chronic low back pain or osteoarthritis pain found no difference between sustained-release tapentadol and sustained- release oxycodone in pain intensity through 1 year.[97] Methodological limitations included open- label design and high attrition. A smaller (n=46), poor-quality trial of patients with various types of chronic noncancer pain (61 percent low back pain) found no clear differences between transdermal buprenorphine versus transdermal fentanyl in pain intensity, pain relief, quality of life, function, or psychological symptoms through 1 year.[96] It was rated poor-quality due to high attrition and open-label design. In addition, statistical analyses comparing results between groups were not reported for most outcomes and the study was not designed to measure efficacy. No deaths were reported in either study, and the studies were not designed to assess risk of addiction, abuse, or misuse. In both trials, opioid doses were titrated to effect.

A fair-quality retrospective cohort study based on national VA system pharmacy data compared all-cause mortality among chronic pain patients prescribed methadone (n=28,554) or long-acting morphine (n=79,938).[98] The study excluded patients prescribed methadone for opioid dependence or in palliative care settings. The mean daily doses of methadone and long acting morphine were 25.4 mg and 67.5 mg, respectively. Compared to the morphine cohort, the methadone group was younger and had fewer comorbid medical conditions, but higher rates of psychiatric conditions, substance use, and back pain. To help control for these and other differences, the study analyzed patients based on their propensity for being prescribed methadone. The baseline characteristics in each propensity quintile were very similar across the two groups. In both groups, all-cause mortality was highest in propensity quintile 1 (patients with the least propensity to receive methadone and most medically ill) and least in quintile 5 (highest propensity to receive methadone). In the propensity-stratified analysis, overall risk of mortality was lower with methadone than with morphine (adjusted HR 0.56, 95 percent CI 0.51 to 0.62).

For propensity quintile 1, the adjusted HR was 0.36 (95 percent CI 0.26 to 0.49); similar trends were observed for quintiles 2 to 4. For quintile 5, there was no difference between methadone and morphine in risk of all-cause mortality (adjusted HR 0.92, 95 percent CI 0.74 to 1.2). The main limitation of this study is the possibility of residual confounding by indication. Although the study stratified patients based on their propensity for being prescribed methadone and performed adjustment on potential confounders, unmeasured confounders could still have been present. The likely effects of residual confounding on estimates is difficult to predict, because people prescribed methadone had features associated both with decreased risk of mortality (younger age and fewer co-morbid medical conditions) as well as with increased risk (more psychiatric conditions and substance abuse).

The SOE was rated Low for no difference between different long-acting opioids in pain or function, Low for mortality risk associated with methadone versus morphine, and Insufficient for abuse and related outcomes.

Table 2. Head-to-head trials and observational studies of different long-acting opioids

Author Year Study Design Duration	Setting/ Data Source Country	Interventions, N	Results	Quality
Allan, 2005[43] Randomized trial 13 months	Multicenter (number of sites not clear) Europe	A: Transdermal fentanyl (titrated from 25 mcg/hr) (Mean dose 57 mcg/hr) (N=338) B: Sustained-release morphine (titrated from 30 mg q 12 hrs) (Mean dose: 140 mg) (N=342)	A vs. B Pain score (mean, 0-100 VAS) at 56 weeks (N=608): 56.0 vs. 55.8 Severe pain at rest (per protocol analyses, N=248 and 162): 22/248 (9%) vs. 20/162 (12%), p=0.030 (no significant differences in ITT analysis, but data not provided) Severe pain on movement (per protocol): 70/248 (28%) vs. 43/162 (27%), p=0.611 Severe pain during the day (per protocol): 48/248 (19%) vs. 40/162 (25%), p=0.385 Severe pain at night (per protocol): 25/248 (10%) vs. 26/162 (16%), p=0.003 (no significant differences in ITT analysis, but data not provided) Rescue strong opioids use: 154/296 (52%) vs. 154/291 (53%) Quality of life (SF-36): No differences between interventions Loss of working days: No differences between interventions Withdrawal due to lack of efficacy: 18/335 (5%) vs.15/342 (4%)	Fair

Table 2. Head-to-head trials and observational studies of different long-acting opioids (continued)

Author Year Study Design Duration	Setting/ Data Source Country	Interventions, N	Results	Quality
Hartung, 2007[95] Retrospective cohort study Duration not applicable	U.S. Medicaid claims	A. Transdermal fentanyl (n=1,546) B. Methadone (n=974) C. ER oxycodone (n=1,866) D. ER morphine (n=1,298)	A vs. B vs. C (reference: D) Mortality: adjusted HR 0.71 (95% CI 0.46 to 1.08) vs. HR 0.71 (95% CI 0.54 to 0.94) vs. 0.80 (95% CI 0.63 to 1.02) ED encounter or hospitalization involving an opioid-related adverse event (HR 0.45, 95% CI 0.26 to 0.77) Among patients with noncancer pain: Fentanyl associated with higher risk of ED encounters than sustained-release morphine (HR 1.27, 95% CI 1.02 to 1.59) Methadone associated with greater risk of overdose symptoms than sustained-release morphine (HR 1.57, 95% CI 1.03 to 2.40) No significant differences between methadone and long-acting morphine in risk of death (adjusted HR 0.71, 95% CI 0.46 to 1.08)	Fair
Krebs, 2011[98] Retrospective cohort study Duration not applicable	U.S. VA	A: Methadone (n=28,554) B: Long-acting morphine sulfate (MS) (n=79,938)	All-cause mortality: Unadjusted: 3,347 (3.4%) patients died; highest mortality within 1st 30 days (1.2% in methadone and 3.7% in MS); raw death rates from MS higher than methadone for all 30-day intervals; Death rate: Quintile #1 (0.042 vs 0.133); Quintile #2 (0.034 vs 0.078); Quintile #3 (0.025 vs 0.053); Quintile #4 (0.022 vs 0.034); Quintile #5 (0.017 vs 0.020); Propensity adjusted mortality (HR): Overall risk of mortality lower with methadone than morphine (adjusted HR 0.56, 95% CI 0.51 to 0.62) Quintile #1: 0.36 (95% CI: 0.26, 0.49); Quintile #2: 0.46 (0.37, 0.56); Quintile #3: 0.50 (0.41, 0.61); Quintile #4: 0.66 (0.54, 0.81); Quintile #5: 0.92 (0.74, 1.16); Results robust in validation dataset	Fair
Mitra, 2013[96] Randomized trial 12 months	Townsville, Australia (1 site)	A: Transdermal buprenorphine (TDB) initial dose=-5 mcg/h (n=22) B: Transdermal fentanyl (TDF) initial dose=12.5 mcg/h (n=24) Both titrated to optimal doses over 4 weeks; increased doses beyond that given as clinically indicated	Sleep quality: No significant difference between groups (data not provided) Pain VAS: 3-point (scale 1-10) reduction in pain in 11% in each treatment group (data not provided) DASS21: TDB had relatively better score at 12 mos (data not provided) PDI: Appears similar (data not provided)	Poor

Table 2. Head-to-head trials and observational studies of different long-acting opioids (continued)

Author Year Study Design Duration	Setting/ Data Source Country	Interventions, N	Results	Quality
Wild, 2010[97] Randomized trial 12 months	53 sites in North America; 36 sites in Europe	A. Tapentadol ER 100-250 mg BID (adjustable) (n=894) B. Oxycodone CR 20-50 mg BID (adjustable) (n=223)	Mean (SE) pain intensity score: decreased from 7.6 (0.05) and 7.6 (0.11) at baseline to 4.4 (0.09) and 4.5 (0.17) Global assessment, very much improved or much improved: 48.1% (394/819) vs 41.2% (73/177) Concomitant nonopioid analgesics (NSAIDS, ASA, acetaminophen): 19.9% (178/894) vs. 17% (38/223)	Fair

Abbreviations: ASA=aspirin, BID=twice daily, CI=confidence interval, CR=controlled release, DASS21=Depression, Anxiety, and Stress Scale-21 Items, ER=extended release, HR=hazard ratio, ITT=intent to treat, MS=long-acting morphine sulfate, NSAID=nonsteroidal anti-inflammatory drug, PDI=Physical Disability Index, q=every, SE=standard error, TDB= transdermal buprenorphine, TDF= transdermal fentanyl, US=United States, VA=Veterans Affairs, VAS=Visual Analogue Scale.

Key Question 3d

In patients with chronic pain, what is the comparative effectiveness of short- plus long-acting opioids versus long-acting opioids alone on outcomes related to pain, function, and quality of life; risk of overdose, addiction, abuse, or misuse; and doses of opioids used?

The APS review identified no trial of short- plus long-acting opioids versus long-acting opioids alone. We also identified no study published since the APS review that addressed this question (SOE: Insufficient).

Key Question 3e

In patients with chronic pain, what is the comparative effectiveness of scheduled, continuous versus as-needed dosing of opioids on outcomes related to pain, function, and quality of life; risk of overdose, addiction, abuse, or misuse; and doses of opioids used?

Key Points
- No study compared long-term opioid therapy using scheduled, continuous dosing versus as-needed dosing (SOE: Insufficient).

Detailed Synthesis

The 2009 APS review included one trial of scheduled, around-the-clock dosing of codeine versus as-needed dosing, but it did not meet inclusion criteria for the current review because duration of followup was five days.[92] In addition, results of this trial were difficult to interpret because the interventions varied on factors other than whether the opioid was dosed around-the-clock, including use of sustained-release versus immediate-release codeine formulations and different doses (200 versus 71 mg/day of codeine).

We identified no study published since the APS review on long-term opioid therapy using scheduled, continuous dosing versus as-needed dosing (SOE: Insufficient).

Key Question 3f

In patients on long-term opioid therapy, what is the comparative effectiveness of dose escalation versus dose maintenance or use of dose thresholds on outcomes related to pain, function, and quality of life?

Key Points
- One fair-quality randomized trial of more liberal dose escalation versus maintenance of current doses found no difference in outcomes related to pain or function, or risk of

withdrawal due to opioid misuse, but achieved limited separation between groups in opioid doses (52 versus 40 mg MED/day at the end of the trial) (SOE: Low).

Detailed Synthesis

The APS review did not address the comparative effectiveness of dose escalation versus dose maintenance or use of dose thresholds. We identified one relevant fair-quality randomized trial (n=140) published since the APS review (Appendix E9 and F4).[99] It compared more liberal dose escalation (doses increased for inadequate pain relief using preset dosing guidelines) versus maintenance of current doses (doses only increased if medically necessary due to clear dosage tolerance or acute injury). The subjects were VA patients with primarily musculoskeletal chronic pain[99] (defined as >6 months duration). Over 90 percent of enrollees were male and initial opioid doses were about 30 mg morphine equivalents/day. Both short- and long-acting opioids were prescribed, with long-acting opioids used more at higher doses. Average pain at baseline was about 7 on a 0 to 10 scale, and mean Oswestry Disability Index (ODI) score was about 48 (indicating moderate functional disability). The trial was fair-quality, primarily due to high attrition. Although doses at the end of the 12-month trial were higher in the dose escalation group, an important limitation of this trial is that the difference in opioid doses prescribed at the end of the trial was relatively small (mean 52 versus 40 mg morphine equivalents/day).

The trial found no difference between groups at 12 months in mean Visual Analogue Scale (VAS) pain ratings (5.6 for escalating dose versus 6.2 for stable dose, p=0.11), proportion with ≥1.5 point improvement in VAS pain rating (28 percent versus 20 percent, RR 1.4, 95 percent CI 1.76 to 2.5), mean ODI scores (46 versus 45, p=0.85), proportion with ≥10 point improvement in ODI score (29 percent versus 23 percent, RR 1.0, 95 percent CI 0.61 to 1.8), or use of various nonopioid medications or physical therapy. There was also no significant difference in all-cause withdrawals (49 percent versus 56 percent, RR 0.88, 95 percent CI 0.64 to 1.2). Withdrawal due to opioid misuse was frequent in both groups, with no difference between groups (24 percent versus 30 percent, RR 0.79, 95 percent 0.46 to 1.4) (SOE: Low).

Key Question 3g

In patients on long-term opioid therapy, what is the comparative effectiveness of opioid rotation versus maintenance of current opioid therapy on outcomes related to pain, function, and quality of life; and doses of opioids used?

Key Points

- No study compared opioid rotation versus maintenance of long-term opioid therapy (SOE: Insufficient).

Detailed Synthesis

The APS review identified no randomized trials or controlled observational studies on opioid rotation versus maintenance of current therapy. We identified no studies published since the APS review that addressed this Key Question (SOE: Insufficient).

Key Question 3h

In patients on long-term opioid therapy, what is the comparative effectiveness of different strategies for treating acute exacerbations of chronic pain on outcomes related to pain, function, and quality of life?

Key Points

- Two good-quality randomized trials found buccal fentanyl more effective than placebo for treating acute exacerbations of pain and three randomized trials found buccal fentanyl or intranasal fentanyl more effective than oral opioids for treating acute exacerbations of pain in patients on long-term opioid therapy, based on outcomes measured up to 2 hours after dosing. (SOE: Moderate).
- No study evaluated long-term benefits or harms (SOE: Insufficient).

Detailed Synthesis

The APS review included two placebo-controlled, randomized trials (n=77 and 79) of buccal fentanyl for acute exacerbations of pain in people prescribed opioid therapy for chronic pain (Table 3 below, Appendix E10 and F4).[100, 101] Both found buccal fentanyl to be more effective than placebo at relieving acute pain exacerbations based on outcomes measured up to 2 hours after dosing, for up to nine episodes over a 3-week period. Neither trial was designed to evaluate benefits or harms associated with longer-term use of buccal fentanyl, including outcomes related to abuse and associated outcomes. Use of a run-in period in both trials could limit generalizability of findings, as about one-quarter of patients were excluded during an open-label run-in period due to lack of efficacy or adverse events.

We identified three subsequent head-to-head trials of buccal or intranasal fentanyl versus oral opioids for acute exacerbations of chronic pain.[102-104] As in the prior trials, all were funded by the manufacturer of buccal or intranasal fentanyl or conducted by researchers affiliated with the manufacturer. All used a double-blind, double-dummy crossover design and enrolled patients prescribed ≥60 mg MED/day and with one to four episodes of pain exacerbations per day. Like the prior trials, they focused on immediate outcomes following administration and used a run-in period. Two good-quality trials (n=183 and 137) found fentanyl buccal tablets to be more effective than oxycodone in reducing pain intensity (pain reduction 0.82 versus 0.60 and 0.88 versus 0.76 on a 0-10 scale; both p<0.001) and meaningful pain relief (undefined) (16 percent versus 12 percent at 15 minutes, p<0.05 and 46 percent versus 38 percent at 30 minutes, p<0.01).[102, 104] The pain condition in most patients in both trials was back or neck pain, osteoarthritis, fibromyalgia, traumatic injury, or complex regional pain syndrome. A fair-quality trial (n=84) of cancer patients found fentanyl pectin nasal spray more effective than immediate-release morphine sulfate at reducing pain intensity by >33 percent at 15 minutes (52 percent versus 44 percent of episodes; p<0.01).[103] It was unclear how many of the patients in the study were at end of life.

The SOE for the effectiveness of buccal or nasal fentanyl for immediate pain relief was rated Moderate.

Table 3. Trials of different strategies for treating acute exacerbations of chronic pain in patients on long-term opioid therapy

Author, Year Study Design Duration	Sample	Interventions, N	Results	Quality
Ashburn, 2011[102] Randomized trial (crossover) Duration: up to 42 days total	n=183 Patients aged 18 to 80 years with >3 months of chronic pain receiving >60 mg/day MED, with 1-4 episodes of breakthrough pain per day Mean age: 48.8 years Female sex: 62% Race: 92% White, 5% Black, 3% other Pain intensity in 24 hours prior to enrollment: 5.1 Indication (most common): 57% back pain, 11% osteoarthritis, 8% neck pain, 9% fibromyalgia, 4% traumatic injury, 4% complex regional pain syndrome	A. Fentanyl buccal tablet (n=183) B. Oxycodone (n=183)	A vs. B Pain intensity difference (from before drug administration; 0-10 scale) at 15 minutes: 0.82 vs. 0.60 (p<0.0001) Pain relief (0-5 scale) at 15 minutes: 0.69 vs. 0.53 (p<0.05) Meaningful pain relief within 15 minutes: 16% vs. 12% of episodes (p<0.05)	Good
Davies, 2011[103] Randomized trial (crossover) 3 to 21 days	n=84 Patients with histologically confirmed cancer, receiving a fixed-schedule opioid regimen at a total daily dose equivalent >60 mg MED, with 1 to 4 episodes of breakthrough pain per day Mean age: 55.9 years Female sex: NR Race: NR	A. Fentanyl pectin nasal spray (n=106 for safety and n=84 for efficacy) B. Immediate-release morphine sulfate (n=106 for safety and n=84 for efficacy)	A vs. B ≥2-point reduction in pain intensity at 10 minutes: 52.4% vs. 45.4% (p<0.05) ≥2 pain relief at 15 minutes: 60.2% vs. 53.4% (p<0.05) Total pain relief ≥33% at 15 minutes: 52.3% vs. 43.5% (p<0.01)	Fair

Table 3. Trials of different strategies for treating acute exacerbations of chronic pain in patients on long-term opioid therapy (continued)

Author, Year Study Design Duration	Sample	Interventions, N	Results	Quality
Portenoy, 2007[100] Randomized trial 3 weeks	n=77 Patients aged 18 to 80 years with chronic low back pain Mean age: 47 years Female gender: 55% Nonwhite race: 12% Baseline pain intensity: 5.1 (10 point scale) Primary etiology of low back pain degenerative disc disease: 68%	A. Buccal fentanyl 100 to 800 mcg for an episode of breakthrough pain B. Placebo (n=77) Dose of buccal fentanyl: 800 mcg 56%; 600 mcg 24%; 400 mcg 15%; 200 mcg 5%	A vs. B Sum of the pain intensity differences from 5 through 60 minutes: 8.3 vs. 3.6 Proportion of breakthrough pain episodes with "meaningful" pain reduction: 70% (289/413) vs. 30% (63/207) (p<0.0001) Proportion of breakthrough pain episodes with ≥33% reduction in pain intensity after 30 minutes: 42% (172/413) vs. 18% (18/207) (p<0.0001) Proportion of breakthrough pain episodes with ≥50% reduction in pain intensity after 30 minutes: 30% (122/413) vs. 13% (27/207) (p<0.0001) Proportion of breakthrough pain episodes with ≥33% reduction in pain intensity after 120 minutes: 65% (269/413) vs. 28% (57/207) (p<0.0001) Proportion of breakthrough pain episodes with ≥50% reduction in pain intensity after 120 minutes: 48% (198/413) vs. 16% (33/207) (p<0.0001)	Good

Table 3. Trials of different strategies for treating acute exacerbations of chronic pain in patients on long-term opioid therapy (continued)

Author, Year Study Design Duration	Sample	Interventions, N	Results	Quality
Simpson, 2007[101] Randomized trial (crossover) 3 weeks	n=79; 18 to 80 years old, >3 months history of chronic neuropathic pain associated with diabetic peripheral neuropathy, postherpetic neuralgia, traumatic injury, or complex regional pain syndrome, on chronic opioids (at least 60 mg/day or morphine or equivalent), pain intensity <7 on a 0 to 10 scale, 1 to 4 daily episodes of breakthrough pain	A. Buccal fentanyl 100 to 800 mcg for an episode of breakthrough pain B. Placebo (n=79) Dose of buccal fentanyl: 800 mcg 54%; 600 mcg 19%; 400 mcg 18%; 200 mcg 5%, 100 mcg 5%	A vs. B Sum of the pain intensity differences from 5 through 60 minutes: 9.63 vs. 5.73 (p<0.001) Proportion of breakthrough pain episodes with 'meaningful' pain reduction: 69% vs. 36% (p<0.0001) Proportion of breakthrough pain episodes with ≥50% reduction in pain intensity after 15 minutes: 12% vs. 5% (p≤0.0001), p<0.0001 for each subsequent time point from 30 to 120 minutes Use of supplemental medication: 14% (59/432) vs. 36% (77/213) (OR 0.28, 95% CI 0.18 to 0.42)	Good
Webster, 2013[104] Randomized trial (crossover) Up to 42 days	N=274 Mean age: 50.8 years Female sex: 58% Race: 91% white, 7% black, 2% other Pain intensity in 24 hours prior to enrollment: 5.1	A. Fentanyl buccal tablet (n=137) B. Oxycodone (n=137)	A vs. B Pain intensity difference (from before drug) at 15 minutes: 0.88 vs. 0.76 (0-10 scale) (p<0.001) Pain relief at 15 minutes: 38% vs. 34% (p<0.05) Meaningful pain relief within 15 minutes: 17% vs. 16% (p=NS) Meaningful pain relief within 30 minutes: 46% vs. 38% (p<0.01)	Good

Abbreviations: CI=confidence interval, MED=morphine equivalent dose, NR=not reported, NS=not significant, OR=odds ratio.

Key Question 3i

In patients on long-term opioid therapy, what are the effects of decreasing opioid doses or of tapering off opioids versus continuation of opioids on outcomes related to pain, function, quality of life, and withdrawal?

Key Points

- One small (n=10), poor-quality crossover trial found abrupt cessation of morphine to be associated with increased pain and decreased function compared to continuation of morphine (SOE: Insufficient).

Detailed Synthesis

The APS review included one small (n=10), poor-quality crossover trial that found abrupt cessation of morphine to be associated with increased pain and decreased function compared to continuation of morphine (Appendix E11 and F4).[105] Three patients (30 percent) reported opioid withdrawal symptoms following abrupt cessation of morphine, though there were no differences in physiologic parameters (vital signs and pupil size). Average dose of morphine prior to entry into was 42 mg/day (range 30 to 120 mg/day). Results of this trial may not apply to the general population of patients with chronic pain, as patients who did not have pain adequately controlled by immobilization and alternative medications were excluded from study entry. We identified no study published since the APS review addressing this question.

Key Question 3j

In patients on long-term opioid therapy, what is the comparative effectiveness of different tapering protocols and strategies on measures related to pain, function, quality of life, withdrawal symptoms, and likelihood of opioid cessation?

Key Points

- Two poor-quality, nonrandomized prospective trials found no clear differences between different methods for opioid discontinuation or tapering (inpatient, patient controlled versus fixed reduction schedule or detoxification plus counseling versus detoxification plus maintenance) in likelihood of opioid abstinence after 3 to 6 months (SOE: Insufficient).

Detailed Synthesis

The APS review included two poor-quality, nonrandomized prospective trials that reported similar rates of opioid abstinence after 3 to 6 months in patients allocated to different methods for opioid discontinuation or tapering (Appendix E12 and F4).[106, 107] In one study (n=108), patients either chose inpatient, patient-controlled reduction of opioids or a fixed reduction schedule.[106] Mean opioid dose on study entry was 36 mg MED/day; duration of opioid therapy was not reported. In the second study, patients (n=42) received detoxification plus counseling or detoxification with maintenance therapy if detoxification was unsuccessful.[107] Mean duration of opioid use was 7.2 years in the detoxification plus counseling group and 9.2 years in the detoxification plus maintenance group; opioid doses ranged widely (e.g., codeine daily doses ranged from 240 to 2400 mg/day). Neither study evaluated effects of different methods for discontinuing opioids on pain, function, quality of life, or withdrawal symptoms.

We identified no study published since the APS review on the comparative effectiveness of different tapering protocols and strategies in chronic pain patients on long-term opioid therapy.

Key Question 4a

In patients with chronic pain being considered for long-term opioid therapy, what is the accuracy of instruments for predicting risk of opioid overdose, addiction, abuse, or misuse?

Key Points

- Three studies (one fair-quality, two poor-quality) evaluated the Opioid Risk Tool (ORT); using a cutoff of ≥4. Estimates of diagnostic accuracy were inconsistent, precluding reliable conclusions. Sensitivities ranged from 0.20 to 0.99; specificities for the two in which this could be calculated were 0.88 and 0.16 (SOE: Insufficient).

- Two studies evaluated the Screening and Opioid Assessment for Patients with Pain (SOAPP) Version 1 instrument. In one fair-quality study, based on a cutoff score of ≥8, sensitivity was 0.68 and specificity was 0.38, for a PLR of 1.11 and NLR of 0.83 for predicting aberrant urine drug test. In one poor-quality study, sensitivity for predicting opioid discontinuation due to aberrant drug-related behavior was 0.73 based on a cutoff score of >6 and other diagnostic accuracy indicators could not be determined. (SOE: Low).
- One poor-quality study evaluated the Diagnosis, Intractability, Risk, and Efficacy Inventory (DIRE), but specificity and other diagnostic accuracy indicators could not be determined as patients who were not discontinued from opioids were not included in this study. (SOE: Insufficient)
- One poor-quality study evaluated the Pain Medication Questionnaire (PMQ), and for a cutoff of scores ≥30, sensitivity was low (0.34), specificity was 0.77, and AUROC was 0.57 for predicting opioid discontinuation due to aberrant drug-related behaviors. (SOE: Insufficient)
- One poor-quality study evaluated the Screening and Opioid Assessment for Patients with Pain-Revised (SOAPP-R). For a cutoff of ≥18, sensitivity was 0.39 and specificity was 0.69 and AUROC was 0.54 for predicting opioid discontinuation and discharge due to aberrant drug-related behavior. (SOE: Insufficient)

Detailed Synthesis

The APS review[108] included two fair-quality prospective studies of instruments to predict risk of opioid abuse or misuse completed by patients before initiation of opioid therapy (Table 4 below; Appendix E13 and F5).[109, 110] One study[109] evaluated the 14-item, patient self-administered Screening and Opioid Assessment for Patients with Pain (SOAPP) Version 1 instrument[111] and the other[110] evaluated the 10-item, self-administered Opioid Risk Tool (ORT). The SOAPP is scored on a scale of 0 to 56, while ORT scores can range from 0 to 25. For both instruments, higher scores indicate greater risk of opioid misuse and patients with scores ≥8 are considered high-risk for abuse. Both studies were performed with samples of patients in pain clinics. Methodological shortcomings of both studies included unclear blinding of outcomes assessors to findings of the screening instrument, use of definitions for aberrant drug-related behaviors that were not well standardized or defined, and failure to distinguish less serious from more serious behaviors. Although the APS review included two other studies used to develop the SOAPP Version 1[111] and the Revised SOAPP,[112] both were conducted using samples of patients already on long-term opioid therapy and did not meet inclusion criteria for the current review. In these studies, sensitivities (0.80 and 0.91) and specificities (0.68 and 0.69) were higher than those reported in the study of the SOAPP Version 1[109] conducted in patients evaluated prior to initiation of treatment.

The study of the SOAPP Version 1 instrument[111] reported a sensitivity of 0.68 (95 percent CI 0.52 to 0.81) and specificity of 0.38 (95 percent CI 0.29 to 0.49) based on a cutoff score of ≥8, for a PLR of 1.11 (95 percent CI 0.86 to 1.43) and NLR of 0.83 (95 percent CI 0.50 to 1.36) (Table 5 below).[109] Results were difficult to interpret because the only outcome reported was aberrant urine drug test, urine drug screens were not obtained in most patients, and duration of followup was unclear.

In the study[110] of the ORT, items in the ORT were chosen and weighted before evaluation of diagnostic test characteristics, and cut-off scores for different risk categories appeared to be selected on an a priori basis. Aberrant drug-related behaviors as documented in medical records over 12 months of follow-up were identified in 6 percent (1/18) of patients categorized as low risk (score 0 to 3), compared with 28 percent (35/123) of patients categorized as moderate risk (score 4 to 7) and 91 percent (41/44) of those categorized as high risk (score ≥8), for PLRs of 0.08 (95 percent CI 0.01 to 0.62) for a low-risk score, 0.57 (95 percent CI 0.44 to 0.74) for a moderate-risk score, and 14.34 (95 percent 5.35 to 38) for a high-risk score (Table 5 below).[110]

We identified two subsequent poor-quality retrospective studies that compared the ability of different risk assessment instruments to predict subsequent opioid abuse or misuse.[113, 114] One study compared the ORT, the Revised (24-item) SOAPP (SOAPP-R), the Pain Medication Questionnaire (PMQ), and a semi-structured clinical interview.[113] SOAPP-R scores range from 0 to 24 (scores ≥18 indicate high risk) and PMQ scores range from 0 to 104 (scores ≥30 indicate high risk.) The other compared the SOAPP Version 1, the ORT, the Diagnosis, Intractability, Risk, and Efficacy Inventory (DIRE) instrument, and a semi-structured clinical interview.[114] DIRE scores range from 7 to 21, and unlike the other risk assessment instruments, lower scores (≤13) indicate high-risk for abuse. Both studies appeared to be conducted in the same pain clinic during different time periods. Methodological shortcomings in both studies included exclusion of patients who were not evaluated with all of the risk assessment instruments (in one study, nearly 300 of 347 patients were excluded for this reason,[113] and in the other the proportion excluded was not reported[114]) and use of a case-control design. In both studies, cases were based on opioid discontinuations due to abuse, without further specification. One study also evaluated aberrant behaviors, but this outcome was not clearly defined.[114]

One poor-quality study found the ORT (cutoff >4), PMQ (cutoff ≥30) and SOAPP-R (cutoff ≥18) associated with sensitivities of 0.20, 0.34, and 0.39, respectively, and specificities of 0.88, 1.77 and 0.69, resulting in weak positive likelihood ratios (PLR; range 1.27 to 1.65) and negative likelihood ratios (NLR; range 0.86 to 0.91).[113] The AUROC ranged from 0.54 to 0.57. Results were similar when cases were based on presence of aberrant behaviors not necessarily resulting in opioid discontinuation. The other poor-quality study reported a higher sensitivity with the SOAPP Version 1 (0.73 at cutoff >6) compared with the ORT (0.45 at cutoff ≥4) or DIRE (0.17 at cutoff <14).[114] Because patients who were not discontinued from opioids were not included in this study, specificity and other diagnostic accuracy indicators could not be determined. Both studies also included a semi-structured clinician interview that addressed many of the components included in the risk prediction instruments (e.g., pain source and duration, history of drug or alcohol abuse, psychiatric symptoms or comorbidities). In both studies, the predictive accuracy of the clinician interview was at least as good as that of formal risk instruments.

The only instruments evaluated in more than one study were the ORT (3 studies[110, 113, 114]) and the SOAPP version 1 (two studies).[109, 114] Across the studies, estimates for diagnostic accuracy were extremely inconsistent. Using a cutoff score of >4, the sensitivity of the ORT ranged from 0.20 to 0.99 in three studies[110, 113, 114] and specificity was 0.88 and 0.16 in two studies and could not be calculated in the third study (SOE: Insufficient).[110, 113] The inconsistency could be due in part to differences in study methods and definitions of opioid abuse or misuse. For the SOAPP, cutoff scores of ≥6 and ≥8 had similar sensitivities (0.73 and 0.68, respectively) (SOE: Low), but other measures of diagnostic accuracy could not be compared because one of the studies only included cases.[114]

Table 4. Studies of risk assessment instrument

Author Year	Population, N	Risk Assessment	Method of Administratio	Reference Standard
Akbik, 2006[109]	n=155 Mean age 43 years (SD 9.6) 33% female 86% White, other races not reported Pain: 39% back	SOAPP (scale 0-56; high risk ≥8)	Self-report	Positive urine drug test
Jones, 2012[113] (Study 2)	n=263 Mean age 48 years (SD 13) 56% female 96% White, other races not reported Pain: 45% low back pain, 21% arthritis or fibromyalgia), 14% joint pain, 10% pelvic or abdominal pain, 7% neck or upper back pain	ORT (scale 0-25; high risk ≥8) PMQ (scale 0-104; high risk ≥30) SOAPP-R (scale 0-24; high risk ≥18) Clinician assessment	Self-report (SOAPP-R, ORT, PMQ); clinician interview	Opioid discontinuation due to abuse
Moore, 2009[114]	n=48 Mean age 44 years (SD 11) 60% female Race not reported Pain not reported	SOAPP (scale 0-56; high risk ≥8) DIRE (scale 7-21; high-risk ≤13) ORT (scale 0-26; high risk ≥8) Clinician assessment	Self-report (SOAPP, DIRE, ORT); clinician interview	Opioid discontinuation due to abuse[a]
Webster, 2005[110]	n=185 Mean age 44 years (SD 13) 58% female Race not reported Pain: 45% back; 18% head; 16% neuropathic; 16% musculoskeletal; 5% visceral	ORT (scale 0-25; high risk ≥8)	Self-report	Documentation in medical record of aberrant behavior during followup

Abbreviations: DIRE= Diagnosis Intractability Risk and Efficacy Inventory, ORT= Opioid Risk Tool, PMQ=Pain Medication Questionnaire,
SD=standard deviation, SOAPP= Screening and Opioid Assessment for Patients with Pain, SOAPP-R= Screening and Opioid Assessment for Patients with Pain-Revised.

Table 5. Predictive value of risk assessment instruments

Scale	Studies	Sensitivity	Specificity	Positive Likelihood Ratio	Negative Likelihood Ratio	AUROC
DIRE	Moore, 2009[114]	Score <14: 0.17	Not calculable[a]	Not calculable[a]	Not calculable[a]	Not calculable[a]
ORT	Jones, 2012[113]	Score >4: 0.20 (95% CI 0.15 to 0.27)	Score >4: 0.88 (95% CI 0.82 to 0.93)	Score >4: 1.65 (95% CI 0.78 to 3.51)	Score >4: 0.91 (95% CI 0.78 to 1.06)	0.54
	Moore, 2009[114]	Score ≥4: 0.45	Not calculable[a]	Not calculable[a]	Not calculable[a]	Not calculable[a]
	Webster, 2005[110]	Score ≥4: 0.99 (95% CI 0.92 to 0.99)	Score ≥4: 0.16 (95% CI 0.10 to 0.24)	Score ≥4: 0.99 (95% CI 0.92 to 0.999) Score 1-3: 0.08 (95% CI 0.01 to 0.62) Score 4-7: 0.57 (95% CI 0.44 to 0.74) Score ≥8: 14.34 (95% CI 5.35 to 38)	Score ≥4: 0.16 (95% CI 0.10 to 0.24)	Not reported
PMQ	Jones, 2012[113]	Score ≥30: 0.34 (95% CI 0.20 to 0.51)	Score ≥30: 0.77 (95% CI 0.69 to 0.80)	Score ≥30: 1.46 (95% CI 0.87 to 2.45)	Score ≥30: 0.86 (95% CI 0.68 to 1.08)	0.57
SOAPP-R	Jones, 2012[113]	Score ≥18: 0.39 (95% CI 0.26 to 0.54)	Score ≥18: 0.69 (95% CI 0.63 to 0.75)	Score ≥18: 1.27 (95% CI 0.86 to 1.90)	Score ≥18: 0.88 (95% CI 0.70 to 1.10)	0.54
SOAPP	Moore, 2009[114]	Score >6: 0.73	Not calculable[a]	Not calculable[a]	Not calculable[a]	Not calculable
	Akbik, 2006[109]	Score ≥8: 0.68 (95% CI 0.52 to 0.81)	Score ≥8: 0.38 (95% CI 0.29 to 0.49)	Score ≥8: 1.11 (95% CI 0.86 to 1.43)	Score ≥8: 0.83 (95% CI 0.50 to 1.36)	Not reported

[a]Retrospective study; only patients who had discontinued opioids due to aberrant drug-related behavior were included.
Abbreviations: CI=confidence interval, DIRE= Diagnosis Intractability Risk and Efficacy Inventory, ORT= Opioid Risk Tool, PMQ=Pain Medication Questionnaire, SOAPP= Screening and Opioid Assessment for Patients with Pain, SOAPP-R=Screening and Opioid Assessment for Patients with Pain-Revised.

Key Question 4b

In patients with chronic pain, what is the effectiveness of use of risk prediction instruments on outcomes related to overdose, addiction, abuse, or misuse?

Key Points

- No study evaluated the effectiveness of risk prediction instruments for reducing outcomes related to overdose, addiction, abuse, or misuse (SOE: Insufficient).

Detailed Synthesis

The APS review identified no studies on the effectiveness of risk prediction instruments in reducing outcomes related to overdose, addiction abuse or misuse. We also did not identify any studies published since the APS review addressing this question.

Key Question 4c

In patients with chronic pain prescribed long-term opioid therapy, what is the effectiveness of risk mitigation strategies, including (1) opioid management plans, (2) patient education, (3) urine drug screening, (4) use of prescription drug monitoring program data, (5) use of monitoring instruments, (6) more frequent monitoring intervals, (pill counts, and (8) use of abuse-deterrent formulations on outcomes related to overdose, addiction, abuse, or misuse?

Key Points

- No study evaluated the effectiveness of risk mitigation strategies for improving outcomes related to overdose, addiction, abuse, or misuse (SOE: Insufficient).

Detailed Synthesis

Like the APS review, we identified no study on the effectiveness of various risk mitigation strategies for improving outcomes related to overdose, addiction, abuse, or misuse.

Key Question 4d

What is the comparative effectiveness of treatment strategies for managing patients with addiction to prescription opioids on outcomes related to overdose, abuse, misuse, pain, function, and quality of life?

Key Points

- No study evaluated the comparative effectiveness of treatment strategies for managing patients with addiction to prescription opioids (SOE: Insufficient).

Detailed Synthesis

Like the APS review, we identified no study on the comparative effectiveness of treatment strategies for managing patients with addiction to prescription opioids. Short-term randomized trials generally excluded patients with a past or current history of addiction.

Discussion

Key Findings and Strength of Evidence

The key findings of this review are summarized in the summary of evidence table (Table 6 below) and the factors used to determine the overall SOE grades are summarized in Appendix G. For a number of Key Questions, we identified no studies meeting inclusion criteria. For Key Questions where studies were available, the SOE was rated no higher than low, due to small numbers of studies and methodological shortcomings, with the exception of buccal or intranasal fentanyl for pain relief outcomes within 2 hours after dosing, for which the SOE was rated moderate.

For effectiveness and comparative effectiveness, we identified no studies of long-term opioid therapy in patients with chronic pain versus no opioid therapy or nonopioid alternative therapies that evaluated outcomes at 1 year or longer. No studies examined how effectiveness varies based on various factors, including type of pain and patient characteristics. Most placebo-controlled randomized trials were shorter than 6 weeks in duration[44] and no cohort studies on the effects of long-term opioid therapy versus no opioid therapy on outcomes related to pain, function, or quality of life were found. Although uncontrolled studies of patients prescribed opioids are available,[8] findings are difficult to interpret due to the lack of a nonopioid comparison group.

Regarding harms, new evidence (published since the APS review) from observational studies suggests that being prescribed long-term opioids for chronic pain is associated with increased risk of abuse,[48] overdose,[61] fractures,[18,71] and myocardial infarction,[80] versus not currently being prescribed opioids. In addition, several recent studies suggest that the risk is dose-dependent, with higher opioid doses associated with increased risk.[11,18,48,61,79,84] Although two studies found an association between opioid dose and increased risk of overdose starting at relatively low doses (20 to 49 mg MED/day), estimates at higher doses were variable (adjusted HR 11.18 at >100 mg MED/day versus adjusted OR 2.88 for ≥200 mg MED/day).[61,84] However, few studies evaluated each outcome and the population evaluated and duration of opioid therapy were not always well characterized. In addition, as in all observational studies, findings are susceptible to residual confounding despite use of statistical adjustment and other techniques such as matching. A study also found long-term opioid therapy associated with increased likelihood of receiving prescriptions for erectile dysfunction or testosterone, which may be markers for sexual dysfunction due to presumed endocrinological effects of opioids.[11] However, it did not directly measure sexual dysfunction, and patients may seek or receive these medications for other reasons.

No study assessed the risk of abuse, addiction, or related outcomes associated with long-term opioid therapy use versus placebo or no opioid therapy. In uncontrolled studies, rates of abuse and related outcomes varied substantially, even after restricting inclusion to studies that evaluated patients on opioid therapy for at least one year and used pre-defined methods for ascertaining these outcomes, and stratifying studies according to whether they evaluated primary care populations or patients evaluated in pain clinic settings.[46,49-58] An important reason for the variability in estimates is differences in patient samples and in how terms such as addiction, abuse, misuse, and dependence were defined in the studies, and in methods used to identify these outcomes (e.g., formal diagnostic interview with patients versus chart review or informal assessment). In one study, estimates of opioid misuse were lower based on independent review than based on assessments by the treating physician.[57] No study evaluated patients with "opioid use disorder" as recently defined in the new DSM-V.[59]

Evidence on the effectiveness of different opioid dosing strategies is also extremely limited. One new trial of a more liberal dose escalation strategy versus maintenance of current doses found no differences in outcomes related to pain, function, or risk of withdrawal from the study due to opioid misuse, but the difference in opioid doses between groups at the end of the trial was small (52 versus 40 mg MED/day).[99] One study from Washington State reported a decrease in the number of opioid-associated overdose deaths after implementing a dose threshold,[115] but did not meet inclusion criteria for this review because it was an ecological, before-after study, and it is not possible to reliably determine whether changes in the number of opioid overdose deaths were related to other factors that could have impacted opioid prescribing practices. Evidence on benefits and harms of different methods for initiating and titrating opioids, short- versus long-acting opioids, scheduled and continuous versus as-needed dosing of opioids, use of opioid rotation, and methods for titrating or discontinuing patients off opioids was not available or too limited to reach reliable conclusions.

We also found limited evidence on the comparative benefits and harms of specific opioids. Three head-to-head trials found few differences in pain relief between various long-acting opioids at 1 year followup,[43, 96, 97] but the usefulness of these studies for evaluating comparative effectiveness may be limited because patients in each arm had doses titrated to achieve adequate pain control. None of the trials was designed to evaluate abuse, addiction, or related outcomes.

Methadone has been an opioid of particular interest because it is disproportionately represented in case series and epidemiological studies of opioid-associated deaths.[116] Characteristics of methadone that may be associated with increased risk of serious harms are its long and variable half-life, which could increase the risk for accidental overdose, and its association with electrocardiographic QTc interval prolongation, which could increase the risk of potentially life-threatening ventricular arrhythmia.[117] However, the highest-quality observational study, which was conducted in VA patients with chronic pain and controlled well for confounders using a propensity-adjusted analysis, found methadone to be associated with lower risk of mortality as compared with sustained-release morphine.[98] These results suggest that in some settings, methadone may not be associated with increased mortality risk, though research is needed to understand the factors that contribute to safer prescribing in different clinical settings.

Although five randomized trials found buccal or intranasal fentanyl more effective than placebo or oral opioids for treating acute exacerbations of chronic pain, all focused on short-term treatment and immediate outcomes in the minutes or hours after administration.[100-104] No study was designed to assess long-term benefits or harms, including accidental overdose, abuse, or addiction. In 2007, the U.S. FDA released a public health advisory due to case reports of deaths and other life-threatening adverse effects in patients prescribed buccal fentanyl.[118]

Evidence also remains limited on the utility of opioid risk assessment instruments, used prior to initiation of opioid therapy, for predicting likelihood of subsequent opioid abuse or misuse. In three studies of the ORT, estimates were extremely inconsistent (sensitivity ranged from 0.20 to 0.99).[110, 114, 119] A study that directly compared the accuracy of the ORT and two other risk assessment instruments reported weak likelihood ratios for predicting future abuse or misuse (PLR 1.27 to 1.65 and NLR 0.86 to 0.91).[119] Risk prediction instruments other than the ORT (such as the SOAPP version 1, revised SOAPP, or DIRE) were only evaluated in one or two studies, and require further validation. Studies on the accuracy of risk instruments for identifying aberrant behavior in patients already prescribed opioids are available,[51, 54, 112, 119-125] but were outside the scope of this review.

No study evaluated the effectiveness of risk mitigation strategies, such as use of risk assessment instruments, opioid management plans, patient education, urine drug screening, prescription drug monitoring program data, monitoring instruments, more frequent monitoring intervals, pill counts, or abuse-deterrent formulations on outcomes related to overdose, addiction, abuse or misuse. Studies on effects of risk mitigation strategies were primarily focused on ability to detect misuse (e.g., urine drug testing and prescription monitoring program data) or on effects on markers of risky prescribing practices or medication-taking behaviors,[126] and did not meet inclusion criteria for this review, which focused on effects on clinical outcomes. One study found that rates of poison center treatment incidents and opioid-related treatment admissions increased at a lower rate in States with a prescription drug monitoring program than in States without one, but used an ecological design, did not evaluate a cohort of patients prescribed opioids for chronic pain, and was not designed to account for other factors that could have impacted opioid prescribing practices.[126]

Although evidence indicates that patients with a history of substance abuse or at higher risk for abuse or misuse due to other risk factors are more likely to be prescribed opioids than patients without these risk factors,[127-130] we identified no study on the effectiveness of methods for mitigating potential harms associated with long-term opioid therapy in high-risk patients.

Table 6. Summary of evidence

Key Question Outcome	Strength of Evidence Grade	Conclusion
1. Effectiveness and comparative effectiveness		
a. In patients with chronic pain, what is the effectiveness of long-term opioid therapy versus placebo or no opioid therapy for long-term (≥1 year) outcomes related to pain, function, and quality of life?		
Pain, function, quality of life	Insufficient	No study of opioid therapy versus placebo or no opioid therapy evaluated long-term (≥1 year) outcomes related to pain, function, or quality of life
b. How does effectiveness vary depending on: 1) the specific type or cause of pain (e.g., neuropathic, musculoskeletal [including low back pain], fibromyalgia, sickle cell disease, inflammatory pain, and headache disorders); 2) patient demographics (e.g., age, race, ethnicity, gender); 3) patient comorbidities (including past or current alcohol or substance use disorders, mental health disorders, medical comorbidities and high risk for addiction)?		
Pain, function, quality of life	Insufficient	No studies
c. In patients with chronic pain, what is the comparative effectiveness of opioids versus nonopioid therapies (pharmacological or nonpharmacological) on outcomes related to pain, function, and quality of life?		

Table 6. Summary of evidence (continued)

Key Question Outcome	Strength of Evidence Grade	Conclusion
Pain, function, quality of life	Insufficient	No studies

Key Question Outcome	Strength of Evidence Grade	Conclusion
d. In patients with chronic pain, what is the comparative effectiveness of opioids plus nonopioid interventions (pharmacological or nonpharmacological) versus opioids or nonopioid interventions alone on outcomes related to pain, function, quality of life, and doses of opioids used?		
Pain, function, quality of life	Insufficient	No studies
2. Harms and adverse events		
a. In patients with chronic pain, what are the risks of opioids versus placebo or no opioid on: 1) opioid abuse, addiction, and related outcomes; 2) overdose; and 3) other harms, including gastrointestinal-related harms, falls, fractures, motor vehicle accidents, endocrinological harms, infections, cardiovascular events, cognitive harms, and psychological harms (e.g., depression)?		
Abuse, addiction	Low	No randomized trial evaluated risk of opioid abuse, addiction, and related outcomes in patients with chronic pain prescribed opioid therapy. One retrospective cohort study found prescribed long-term opioid use associated with significantly increased risk of abuse or dependence versus no opioid use.
Abuse, addiction	Insufficient	In 10 uncontrolled studies, estimates of opioid abuse, addiction, and related outcomes varied substantially even after stratification by clinic setting
Overdose	Low	Current opioid use was associated with increased risk of any overdose events (adjusted HR 5.2, 95% CI 2.1 to 12) and serious overdose events (adjusted HR 8.4, 95% CI 2.5 to 28) versus current nonuse
Fractures	Low	Opioid use associated with increased risk of fracture in 1 cohort study (adjusted HR 1.28, 95% CI 0.99 to 1.64) and 1 case-control study (adjusted OR 1.27, 95% CI 1.21 to 1.33)
Myocardial infarction	Low	Current opioid use associated with increased risk of myocardial infarction versus nonuse (adjusted OR 1.28, 95% CI 1.19 to 1.37 and incidence rate ratio 2.66, 95% CI 2.30 to 3.08)
Endocrine	Low	Long-term opioid use associated with increased risk of use of medications for erectile dysfunction or testosterone replacement versus nonuse (adjusted OR 1.5, 95% CI 1.1 to 1.9)

Table 6. Summary of evidence (continued)

Key Question Outcome	Strength of Evidence Grade	Conclusion
Gastrointestinal harms, motor vehicle accidents, infections, psychological harms, cognitive harms	Insufficient	No studies
b. How do harms vary depending on: 1) the specific type or cause of pain (e.g., neuropathic, musculoskeletal [including back pain], fibromyalgia, sickle cell disease, inflammatory pain, headache disorders); 2) patient demographics; 3) patient comorbidities (including past or current substance use disorder or at high risk for addiction)?		
Various harms	Insufficient	No studies
b. How do harms vary depending on the dose of opioids used?		
Abuse, addiction	Low	One retrospective cohort study found higher doses of long-term opioid therapy associated with increased risk of opioid abuse or dependence than lower doses. Compared to no opioid prescription, the adjusted odds ratios were 15 (95 percent CI 10 to 21) for 1-36 MED/day, 29 (95 percent CI 20 to 41) for 36-120 MED/day, and 122 (95 percent CI 73 to 205) for ≥120 MED/day.
Overdose	Low	Versus 1 to 19 mg MED/day, 1 cohort study found an adjusted HR for an overdose event of 1.44 (95% CI 0.57 to 3.62) for 20 to 49 mg MED/day that increased to 11.18 (95% CI 4.80 to 26.03) at >100 mg MED/day; 1 case-control study found an adjusted OR for an opioid-related death of 1.32 (95% CI 0.94 to 1.84) for 20 to 49 mg MED/day that increased to 2.88 (95% CI 1.79 to 4.63) at ≥200 mg MED/day
Fracture	Low	Risk of fracture increased from an adjusted HR of 1.20 (95% CI 0.92 to 1.56) at 1 to <20 mg MED/day to 2.00 (95% CI 1.24 to 3.24) at ≥50 mg MED/day; the trend was of borderline statistical significance
Myocardial infarction	Low	Relative to a cumulative dose of 0 to 1350 mg MED over 90 days, the incidence rate ratio for myocardial infarction for 1350 to <2700 mg was 1.21 (95% CI 1.02 to 1.45), for 2700 to <8100 mg was 1.42 (95% CI 1.21 to 1.67), for 8100 to <18,000 mg was 1.89 (95% CI 1.54 to 2.33), and for >18,000 mg was 1.73 (95% CI 1.32 to 2.26)
Motor vehicle accidents	Low	No association between opioid dose and risk of motor vehicle accidents
Endocrine	Low	Relative to 0 to <20 mg MED/day, the adjusted OR for daily opioid dose of ≥120 mg MED/day for use of medications for erectile dysfunction or testosterone replacement was 1.6 (95% CI 1.0 to 2.4)

Table 6. Summary of evidence (continued)

Key Question Outcome	Strength of Evidence Grade	Conclusion
3. Dosing strategies		
a. In patients with chronic pain, what is the comparative effectiveness of different methods for initiating and titrating opioids for outcomes related to pain, function, and quality of life; risks of overdose, addiction, abuse, or misuse; and doses of opioids used?		
Pain	Insufficient	Evidence from three trials on effects of titration with immediate-release versus sustained-release opioids reported inconsistent results on outcomes related to pain and are difficult to interpret due to additional differences between treatment arms in dosing protocols (titrated vs. fixed dosing) and doses of opioids used
Function, quality of life, outcomes related to abuse	Insufficient	No studies
b. In patients with chronic pain, what is the comparative effectiveness of short- versus long-acting opioids on outcomes related to pain, function, and quality of life; risk of overdose, addiction, abuse, or misuse; and doses of opioids used?		
Pain, function, quality of life, outcomes related to abuse	Insufficient	No studies
c. In patients with chronic pain, what is the comparative effectiveness of different long-acting opioids on outcomes related to pain, function, and quality of life; and risk of overdose, addiction, abuse, or misuse?		
Pain and function	Low	No difference between various long-acting opioids
Assessment of risk of overdose, addiction, abuse, or misuse	Insufficient	No studies were designed to assess risk of overdose, addiction, abuse, or misuse
Overdose (as indicated by all-cause mortality)	Low	One cohort study found methadone to be associated with lower all-cause mortality risk than sustained-release morphine in a propensity adjusted analysis
Abuse and related outcomes	Insufficient	Another cohort study found some differences between long-acting opioids in rates of adverse outcomes related to abuse, but outcomes were nonspecific for opioid-related adverse events, precluding reliable conclusions
d. In patients with chronic pain, what is the comparative effectiveness of short- plus long-acting opioids vs. long-acting opioids alone on outcomes related to pain, function, and quality of life; risk of overdose, addiction, abuse, or misuse; and doses of opioids used?		
Pain, function, quality of life, outcomes related to abuse	Insufficient	No studies
e. In patients with chronic pain, what is the comparative effectiveness of scheduled, continuous versus as-needed dosing of opioids on outcomes related to pain, function, and quality of life; risk of overdose, addiction, abuse, or misuse; and doses of opioids used?		

Table 6. Summary of evidence (continued)

Key Question Outcome	Strength of Evidence Grade	Conclusion
Pain, function, quality of life, outcomes related to abuse	Insufficient	No studies
f. In patients with chronic pain on long-term opioid therapy, what is the comparative effectiveness of dose escalation versus dose maintenance or use of dose thresholds on outcomes related to pain, function, and quality of life?		
Pain, function, withdrawal due to opioid misuse	Low	No difference between more liberal dose escalation versus maintenance of current doses in pain, function, or risk of withdrawal due to opioid misuse, but there was limited separation in opioid doses between groups (52 vs. 40 mg MED/day at the end of the trial)
g. In patients on long-term opioid therapy, what is the comparative effectiveness of opioid rotation versus maintenance of current opioid therapy on outcomes related to pain, function, and quality of life; and doses of opioids used?		
Pain, function, quality of life, outcomes related to abuse	Insufficient	No studies
h. In patients on long-term opioid therapy, what is the comparative effectiveness of different strategies for treating acute exacerbations of chronic pain on outcomes related to pain, function, and quality of life?		
Pain	Moderate	Two randomized trials found buccal fentanyl more effective than placebo for treating acute exacerbations of pain and three randomized trials found buccal fentanyl or intranasal fentanyl more effective than oral opioids for treating acute exacerbations of pain in patients on long-term opioid therapy, based on outcomes measured up to 2 hours after dosing
Abuse and related outcomes	Insufficient	No studies
i. In patients on long-term opioid therapy, what are the effects of decreasing opioid doses or of tapering off opioids versus continuation of opioids on outcomes related to pain, function, quality of life, and withdrawal?		
Pain, function	Insufficient	Abrupt cessation of morphine was associated with increased pain and decreased function compared to continuation of morphine
j. In patients on long-term opioid therapy, what is the comparative effectiveness of different tapering protocols and strategies on measures related to pain, function, quality of life, withdrawal symptoms, and likelihood of opioid cessation?		
Opioid abstinence	Insufficient	No clear differences between different methods for opioid discontinuation or tapering in likelihood of opioid abstinence after 3 to 6 months

Table 6. Summary of evidence (continued)

Key Question Outcome	Strength of Evidence Grade	Conclusion
4. Risk assessment and risk mitigation strategies		
a. In patients with chronic pain being considered for long-term opioid therapy, what is the accuracy of instruments for predicting risk of opioid overdose, addiction, abuse, or misuse?		
Diagnostic accuracy: Opioid Risk Tool	Insufficient	Based on a cutoff of >4, three studies (one poor-quality, two poor-quality) reported very inconsistent estimates of diagnostic accuracy, precluding reliable conclusions
Diagnostic accuracy: Screening and Opioid Assessment for Patients with Pain (SOAPP) version 1	Low	Based on a cutoff score of ≥ 8, sensitivity was 0.68 and specificity of 0.38 in 1 study, for a PLR of 1.11 and NLR of 0.83. Based on a cutoff score of >6, sensitivity was 0.73 in 1 study.
b. In patients with chronic pain, what is the effectiveness of use of risk prediction instruments on outcomes related to overdose, addiction, abuse, or misuse?		
Outcomes related to abuse	Insufficient	No study evaluated the effectiveness of risk prediction instruments for reducing outcomes related to overdose, addiction, abuse, or misuse
c. In patients with chronic pain prescribed long-term opioid therapy, what is the effectiveness of risk mitigation strategies, including 1) opioid management plans, 2) patient education, 3) urine drug screening, 4) use of prescription drug monitoring program data, 5) use of monitoring instruments, 6) more frequent monitoring intervals, 7) pill counts, and 8) use of abuse-deterrent formulations on outcomes related to overdose, addiction, abuse, or misuse?		
Outcomes related to abuse	Insufficient	No studies
d. What is the comparative effectiveness of treatment strategies for managing patients with addiction to prescription opioids on outcomes related to overdose, abuse, misuse, pain, function, and quality of life?		
Outcomes related to abuse	Insufficient	No studies

Abbreviations: CI=confidence interval, HR=hazard ratio, MED= morphine equivalent dose, NLR=negative likelihood ratio, OR=odds ratio,
PLR=positive likelihood ratio, SOAPP= Screening and Opioid Assessment for Patients with Pain.

Findings in Relationship to What is Already Known

Our findings are generally consistent with prior systematic reviews of opioid therapy for chronic pain that also found no long-term, placebo-controlled randomized trials.[8, 44] One systematic review of outcomes associated with long-term opioid therapy concluded that many patients discontinue treatment due to adverse events or insufficient pain relief, though patients who continue opioid therapy experience clinically significant pain relief.[8] However, results of the studies included in this review are difficult to interpret because the studies had no nonopioid therapy control group, reported substantial between-study heterogeneity, and were susceptible to potential attrition and selection bias. Our findings are also consistent with a systematic review on comparative benefits and harms of various long-acting opioids and short- versus long-acting opioids, which found no clear differences, primarily based on short-term randomized trials.[131]

Our review reported rates of abuse and related outcomes that are higher than a previously published systematic review of long-term opioid therapy that reported a very low rate of opioid addiction (0.27 percent).[8] Factors that may explain this discrepancy are that the prior review included studies that did not report predefined methods for ascertaining opioid addiction, potentially resulting in underreporting, and primarily included studies that excluded high-risk patients. Like a previous systematic review, we found variability in estimates of abuse and related outcomes, with some potential differences in estimates based on clinical setting (primary care versus pain clinic) and patient characteristics (e.g., exclusion of high-risk patients).[132]

Regarding risk mitigation strategies, our findings were similar to a previously published systematic review that found weak evidence with which to evaluate risk prediction instruments.[133] Unlike our review, which found no evidence on effects of risk mitigation strategies on risk of abuse, addiction, or related outcomes, a previously published review found use of opioid management plans and urine drug screens to be associated with decreased risk of misuse behaviors.[14] However, this conclusion was based on four studies that did not meet inclusion criteria for our review because effects of opioid management plans and urine drug screens could not be separated from other concurrent opioid prescribing interventions,[134, 135] use of a historical control group,[136, 137] or before-after study design.[134]

Applicability

A number of issues could impact the applicability of our findings. One challenge was difficulty in determining whether studies focused on patients with chronic pain. Although a number of large observational studies reported harms based on analyses of administrative databases, they were frequently limited in their ability to assess important clinical factors such as the duration or severity of pain. For some of these studies, we inferred the presence of chronic pain from prescribing data, such as the number of prescriptions over a defined period or the use of long-acting opioid preparations. Some potentially relevant studies were excluded because it was not possible to determine whether the sample evaluated had chronic pain or received long- term therapy.[16, 74-78, 85]

Another issue that could impact applicability is the type of opioid used in the studies. Both long-acting and short-acting opioids are often prescribed for chronic pain. In some studies, use of short-acting opioids predominated.[11, 18, 84] Results of studies of short-acting opioids may not generalize to patients prescribed long-acting opioids.

Selection of patients could also impact applicability. The few randomized trials that met inclusion criteria typically excluded patients at high risk of abuse or misuse and frequently used run-in periods prior to allocating treatments. The use of a run-in period preselects patients who respond to and tolerate initial exposure to the studied treatment. Therefore, benefits observed in the trials might be greater and harms lower than seen in actual clinical practice.[138]

Another factor impacting applicability is that most trials were not designed or powered to assess risk of abuse, addiction, or related outcomes. For example, trials of buccal fentanyl for acute exacerbations of chronic pain focused exclusively on immediate (episode-based) outcomes and were not designed to assess long-term outcomes, including outcomes related to the potential for abuse.[100-104] Long-term head-to-head trials of long-acting opioids excluded patients at high risk for these outcomes and reported no events.[43, 96, 97]

The setting in which studies were conducted could also impact applicability. As noted in other sections of this report, rates of overdose, abuse, addiction, and related outcomes are likely to vary based on the clinical setting. Therefore, we stratified studies reporting rates of abuse according to whether they were performed in primary care or pain clinic settings. The highest-quality comparative study of methadone versus another opioid (long-acting morphine) found decreased mortality risk but was conducted in a VA setting,[98] which could limit applicability to other settings, due to factors such as how clinicians were trained in methadone use, policies on opioid prescribing, availability of resources to manage opioid prescribing, or other factors.

Implications for Clinical and Policy Decisionmaking

Our review has important implications for clinical and policy decisionmaking. Based on our review, most clinical and policy decisions regarding use of long-term opioid therapy must necessarily still be made on the basis of weak or insufficient evidence. This is in accordance with findings from a 2009 U.S. guideline on use of opioids for chronic pain, which found 21 of 25 recommendations supported by only low-quality evidence,[108] and a 2010 Canadian guideline,[139] which classified 3 of 24 recommendations as based on (short-term) randomized trials and 19 recommendations as based solely or partially on consensus opinion. Although randomized trials show short-term, moderate improvements in pain in highly selected, low-risk populations with chronic pain, such efficacy-based evidence is of limited usefulness for informing long-term opioid prescribing decisions in clinical practice.

Given the marked increase in numbers of overdose deaths and other serious adverse events that have occurred following the marked increase in opioid prescribing for chronic pain, recent policy efforts have focused on safer prescribing of opioids. A recent review of opioid guidelines found broad agreement regarding a number of risk mitigation strategies despite weak evidence, such as risk-assessment guided patient assessment for opioid therapy, urine drug testing, use of prescription monitoring program data, abuse-deterrent formulations, and opioid management plans.[140] Based on low-quality evidence regarding harms associated with long-term opioid therapy, our review provides some limited support for clinical policy efforts aimed at reducing harms. One area in which there has been less agreement across guidelines is whether dose thresholds that warrant more intense monitoring or used to define maximum ceiling doses should be implemented, and if so, what is the appropriate threshold. Some evidence is now available on dose-dependent harms associated with opioids,[61, 84] which could help inform policies related to dose thresholds. However, research on the effects of implementing dose thresholds on clinical outcomes is limited to a single ecological study.[115] In addition, although two observational studies were consistent in reporting a relationship between higher opioid dose and risk of overdose, estimates were highly variable at similar doses.[61, 84] This makes it difficult to determine an optimal maximum dose threshold based on an objective parameter, such as a dose inflection point where risk rises markedly. Other studies have begun to characterize cardiovascular, endocrinological, and injury-related harms associated with long-term opioid therapy and could be used to inform clinical decisions, though using such information in balanced assessments to inform clinical and policy decision-making remains a challenge given the lack of evidence regarding long-term benefits.

Limitations of the Review Process

We excluded non-English language articles and did not search for studies published only as abstracts. We did not attempt meta-analysis or assess for publication bias using graphical or statistical methods to detect small sample effects due to the paucity of evidence. Although we found no evidence of unpublished studies through searches on clinical trial registries and regulatory documents and solicitation of unpublished studies through SIP requests, the usefulness of such methods for identifying unpublished observational studies may be limited, as such studies are often not registered. We identified no unpublished randomized trials meeting inclusion criteria. We focused on studies that reported outcomes after at least one year of opioid therapy, though applying a shorter duration threshold for inclusion could have provided additional evidence. However, we identified no placebo-controlled trials of opioid therapy for at least 6 months.

Limitations of the Evidence Base

As noted previously, the critical limitation of our review is the lack of evidence in the target population (patients with chronic pain) and intervention (long-term opioid therapy), despite broadening of inclusion criteria to incorporate studies in which we assumed that patients were being treated for chronic pain due to the type of opioid prescribed (long-acting opioid) or number of prescriptions. We were also unable to determine how benefits and harms vary in subgroups, such as those defined by demographic characteristics, characteristics of the pain condition, and other patient characteristics (e.g., medical or psychological comorbidities). Due to the lack of evidence and methodological shortcomings in the available studies, no body of evidence (with

the exception of buccal or intranasal fentanyl for immediate pain relief) was rated higher than low, meaning that conclusions are highly uncertain.

Research Gaps

Many research gaps limit the full understanding of the effectiveness, comparative effectiveness, and harms of long-term opioid therapy, as well as of the effectiveness of different dosing methods and risk mitigation strategies, and effectiveness in special populations. Longer-term studies of patients clearly with chronic pain comparing those who are prescribed long-term opioid therapy with those receiving other pharmacological and non-pharmacological therapies are needed. Studies that include higher-risk patients, commonly treated with opioids in clinical practice, and that measure multiple important outcomes, including pain, physical and psychological functioning, as well as misuse and abuse, would be more helpful than efficacy studies focused solely on pain intensity. Greater standardization of methods for defining and identifying abuse-related outcomes in studies that report these outcomes are needed. The Initiative on Methods, Measurement, and Pain Assessment in Clinical Trials (IMMPACT) group recently issued recommendations on measuring abuse liability in analgesic clinical trials.[141]

Additional research is also needed to develop and validate risk prediction instruments, and to determine how using them impacts treatment decisions and, ultimately, patient outcomes. More research is needed on the comparative benefits and harms of different opioids or formulations and different prescribing methods. Studies comparing effectiveness and harms of methadone versus other long-acting opioids, to determine if findings from a study[98] conducted in a VA setting are reproducible in other settings, and to better understand factors associated with safer methadone prescribing.

Research is also needed to understand the effects of risk mitigation strategies such as urine drug screening, use of prescription drug monitoring program data, and abuse-deterrent formulations on clinical outcomes such as rates of overdose, abuse, addiction, and misuse. In one before-after study, the introduction of an abuse-deterrent opioid was followed by patients switching to other prescription opioids or illicit opioids,[142] underscoring the need for research to understand both the positive and negative clinical effects of risk mitigation strategies.

Long-term randomized trials of opioid therapy are difficult to implement due to attrition, challenges in recruitment, or ethical factors (e.g., long-term allocation of patients with pain to placebo or allocation to non-use of risk mitigation strategies recommended in clinical practice guidelines). Nonetheless, pragmatic and other non-traditional randomized trial approaches could be used to address these challenges.[143] Observational studies could also help address a number of these research questions, but should be specifically designed to evaluate patients with chronic pain prescribed long-term opioid therapy and appropriately measure and address potential confounders. Well-designed clinical registries that enroll patients with chronic pain prescribed and not prescribed chronic opioids could help address the limitations of studies based solely or primarily on administrative databases, which are often unable to fully characterize the pain condition (e.g., duration, type, and severity) or other clinical characteristics and frequently do not have information regarding outcomes related to pain, function, and quality of life. Such registry studies could be designed to extend the observations from randomized trials of opioids versus placebo or other treatments, but would differ from currently available studies by following patients who discontinue or do not start opioids, in addition to those who continue on or start opioid therapy.

Conclusions

Evidence on long-term opioid therapy for chronic pain is very limited, but suggests an increased risk of serious harms that appears to be dose-dependent. Based on our review, most clinical and policy decisions regarding use of long-term opioid therapy must necessarily still be made on the basis of weak or insufficient evidence. More research is needed to understand long-term benefits, risk of abuse and related outcomes, and effectiveness of different opioid prescribing methods and risk mitigation strategies.

References

1. International Association for the Study of Pain. Classification of chronic pain: Descriptions of chronic pain syndromes and definitions of pain terms. Pain. 1986;3:S1-226. PMID: 3461421.
2. Institute of Medicine (U.S.) Committee on Advancing Pain Research Care and Education. Relieving Pain in America: A Blueprint for Transforming Prevention, Care, Education, and Research. National Academies Press. Washington, DC: 2011. PMID: 22553896.
3. Ballantyne JC, Shin NS. Efficacy of opioids for chronic pain: A review of the evidence. Clinical J Pain. 2008;24(6):469-78. PMID: PMID: 18574357.
4. Eriksen J, Sjogren P, Bruera E, et al. Critical issues on opioids in chronic non-cancer pain: an epidemiological study. Pain. 2006;125(1-2):172-9. PMID: 16842922.
5. Sullivan MD, Edlund MJ, Fan M-Y, et al. Trends in use of opioids for non-cancer pain conditions 2000–2005 in Commercial and Medicaid insurance plans: The TROUP study. Pain. 2008;138(2):440-9. PMID: 18547726.
6. Boudreau D, Von Korff M, Rutter CM, et al. Trends in long-term opioid therapy for chronic non-cancer pain. Pharmacoepidemiol Drug Saf. 2009;18(12):1166-75. PMID: 19718704.
7. Olsen Y, Daumit GL, Ford DE. Opioid prescriptions by U.S. primary care physicians from 1992 to 2001. J Pain. 2006;7(4):225-35. PMID: 16618466.
8. Noble M, Treadwell JR, Tregear SJ, et al. Long-term opioid management for chronic noncancer pain. Cochrane Database Syst Rev. 2010(11):CD006605. doi: 10.1002/14651858.CD006605.pub2. PMID 20091598.
9. Chou R, Fanciullo GJ, Fine PG, et al. Clinical guidelines for the use of chronic opioid therapy in chronic noncancer pain. J Pain. 2009;10(2):113-30. PMID: 19187889.
10. Starrels JL, Becker WC, Weiner MG, et al. Low use of opioid risk reduction strategies in primary care even for high-risk patients with chronic pain. J Gen Intern Med. 2011;26(9):958-64. PMID: 21347877.
11. Deyo RA, Smith DH, Johnson ES, et al. Prescription opioids for back pain and use of medications for erectile dysfunction. Spine. 2013;38(11):909-15. PMID: 23459134.
12. Substance Abuse and Mental Health Services Administration. Treatment Episode Data Set (TEDS). 1999–2009. National Admissions to Substance Abuse Treatment Services, DASIS Series: S-56. Substance Abuse and Mental Health Services Administration. Rockville, MD: 2011.
13. Substance Abuse and Mental Health Services Administration. The DAWN Report: Highlights of the 2010 Drug Abuse Warning Network (DAWN) Findings on Drug-Related Emergency Department Visits. Center for Behavioral Health Statistics and Quality. Rockville, MD: 2012.
14. Starrels JL, Becker WC, Alford DP, et al. Systematic review: treatment agreements and urine drug testing to reduce opioid misuse in patients with chronic pain. Ann Intern Med. 2010;152:712-20. PMID: 20513829.
15. Warner M, Chen LH, Makuc DM, et al. Drug poisoning deaths in the United States, 1980–2008. NCHS Data Brief. 2011;81:1-8. PMID: 22617462.
16. Bohnert ASB VM, Bair MJ, et al. Association between opioid prescribing patterns and opioid overdose-related deaths. JAMA. 2011;305(13):1315-21. PMID: 21467284.
17. Volkow ND, McLellan TA. Curtailing diversion and abuse of opioid analgesics without jeopardizing pain treatment. JAMA. 2011;305(13):1346-7. PMID: 21467287.
18. Saunders KW, Dunn KM, Merrill JO, et al. Relationship of opioid use and dosage levels to fractures in older chronic pain patients. J Gen Intern Med. 2010;25(4):310-5. PMID: 20049546.
19. Rolita L, Spegman A, Tang X, et al. Greater number of narcotic analgesic prescriptions for osteoarthritis is associated with falls and fractures in elderly adults. J Am Geriatr Soc. 2013;61(3):335-40. PMID: 23452054.
20. Gomes T, Redelmeier DA, Juurlink DN, et al. Opioid dose and risk of road trauma in Canada: a population-based study. JAMA Intern Med. 2013;173(3):196-201. PMID: 23318919.
21. Centers for Disease Control and Prevention. Prescription Drug Overdose in the United

States: Fact Sheet. Atlanta, GA: Centers for Disease Control and Prevention; 2014. Available at: http://www.cdc.gov/homeandrecreationalsafety/overdose/facts.html. Accessed on July 17 2014.
22. Furlan AD, Sandoval JA, Mailis-Gagnon A, et al. Opioids for chronic noncancer pain: a meta-analysis of effectiveness and side effects. CMAJ. 2006;174(11):1589-94. PMID: 16717269.
23. Daniell HW. Hypogonadism in men consuming sustained-action oral opioids. J Pain. 2002;3:377-84. PMID: 14622741.
24. Daniell HW. Opioid endocrinopathy in women consuming prescribed sustained-action opioids for control of nonmalignant pain. J Pain. 2008;9:28-36. PMID: 14622741.
25. Angst MS, Clark JD. Opioid-induced hyperalgesia: a qualitative systematic review. Anesthesiology. 2006;104(3):570-87. PMID: 16508405.
26. Chou R, Ballantyne JC, Fanciullo GJ, et al. Research gaps on use of opioids for chronic noncancer pain: findings from a review of the evidence for an American Pain Society and American Academy of Pain Medicine clinical practice guideline. J Pain. 2009;10(2):147-59. PMID: 19187891.
27. Furlan AD, Reardon R, Weppler C, et al. Opioids for chronic noncancer pain: a new Canadian practice guideline. CMAJ. 2011;182(9):923-30. PMID: 20439443.
28. United States Department of Veterans Affairs, The Management of Opioid Therapy for Chronic Pain Working Group. VA/DoD Clinical Practice Guideline for Management of Opioid Therapy for Chronic Pain; 2010. Available at: http://www.healthquality.va.gov/Chronic_Opioid_Therapy_COT.asp. Accessed September 19, 2014.
29. American Pain Society-American Academy of Pain Medicine Opioids Guidelines Panel. Guideline for the Use of Chronic Opioid Therapy in Chronic Noncancer Pain: Evidence Review; 2009. Available at: http://www.americanpainsociety.org/uploads/pdfs/Opioid_Final_Evidence_Report.pdf. Accessed September 19, 2014.
30. Owens D, Lohr KN, Atkins D, et al. Methods Guide for Effectiveness and Comparative Effectiveness Reviews. Rockville, MD: Agency for Healthcare Research and Quality. 2011.
31. Chou R. The effectiveness and risks of long-term opioid treatment of chronic pain. PROSPERO 2014:CRD42014007016 Available at: http://www.crd.york.ac.uk/PROSPERO/display_record.asp?ID=CRD42014007016. Accessed September 19, 2014.
32. U.S. Food and Drug Administration. Extended-Release and Long-Acting (ER/LA) Opioid Analgesics Risk Evaluation and Mitigation Strategy (REMS) a single shared system - Current Application Holders; 2014. Available at: http://www.fda.gov/downloads/Drugs/DrugSafety/InformationbyDrugClass/UCM348818.pdf. Accessed September 19, 2014.
33. Hall AJ, Logan JE, Toblin RL, et al. Patterns of abuse among unintentional pharmaceutical overdose fatalities. JAMA. 2008;300(22):2613-20. PMID: 19066381.
34. Altman DG, Bland JM. Diagnostic tests 3: receiver operating characteristic plots. BMJ. 1994;309(6948):188. PMID: 8044101.
35. Zweig MH, Campbell G. Receiver-operating characteristic (ROC) plots: a fundamental evaluation tool in clinical medicine. Clin Chem. 1993;39(4):561-77. PMID: 8472349.
36. Furlan AD, Pennick V, Bombardier C, et al. 2009 updated methods guidelines for systematic reviews in the Cochrane Back Review Group. Spine. 2009;24:1929-41. PMID: 19680101.
37. U.S. Preventive Services Task Force. U.S. Preventive Services Task Force Procedure Manual. AHRQ Publication No. 08-05118-EF, July 2008. Available at: http://www.uspreventiveservicestaskforce.org/uspstf08/methods/procmanual.htm. Accessed September 19, 2014.
38. Quality AfHRa. Methods Guide for Medical Test Reviews. Rockville, MD: 2010. Avaiable at: http://www.effectivehealthcare.ahrq.gov/tasks/sites/ehc/assets/File/methods_guide_for_medical_tests.pdf. Accessed September 19, 2014.
39. Whiting PF, Rutjes AWS, Westwood ME, et al. QUADAS-2: A revised tool for the Quality Assessment of Diagnostic Accuracy Studies. Ann Intern Med. 2011;155(8):529-36. PMID: 22007046.
40. McGinn TG, Guyatt GH, Wyer PC, et al. Users' guides to the medical literature: XXII: how to use articles about clinical decision rules. JAMA. 2000;284(1):79-84. PMID: 10872017.

41. Agency for Healthcare Research and Quality. Methods guide for Effectiveness and Comparative Effectiveness Reviews. AHRQ Publication No. 10(13)-EHC063-EF. Rockville, MD: Agency for Healthcare Research and Quality. November 2013. Chapters available at: www.effectivehealthcare.ahrq.gov. Accessed September 19, 2014.

42. Atkins D, Chang SM, Gartlehner G, et al. Assessing applicability when comparing medical interventions: AHRQ and the Effective Health Care Program. J Clin Epidemiol. 2011;64(11):1198-207. PMID: 21463926.

43. Allan L, Richarz U, Simpson K, et al. Transdermal fentanyl versus sustained release oral morphine in strong-opioid naive patients with chronic low back pain. Spine. 2005;30(22):2484-90. PMID: 16284584.

44. Furlan A, Chaparro LE, Irvin E, et al. A comparison between enriched and nonenriched enrollment randomized withdrawal trials of opioids for chronic noncancer pain. Pain Res Manag. 2011;16(5):337-51. PMID: 22059206.

45. Noble M, Tregear SJ, Treadwell JR, et al. Long-term opioid therapy for chronic noncancer pain: a systematic review and meta-analysis of efficacy and safety. J Pain Symptom Manag. 2008;35(2):214-28. PMID: 18178367.

46. Martell BA, O'Connor PG, Kerns RD, et al. Systematic review: opioid treatment for chronic back pain: prevalence, efficacy, and association with addiction. Ann Intern Med. 2007;146(2):116-27. PMID: 17227935.

47. Carrington Reid M, Engles-Horton LL, Weber MB, et al. Use of opioid medications for chronic noncancer pain syndromes in primary care. J Gen Intern Med. 2002;17(3):173-9. PMID: 11929502.

48. Edlund MJ, Martin BC, Russo JE, et al. The role of opioid prescription in incident opioid abuse and dependence among individuals with chronic noncancer pain. Clin J Pain. 2014;30(7):557-64.

49. Banta-Green CJ, Merrill JO, Doyle SR, et al. Opioid use behaviors, mental health and pain--development of a typology of chronic pain patients. Drug Alcohol Depend. 2009;104(1-2):34-42. PMID: 19473786.

50. Boscarino JA, Rukstalis M, Hoffman SN, et al. Risk factors for drug dependence among out-patients on opioid therapy in a large U.S. health-care system. Addiction. 2010;105(10):1776-82. PMID: 20712819.

51. Compton PA, Wu SM, Schieffer B, et al. Introduction of a self-report version of the Prescription Drug Use Questionnaire and relationship to medication agreement noncompliance. J Pain Symptom Manage. 2008;36(4):383-95. PMID: 18508231.

52. Cowan DT, Wilson-Barnett J, Griffiths P, et al. A survey of chronic noncancer pain patients prescribed opioid analgesics. Pain Med. 2003;4(4):340-51. PMID: 14750910.

53. Fleming MF, Balousek SL, Klessig CL, et al. Substance use disorders in a primary care sample receiving daily opioid therapy. J Pain. 2007;8(7):573-82. PMID: 17499555.

54. Hojsted J, Nielsen PR, Guldstrand SK, et al. Classification and identification of opioid addiction in chronic pain patients. Eur J Pain. 2010;14(10):1014-20. PMID: 20494598.

55. Portenoy RK, Farrar JT, Backonja MM, et al. Long-term use of controlled-release oxycodone for noncancer pain: results of a 3-year registry study. Clin J Pain. 2007;23(4):287-99. PMID: 17449988.

56. Saffier K, Colombo C, Brown D, et al. Addiction Severity Index in a chronic pain sample receiving opioid therapy. J Subst Abuse Treat. 2007;33(3):303-11. PMID: 17376639.

57. Schneider JP, Kirsh KL. Defining clinical issues around tolerance, hyperalgesia, and addiction: a quantitative and qualitative outcome study of long-term opioid dosing in a chronic pain practice. J Opioid Manag. 2010;6(6):385-95. PMID: 21268999.

58. Wasan AD, Butler SF, Budman SH, et al. Does report of craving opioid medication predict aberrant drug behavior among chronic pain patients? Clin J Pain. 2009;25(3):193-8. PMID: 19333168.

59. American Psychiatric Association. Diagnostic and statistical manual of mental disorders, fifth edition. Arlington, VA: American Psychiatric Association; 2013.

60. Chou R. 2009 Clinical Guidelines from the American Pain Society and the American Academy of Pain Medicine on the use of chronic opioid therapy in chronic noncancer pain: what are the key messages for clinical practice? Pol Arch Med Wewn. 2009;119(7-8):469-77. PMID: 19776687.

61. Dunn KM, Saunders KW, Rutter CM, et al. Opioid prescriptions for chronic pain and

62. Kalso E, Edwards JE, Moore RA, et al. Opioids in chronic non-cancer pain: systematic review of efficacy and safety. Pain. 2004;112(3):372-80. PMID: 15561393.
63. Moore RA, McQuay HJ. Prevalence of opioid adverse events in chronic non-malignant pain: systematic review of randomised trials of oral opioids. Arthritis Res Ther. 2005;7(5):R1046-51. PMID: 16207320.
64. Takkouche B, Montes-Martinez A, Gill SS, et al. Psychotropic medications and the risk of fracture: a meta-analysis. Drug Saf. 2007;30(2):171-84. PMID: 17253881.
65. Vestergaard P, Rejnmark L, Mosekilde L. Fracture risk associated with the use of morphine and opiates. J Intern Med. 2006;260(1):76-87. PMID: 16789982.
66. Miller M, Sturmer T, Azrael D, et al. Opioid analgesics and the risk of fractures in older adults with arthritis. J Am Ger Soc. 2011;59(3):430-8. PMID: 21391934.
67. Solomon DH, Rassen JA, Glynn RJ, et al. The comparative safety of opioids for nonmalignant pain in older adults. Arch Intern Med. 2010;170(22):1979-86. PMID: 21149754.
68. Solomon DH, Rassen JA, Glynn RJ, et al. The comparative safety of analgesics in older adults with arthritis. Arch Intern Med. 2010;170(22):1968-76. PMID: 21149752.
69. Spector W, Shaffer T, Potter DE, et al. Risk factors associated with the occurrence of fractures in U.S. nursing homes: resident and facility characteristics and prescription medications. J Am Geriatr Soc. 2007;55(3):327-33. PMID: 17341233.
70. Abrahamsen B, Brixen K. Mapping the prescriptiome to fractures in men--a national analysis of prescription history and fracture risk. Osteoporos Int. 2009;20(4):585-97. PMID: 18690484.
71. Li L, Setoguchi S, Cabral H, et al. Opioid use for noncancer pain and risk of fracture in adults: a nested case-control study using the general practice research database. Am J Epidemiol. 2013;178(4):559-69. PMID: 23639937.
72. Fishbain DA, Cutler RB, Rosomoff HL, et al. Can patients taking opioids drive safely? A structured evidence-based review. J Pain Palliat Care Pharmacother. 2002;16(1):9-28. PMID: 14650448.
73. Fishbain DA, Cutler RB, Rosomoff HL, et al. Are opioid-dependent/tolerant patients impaired in driving-related skills? A structured evidence-based review. J Pain Symptom Manag. 2003;25(6):559-77. PMID: 12782437.
74. Byas-Smith MG, Chapman SL, Reed B, et al. The effect of opioids on driving and psychomotor performance in patients with chronic pain. Clin J Pain. 2005;21(4):345-52. PMID: 15951653.
75. Gaertner J, Frank M, Bosse B, et al. [Oral controlled-release oxycodone for the treatment of chronic pain. Data from 4196 patients]. Schmerz. 2006;20(1):61-8. PMID: 15926076.
76. Galski T, Williams JB, Ehle HT. Effects of opioids on driving ability. J Pain Symptom Manag. 2000;19(3):200-8. PMID: 10760625.
77. Sabatowski R, Schwalen S, Rettig K, et al. Driving ability under long-term treatment with transdermal fentanyl. J Pain Symptom Manag. 2003;25(1):38-47. PMID: 12565187.
78. Menefee LA, Frank ED, Crerand C, et al. The effects of transdermal fentanyl on driving, cognitive performance, and balance in patients with chronic nonmalignant pain conditions. Pain Med. 2004;5(1):42-9. PMID: 14996236.
79. Carman WJ, Su S, Cook SF, et al. Coronary heart disease outcomes among chronic opioid and cyclooxygenase-2 users compared with a general population cohort. Pharmacoepidemiol Drug Saf. 2011;20(7):754-62. PMID: 21567652.
80. Li L, Setoguchi S, Cabral H, et al. Opioid use for noncancer pain and risk of myocardial infarction amongst adults. J Intern Med. 2013;273(5):511-26. PMID: 23331508.
81. Merza Z, Edwards N, Walters S, et al. Patients with chronic pain and abnormal pituitary function require investigation. The Lancet. 2003;361(9376):2203-4. PMID: 12842375.
82. Daniell HW. DHEAS deficiency during consumption of sustained-action prescribed opioids: evidence for opioid-induced inhibition of adrenal androgen production. J Pain. 2006;7(12):901-7. PMID: 17157776.
83. Rhodin A, Stridsberg M, Gordh T. Opioid endocrinopathy: a clinical problem in patients with chronic pain and long-term

84. Gomes T, Mamdani MM, Dhalla IA, et al. Opioid dose and drug-related mortality in patients with nonmalignant pain. Arch Intern Med. 2011;171(7):686-91. PMID: 21482846.
85. Paulozzi LJ, Kilbourne EM, Shah NG, et al. A history of being prescribed controlled substances and risk of drug overdose death. Pain Med. 2012;13(1):87-95. PMID: 22026451.
86. Braden JB, Russo J, Fan MY, et al. Emergency department visits among recipients of chronic opioid therapy. Arch Intern Med. 2010;170(16):1425-32. PMID: 20837827.
87. Salzman RT, Roberts MS, Wild J, et al. Can a controlled-release oral dose form of oxycodone be used as readily as an immediate-release form for the purpose of titrating to stable pain control? J Pain Symptom Manag. 1999;18(4):271-9. PMID: 10534967.
88. Jamison RN, Raymond SA, Slawsby EA, et al. Opioid therapy for chronic noncancer back pain. A randomized prospective study. Spine. 1998;23(23):2591-600. PMID: 9854758.
89. Chou R, Clark E, Helfand M. Comparative efficacy and safety of long-acting oral opioids for chronic non-cancer pain: a systematic review. J Pain Symptom Manag. 2003;26(5):1026-48. PMID: 14585554.
90. Caldwell JR, Hale ME, Boyd RE, et al. Treatment of osteoarthritis pain with controlled release oxycodone or fixed combination oxycodone plus acetaminophen added to nonsteroidal anti-inflammatory drugs: a double blind, randomized, multicenter, placebo controlled trial. J Rheumatol. 1999;26(4):862-9. PMID: 10229408.
91. Gostick N, Allen J, Cranfield R, et al. A comparison of the efficacy and adverse effects of controlled-release dihydrocodeine and immediate-release dihydrocodeine in the treatment of pain in osteoarthritis and chronic back pain. Proceedings of The Edinburgh Symposium on Pain Control and Medical Education; 1989.
92. Hale M, Speight K, Harsanyi Z, et al. Efficacy of 12 hourly controlled-release codeine compared with as required dosing of acetaminophen plus codeine in patients with chronic low back pain. Pain Res Manag. 1997;2(1):33-8. PMID: 10524470.
93. Hale ME, Fleischmann R, Salzman R, et al. Efficacy and safety of controlled-release versus immediate-release oxycodone: randomized, double-blind evaluation in patients with chronic back pain. Clin J Pain. 1999;15(3):179-83. PMID: 10524470.
94. Lloyd R, Costello F, Eves M, et al. The efficacy and tolerability of controlled-release dihydrocodeine tablets and combination dextro-propoxyphene/paracetamol tablets in patients with severe osteoarthritis of the hips. Curr Med Res Op. 1992;13(1):37-48. PMID: 1468244.
95. Hartung DM, Middleton L, Haxby DG, et al. Rates of Adverse Events of Long-Acting Opioids in a State Medicaid Program. Ann Pharmacother. 2007;41(6):921-8. PMID: 17504834.
96. Mitra F, Chowdhury S, Shelley M, et al. A feasibility study of transdermal buprenorphine versus transdermal fentanyl in the long-term management of persistent non-cancer pain. Pain Med. 2013;14(1):75-83. PMID: 23320402.
97. Wild JE, Grond S, Kuperwasser B, et al. Long-term safety and tolerability of tapentadol extended release for the management of chronic low back pain or osteoarthritis pain. Pain Pract. 2010;10(5):416-27. PMID: 20602712.
98. Krebs EE, Becker WC, Zerzan J, et al. Comparative mortality among Department of Veterans Affairs patients prescribed methadone or long-acting morphine for chronic pain. Pain. 2011;152(8):1789-95. PMID: 21524850.
99. Naliboff BD, Wu SM, Schieffer B, et al. A randomized trial of 2 prescription strategies for opioid treatment of chronic nonmalignant pain. J Pain. 2011;12(2):288-96. PMID: 21111684.
100. Portenoy RK, Messina J, Xie F, et al. Fentanyl buccal tablet (FBT) for relief of breakthrough pain in opioid-treated patients with chronic low back pain: a randomized, placebo-controlled study. Curr Med Res Opin. 2007;23(1):223-33. PMID: 17207304.
101. Simpson DM, Messina J, Xie F, et al. Fentanyl buccal tablet for the relief of breakthrough pain in opioid-tolerant adult patients with chronic neuropathic pain: a multicenter, randomized, double-blind,

102. Ashburn MA, Slevin KA, Messina J, et al. The efficacy and safety of fentanyl buccal tablet compared with immediate-release oxycodone for the management of breakthrough pain in opioid-tolerant patients with chronic pain. Anesth Analg. 2011;112(3):693-702. PMID: 21304148.
103. Davies A, Sitte T, Elsner F, et al. Consistency of efficacy, patient acceptability, and nasal tolerability of fentanyl pectin nasal spray compared with immediate-release morphine sulfate in breakthrough cancer pain. J Pain Symptom Manag. 2011;41(2):358-66. PMID: 21334555.
104. Webster LR, Slevin KA, Narayana A, et al. Fentanyl buccal tablet compared with immediate-release oxycodone for the management of breakthrough pain in opioid-tolerant patients with chronic cancer and noncancer pain: a randomized, double-blind, crossover study followed by a 12-week open-label phase to evaluate patient outcomes. Pain Med. 2013;14(9):1332-45. PMID: 23855816.
105. Cowan DT, Wilson-Barnett J, Griffiths P, et al. A randomized, double-blind, placebo-controlled, cross-over pilot study to assess the effects of long-term opioid drug consumption and subsequent abstinence in chronic noncancer pain patients receiving controlled-release morphine. Pain Med. 2005;6(2):113-21. PMID: 15773875.
106. Ralphs JA, Williams AC, Richardson PH, et al. Opiate reduction in chronic pain patients: a comparison of patient-controlled reduction and staff controlled cocktail methods. Pain. 1994;56(3):279-88. PMID: 8022621.
107. Tennant FS, Jr., Rawson RA. Outpatient treatment of prescription opioid dependence: comparison of two methods. Arch Intern Med. 1982;142(10):1845-7. PMID: 6181749.
108. Chou R, Fanciullo GJ, Fine PG, et al. Opioids for chronic noncancer pain: prediction and identification of aberrant drug-related behaviors: a review of the evidence for an American Pain Society and American Academy of Pain Medicine clinical practice guideline. J Pain. 2009;10(2):131-46. PMID: 19187890.
109. Akbik H, Butler SF, Budman SH, et al. Validation and clinical application of the Screener and Opioid Assessment for Patients with Pain (SOAPP). J Pain Symptom Manag. 2006;32(3):287-93. PMID: 16939853.
110. Webster LR, Webster RM. Predicting aberrant behaviors in opioid-treated patients: preliminary validation of the Opioid Risk Tool. Pain Med. 2005;6(6):432-42. PMID: 16336480.
111. Butler SF, Budman SH, Fernandez K, et al. Validation of a screener and opioid assessment measure for patients with chronic pain. Pain. 2004;112(1-2):65-75. PMID: 15494186.
112. Butler SF, Fernandez K, Benoit C, et al. Validation of the revised Screener and Opioid Assessment for Patients with Pain (SOAPP-R). J Pain. 2008;9(4):360-72. PMID: 18203666.
113. Jones T, Moore T, Levy JL, et al. A comparison of various risk screening methods in predicting discharge from opioid treatment. Clin J Pain. 2012;28(2):93-100. PMID: 21750461.
114. Moore TM, Jones T, Browder JH, et al. A comparison of common screening methods for predicting aberrant drug-related behavior among patients receiving opioids for chronic pain management. Pain Med. 2009;10(8):1426-33. PMID: 20021601.
115. Franklin GM, Mai J, Turner J, et al. Bending the prescription opioid dosing and mortality curves: impact of the Washington State opioid dosing guideline. Am J Ind Med. 2012;55(4):325-31. PMID: 22213274.
116. Chou R, Cruciani RA, Fiellin DA, et al. Methadone safety: a clinical practice guideline from the American Pain Society and College on Problems of Drug Dependence, in collaboration with the Heart Rhythm Society. J Pain. 2014;15(4):321-37. PMID: 24685458.
117. Chou R, Weimer MB, Dana T. Methadone overdose and cardiac arrhythmia potential: findings from a review of the evidence for an American Pain Society and College on Problems of Drug Dependence clinical practice guideline. J Pain. 2014;15(4):338-65. PMID: 24685459.
118. U.S. Food and Drug Administration. Public Health Advisory: Important Information for the Safe Use of Fentora (fentanyl buccal tablets). Silver Springs, MD; 2013. Available at: http://www.fda.gov/Drugs/DrugSafety/PostmarketDrugSafetyInformationforPatientsandProviders/DrugSafetyInformationforHeat

hcareProfessionals/PublicHealthAdvisories/ucm051273.htm. Accessed on May 22 2014.
119. Jones T, Moore T. Preliminary data on a new opioid risk assessment measure: the Brief Risk Interview. J Opioid Manag. 2013;9(1):19-27. PMID: 23709300.
120. Butler SF, Budman SH, Fanciullo GJ, et al. Cross validation of the current opioid misuse measure to monitor chronic pain patients on opioid therapy. Clin J Pain. 2010;26(9):770-6. PMID: 20842012.
121. Butler SF, Budman SH, Fernandez KC, et al. Cross-validation of a screener to predict opioid misuse in chronic pain patients (SOAPP-R). J Addict Med. 2009;3(2):66-73. PMID: 20161199.
122. Fleming MF, Davis J, Passik SD. Reported lifetime aberrant drug-taking behaviors are predictive of current substance use and mental health problems in primary care patients. Pain Med. 2008;9(8):1098-106. PMID: 18721174.
123. Meltzer EC, Rybin D, Saitz R, et al. Identifying prescription opioid use disorder in primary care: diagnostic characteristics of the Current Opioid Misuse Measure (COMM). Pain. 2011;152(2):397-402. PMID: 21177035.
124. Butler SF, Budman SH, Fernandez KC, et al. Development and validation of the Current Opioid Misuse Measure. Pain. 2007;130(1-2):144-56. PMID: 17493754.
125. Holmes CP, Gatchel RJ, Adams LL, et al. An Opioid Screening Instrument: Long-Term Evaluation of the Utility of the Pain Medication Questionnaire. Pain Pract. 2006;6(2):74-88. PMID: 17309714.
126. Reifler LM, Droz D, Bailey JE, et al. Do Prescription Monitoring Programs Impact State Trends in Opioid Abuse/Misuse? Pain Med. 2012;13(3):434-42. PMID: 22299725.
127. Deyo RA, Smith DH, Johnson ES, et al. Opioids for back pain patients: primary care prescribing patterns and use of services. J Am Board Fam Med. 2011;24(6):717-27. PMID: 22086815.
128. Seal KH, Shi Y, Cohen G, et al. Association of mental health disorders with prescription opioids and high-risk opioid use in us veterans of Iraq and Afghanistan. JAMA. 2012;307(9):940-7. PMID: 22396516.
129. Sullivan MD, Edlund MJ, Zhang L, et al. Association between mental health disorders, problem drug use, and regular prescription opioid use. Arch Intern Med. 2006;166(19):2087-93. PMID: 17060538.
130. Morasco BJ, Duckart JP, Carr TP, et al. Clinical characteristics of veterans prescribed high doses of opioid medications for chronic non-cancer pain. Pain. 2010;151(3):625-32. PMID: 20801580.
131. Carson S, Thakurta S, Low A, et al. Drug Class Review: Long-Acting Opioid Analgesics: Final Update 6 Report Oregon Health & Science University. Portland, OR: Jul 2011. PMID: 21977550.
132. Fishbain DA, Cole B, Lewis J, et al. What percentage of chronic nonmalignant pain patients exposed to chronic opioid analgesic therapy develop abuse/addiction and/or aberrant drug-related behaviors? A structured evidence-based review. Pain Med. 2008;9(4):444-59. PMID: 18489635.
133. Turk DC, Swanson KS, Gatchel RJ. Predicting opioid misuse by chronic pain patients: a systematic review and literature synthesis. Clin J Pain. 2008;24(6):497-508. PMID: 18574359.
134. Wiedemer NL, Harden PS, Arndt IO, et al. The opioid renewal clinic: a primary care, managed approach to opioid therapy in chronic pain patients at risk for substance abuse. Pain Med. 2007;8(7):573-84. PMID: 17883742.
135. Goldberg KC, Simel DL, Oddone EZ. Effect of an opioid management system on opioid prescribing and unscheduled visits in a large primary care clinic. J Clin Outcome Manag. 2005;12(12)
136. Manchikanti L, Manchukonda R, Damron KS, et al. Does adherence monitoring reduce controlled substance abuse in chronic pain patients? Pain Physician. 2006;9(1):57-60. PMID: 16700282.
137. Manchikanti L, Manchukonda R, Pampati V, et al. Does random urine drug testing reduce illicit drug use in chronic pain patients receiving opioids? Pain Physician. 2006;9(2):123-9. PMID: 16703972.
138. Pablos-Mendez A, Barr RG, Shea S. Run-in periods in randomized trials: implications for hte application of results in clinical practice. JAMA. 1998;279(3):222-5. PMID: 9438743.
139. Furlan AD, Reardon R, Weppler C. Opioids for chronic noncancer pain: a new Canadian practice guideline. CMAJ. 2010;182(9):923-30. PMID: 20439443.
140. Nuckols TK, Anderson L, Popescu I, et al. Opioid prescribing: a systematic review and critical appraisal of guidelines for chronic

pain. Ann Intern Med. 2014;160(1):38-47. PMID: 24217469.

141. O'Connor AB, Turk DC, Dworkin RH, et al. Abuse liability measures for use in analgesic clinical trials in patients with pain: IMMPACT recommendations. Pain. 2013;154(11):2324-34. PMID: 24148704.

142. Cicero TJ, Ellis MS, Surratt HL. Effect of abuse-deterrent formulation of OxyContin. N Engl J Med. 2012;367(2):187-9. PMID: 22784140.

143. Roland M, Torgerson DJ. Understanding controlled trials: What are pragmatic trials? BMJ. 1998;316:285. PMID: 9472515.

Abbreviations and Acronyms

AUROC	area under receiver operating characteristic curve
ASA	aspirin
ASI	Addiction Severity Index
APS	American Pain Society
BID	twice daily
CI	confidence interval
CIDI	Composite International Diagnostic Interview
CR	controlled release
DASS21	Depression, Anxiety, and Stress Scale-21 Items
DIRE	Diagnosis, Intractability, Risk, and Efficacy Inventory
DSM-V	Diagnostic and Statistical Manual, Fourth Edition DSM-
IV	Diagnostic and Statistical Manual, Fifth Edition
ER	extended release
GC/M	gas chromatography mass spectrometry
HR	hazard ratio
ICD-10	International Statistical Classification of Diseases and Related Health Problems Version 10 IRR incidence rate ratio
ITT	intent to treat
MED	morphine equivalent dose
MS	long-acting morphine sulfate
NA	not applicable
NLR	negative likelihood ratio
NR	not reported
NSAID	nonsteroidal anti-inflammatory drug
ODI	Oswestry Disability Index
OR	odds ratio
ORT	Opioid Risk Tool
PDI	Physical Disability Index
PDUQ	Prescription Drug Use Questionnaire
PLR	positive likelihood ratio
PMQ	Pain Medication Questionnaire
POTQ	Prescription Opioid Therapy Questionnaire
RCT	randomized controlled trial
SE	standard error
SDSS	Dependence Severity Scale
SOAPP	Screening and Opioid Assessment for Patients with Pain
SOAPP-R	Screening and Opioid Assessment for Patients with Pain-Revised
SOE	strength of evidence
SUQ	Self-report Substance Use Questionnaire
TDB	transdermal buprenorphine
TDF	transdermal fentanyl
U.S.	United States
UDT	urine drug test
VA	Veterans Affairs
VAS	Visual Analogue Scale

Appendix A. Search Strategies

Database: Ovid MEDLINE(R) Without Revisions

KQ 1 and 2: Comparative Effectiveness and Harms
1. exp Analgesics, Opioid/
2. opioid*.mp.
3. (alfentanil or alphaprodine or beta-casomorphin$ or buprenorphine or carfentanil or codeine or deltorphin or dextromethorphan or dezocine or dihydrocodeine or dihydromorphine or enkephalin$ or ethylketocyclazocine or ethylmorphine or etorphine or fentanyl or heroin or hydrocodone or hydromorphone or ketobemidone or levorphanol or lofentanil or meperidine or meptazinol or methadone or methadyl acetate or morphine or nalbuphine or opium or oxycodone or oxymorphone or pentazocine or phenazocine or phenoperidine or pirinitramide or promedol or propoxyphene or remifentanil or sufentanil or tilidine or tapentadol).mp.
4. or/1-3
5. exp Chronic Pain/
6. (chronic adj2 pain).mp.
7. 5 or 6
8. 4 and 7
9. limit 8 to yr="2008 - 2013"
10. limit 9 to (clinical trial, all or clinical trial or comparative study or controlled clinical trial or multicenter study or randomized controlled trial)
11. 9 and random$.mp.
12. 10 or 11

KQ 2a: Supplemental Search – Abuse and Addiction Detection
1. Analgesics, Opioid/
2. 1 and 2
3. Substance Abuse Detection/
4. Opioid-Related Disorders/ or Substance-Related Disorders/
5. 3 and (4 or 5)
6. (chronic adj3 pain).mp.
7. 1 and 7
8. 8 not 3
9. 9 and (4 or 5)
10. 6 or 10

KQ 3a-3g; 3i: Dosing Strategies
1. exp Analgesics, Opioid/
2. opioid*.mp. (alfentanil or alphaprodine or beta-casomorphins or buprenorphine or carfentanil or codeine or deltorphin or dextromethorphan or dezocine or dihydrocodeine or dihydromorphine or enkephalin$ or ethylketocyclazocine or ethylmorphine or etorphine or fentanyl or heroin or hydrocodone or hydromorphone or ketobemidone or levorphanol or lofentanil or meperidine or meptazinol or methadone or methadyl acetate or morphine or nalbuphine or opium or oxycodone or oxymorphone or pentazocine or

phenazocine or phenoperidine or pirinitramide or promedol or propoxyphene or remifentanil or sufentanil or tilidine or tapentadol).mp.
3. or/1-3
4. Opioid-Related Disorders/
5. (opioid adj2 (abuse or addict* or misuse or diversion)).mp.
6. Drug Administration Schedule/
7. Pain Management/
8. Clinical Protocols/
9. Breakthrough Pain/
10. Dose-Response Relationship, Drug/
11. ((dose$ or dosing) adj7 (strateg$ or adjust$ or titrat$ or taper$)).mp.
12. exp Chronic Pain/
13. (chronic adj2 pain).mp.
14. or/4-6
15. or/7-12
16. 15 and 16
17. (or/13-14) and 17
18. 18 and (random$ or control$ or trial or cohort or prospective or retrospective).mp.
19. limit 19 to yr="2008 - 2013"

KQ 3h: Dosing Strategies – Tapered Dosing

1. exp Analgesics, Opioid/
2. opioid*.mp.
3. (alfentanil or alphaprodine or beta-casomorphins or buprenorphine or carfentanil or codeine or deltorphin or dextromethorphan or dezocine or dihydrocodeine or dihydromorphine or enkephalin$ or ethylketocyclazocine or ethylmorphine or etorphine or fentanyl or heroin or hydrocodone or hydromorphone or ketobemidone or levorphanol or lofentanil or meperidine or meptazinol or methadone or methadyl acetate or morphine or nalbuphine or opium or oxycodone or oxymorphone or pentazocine or phenazocine or phenoperidine or pirinitramide or promedol or propoxyphene or remifentanil or sufentanil or tilidine or tapentadol).mp.
4. or/1-3
5. Opioid-Related Disorders/
6. (opioid adj2 (abuse or addict* or misuse or diversion)).mp.
7. Drug Administration Schedule/
8. Pain Management/
9. Clinical Protocols/
10. Breakthrough Pain/
11. Dose-Response Relationship, Drug/
12. ((dose$ or dosing) adj7 (strateg$ or adjust$ or titrat$ or taper$)).mp.
13. exp Chronic Pain/
14. (chronic adj2 pain).mp.
15. or/4-6
16. or/7-12
17. 15 and 16
18. (or/13-14) and 17

19. 18 and (random$ or control$ or trial or cohort or prospective or retrospective).mp.
20. 19 and (taper$ or decreas$ or reduc$).mp.
21. limit 20 to yr="1902 - 2007"

KQ 4a-4b: Risk Prediction
1. exp Analgesics, Opioid/
2. opioid*.mp.
3. (alfentanil or alphaprodine or beta-casomorphins or buprenorphine or carfentanil or codeine or deltorphin or dextromethorphan or dezocine or dihydrocodeine or dihydromorphine or enkephalin$ or ethylketocyclazocine or ethylmorphine or etorphine or fentanyl or heroin or hydrocodone or hydromorphone or ketobemidone or levorphanol or lofentanil or meperidine or meptazinol or methadone or methadyl acetate or morphine or nalbuphine or opium or oxycodone or oxymorphone or pentazocine or phenazocine or phenoperidine or pirinitramide or promedol or propoxyphene or remifentanil or sufentanil or tilidine or tapentadol).mp.
4. or/1-3
5. exp Chronic Pain/
6. (chronic adj2 pain).mp.
7. Opioid-Related Disorders/
8. (opioid adj2 (abuse or addict* or misuse or diversion)).mp.
9. 4 and (5 or 6)
10. 7 or 8
11. 9 or 10
12. Decision Support Techniques/
13. "Predictive Value of Tests"/
14. Prognosis/
15. Risk Assessment/
16. Risk Factors/
17. Proportional Hazards Models/
18. "Reproducibility of Results"/
19. "Sensitivity and Specificity"/
20. (sensitivity or specificity).mp.
21. (risk and (predict$ or assess$)).mp.
22. or/12-21
23. 11 and 22
24. limit 23 to yr="2008 - 2013"

KQ 4c: Risk Mitigation
1. exp Analgesics, Opioid/
2. opioid*.mp.
3. (alfentanil or alphaprodine or beta-casomorphins or buprenorphine or carfentanil or codeine or deltorphin or dextromethorphan or dezocine or dihydrocodeine or dihydromorphine or enkephalin$ or ethylketocyclazocine or ethylmorphine or etorphine or fentanyl or heroin or hydrocodone or hydromorphone or ketobemidone or levorphanol or lofentanil or meperidine or meptazinol or methadone or methadyl acetate or morphine or nalbuphine or opium or oxycodone or oxymorphone or pentazocine or phenazocine or

phenoperidine or pirinitramide or promedol or propoxyphene or remifentanil or sufentanil or tilidine or tapentadol).mp.
4. or/1-3
5. exp Chronic Pain/
6. (chronic adj2 pain).mp.
7. Opioid-Related Disorders/
8. (opioid adj2 (abuse or addict* or misuse or diversion)).mp.
9. 4 and (5 or 6)
10. 7 or 8
11. 9 or 10
12. Patient Compliance/
13. Health Services Misuse/
14. Substance Abuse Detection/
15. Drug Monitoring/
16. (urine adj7 (screen$ or test$ or detect$)).mp.
17. (abus$ or misus$ or diversion$ or divert$).mp.
18. (opioid$ adj7 (contract$ or agree$)).mp.
19. Contracts/
20. Patient Education as Topic/
21. Drug Overdose/
22. or/12-21
23. ((risk$ adj7 mitigat$) or reduc$).mp.
24. ("risk evaluation and mitigation" or "rems").mp.
25. Risk Reduction Behavior/ or Risk/
26. or/23-25
27. 11 and 22 and 26
28. limit 27 to yr="2008 - 2013"

KQ 4d: Treatment Strategies
1. exp Analgesics, Opioid/
2. opioid*.mp.
3. (alfentanil or alphaprodine or beta-casomorphins or buprenorphine or carfentanil or codeine or deltorphin or dextromethorphan or dezocine or dihydrocodeine or dihydromorphine or enkephalin$ or ethylketocyclazocine or ethylmorphine or etorphine or fentanyl or heroin or hydrocodone or hydromorphone or ketobemidone or levorphanol or lofentanil or meperidine or meptazinol or methadone or methadyl acetate or morphine or nalbuphine or opium or oxycodone or oxymorphone or pentazocine or phenazocine or phenoperidine or pirinitramide or promedol or propoxyphene or remifentanil or sufentanil or tilidine or tapentadol).mp.
4. or/1-3
5. Opioid-Related Disorders/
6. (opioid adj2 (abuse or addict* or misuse or diversion)).mp.
7. Patient Compliance/
8. Health Services Misuse/
9. Substance Abuse Detection/
10. Drug Monitoring/

11. (urine adj7 (screen$ or test$ or detect$)).mp.
12. (abus$ or misus$ or diversion$ or divert$)).mp.
13. opioid$ adj7 (contract$ or agree$)).mp.
14. Contracts/
15. Patient Education as Topic/
16. Drug Overdose/
17. or/7-16
18. Substance Abuse Detection/
19. Opiate Substitution Treatment/
20. Risk Management/
21. or/18-20
22. or/4-6
23. 17 and 21 and 22
24. treatment outcome.mp. or Treatment Outcome/
25. (treatment and (strateg$ or plan$)).mp.
26. 23 and (24 or 25)

All KQs: Systematic Reviews
1. meta-analysis.mp. or exp Meta-Analysis/
2. (cochrane or medline).tw.
3. search$.tw.
4. 1 or 2 or 3
5. "Review Literature as Topic"/ or systematic review.mp.
6. 4 or 5
7. exp Analgesics, Opioid/
8. opioid*.mp.
9. (alfentanil or alphaprodine or beta-casomorphins or buprenorphine or carfentanil or codeine or deltorphin or dextromethorphan or dezocine or dihydrocodeine or dihydromorphine or enkephalin$ or ethylketocyclazocine or ethylmorphine or etorphine or fentanyl or heroin or hydrocodone or hydromorphone or ketobemidone or levorphanol or lofentanil or meperidine or meptazinol or methadone or methadyl acetate or morphine or nalbuphine or opium or oxycodone or oxymorphone or pentazocine or phenazocine or phenoperidine or pirinitramide or promedol or propoxyphene or remifentanil or sufentanil or tilidine or tapentadol).mp.
10. 10   (chronic and pain).mp.
11. or/7-9
12. 6 and 10 and 11
13. limit 12 to yr="2008 - 2013"

Database: EBM Reviews - Cochrane Central Register of Controlled Trials

KQ 1 and 2: Comparative Effectiveness and Harms
1. exp Analgesics, Opioid/
2. opioid*.mp.

3. (alfentanil or alphaprodine or beta-casomorphin$ or buprenorphine or carfentanil or codeine or deltorphin or dextromethorphan or dezocine or dihydrocodeine or dihydromorphine or enkephalin$ or ethylketocyclazocine or ethylmorphine or etorphine or fentanyl or heroin or hydrocodone or hydromorphone or ketobemidone or levorphanol or lofentanil or meperidine or meptazinol or methadone or methadyl acetate or morphine or nalbuphine or opium or oxycodone or oxymorphone or pentazocine or phenazocine or phenoperidine or pirinitramide or promedol or propoxyphene or remifentanil or sufentanil or tilidine or tapentadol).mp.
4. or/1-3
5. exp Chronic Pain/
6. (chronic adj2 pain).mp.
7. 5 or 6
8. 4 and 7
9. limit 8 to yr="2008 - 2013"

KQ 3a-3g, 3i: Dosing Strategies

1. exp Analgesics, Opioid/
2. opioid*.mp.
3. (alfentanil or alphaprodine or beta-casomorphins or buprenorphine or carfentanil or codeine or deltorphin or dextromethorphan or dezocine or dihydrocodeine or dihydromorphine or enkephalin$ or ethylketocyclazocine or ethylmorphine or etorphine or fentanyl or heroin or hydrocodone or hydromorphone or ketobemidone or levorphanol or lofentanil or meperidine or meptazinol or methadone or methadyl acetate or morphine or nalbuphine or opium or oxycodone or oxymorphone or pentazocine or phenazocine or phenoperidine or pirinitramide or promedol or propoxyphene or remifentanil or sufentanil or tilidine or tapentadol).mp.
4. or/1-3
5. Opioid-Related Disorders/
6. (opioid adj2 (abuse or addict* or misuse or diversion)).mp.
7. Drug Administration Schedule/
8. Pain Management/
9. Clinical Protocols/
10. Breakthrough Pain/
11. Dose-Response Relationship, Drug/
12. ((dose$ or dosing) adj7 (strateg$ or adjust$ or titrat$ or taper$)).mp.
13. exp Chronic Pain/
14. (chronic adj2 pain).mp.
15. or/4-6
16. or/7-12
17. 15 and 16
18. (or/13-14) and 17
19. limit 18 to yr="2008 - 2013"

KQ 3h: Tapered Dosing

1. exp Analgesics, Opioid/
2. opioid*.mp.

3. (alfentanil or alphaprodine or beta-casomorphins or buprenorphine or carfentanil or codeine or deltorphin or dextromethorphan or dezocine or dihydrocodeine or dihydromorphine or enkephalin$ or ethylketocyclazocine or ethylmorphine or etorphine or fentanyl or heroin or hydrocodone or hydromorphone or ketobemidone or levorphanol or lofentanil or meperidine or meptazinol or methadone or methadyl acetate or morphine or nalbuphine or opium or oxycodone or oxymorphone or pentazocine or phenazocine or phenoperidine or pirinitramide or promedol or propoxyphene or remifentanil or sufentanil or tilidine or tapentadol).mp.
4. or/1-3
5. Opioid-Related Disorders/
6. (opioid adj2 (abuse or addict* or misuse or diversion)).mp.
7. Drug Administration Schedule/
8. Pain Management/
9. Clinical Protocols/
10. Breakthrough Pain/
11. Dose-Response Relationship, Drug/
12. ((dose$ or dosing) adj7 (strateg$ or adjust$ or titrat$ or taper$)).mp.
13. exp Chronic Pain/
14. (chronic adj2 pain).mp.
15. or/4-6
16. or/7-12
17. 15 and 16
18. (or/13-14) and 17
19. 18 and (random$ or control$ or trial or cohort or prospective or retrospective).mp.
20. 19 and (taper$ or decreas$ or reduc$).mp.
21. limit 20 to yr="1902 - 2007"

KQ 4a-b: Risk Prediction

1. exp Analgesics, Opioid/
2. opioid*.mp.
3. (alfentanil or alphaprodine or beta-casomorphins or buprenorphine or carfentanil or codeine or deltorphin or dextromethorphan or dezocine or dihydrocodeine or dihydromorphine or enkephalin$ or ethylketocyclazocine or ethylmorphine or etorphine or fentanyl or heroin or hydrocodone or hydromorphone or ketobemidone or levorphanol or lofentanil or meperidine or meptazinol or methadone or methadyl acetate or morphine or nalbuphine or opium or oxycodone or oxymorphone or pentazocine or phenazocine or phenoperidine or pirinitramide or promedol or propoxyphene or remifentanil or sufentanil or tilidine or tapentadol).mp.
4. or/1-3
5. exp Chronic Pain/
6. (chronic adj2 pain).mp.
7. Opioid-Related Disorders/
8. (opioid adj2 (abuse or addict* or misuse or diversion)).mp.
9. 4 and (5 or 6)
10. 7 or 8
11. 9 or 10

12. Decision Support Techniques/
13. "Predictive Value of Tests"/
14. Prognosis/
15. Risk Assessment/
16. Risk Factors/
17. Proportional Hazards Models/
18. "Reproducibility of Results"/
19. "Sensitivity and Specificity"/
20. (sensitivity or specificity).mp.
21. (risk and (predict$ or assess$)).mp.
22. or/12-21
23. 11 and 22
24. limit 23 to yr="2008 - 2013"

KQ 4c: Risk Mitigation

1. exp Analgesics, Opioid/
2. opioid*.mp.
3. (alfentanil or alphaprodine or beta-casomorphins or buprenorphine or carfentanil or codeine or deltorphin or dextromethorphan or dezocine or dihydrocodeine or dihydromorphine or enkephalin$ or ethylketocyclazocine or ethylmorphine or etorphine or fentanyl or heroin or hydrocodone or hydromorphone or ketobemidone or levorphanol or lofentanil or meperidine or meptazinol or methadone or methadyl acetate or morphine or nalbuphine or opium or oxycodone or oxymorphone or pentazocine or phenazocine or phenoperidine or pirinitramide or promedol or propoxyphene or remifentanil or sufentanil or tilidine or tapentadol).mp. (20690)
4. or/1-3 (22725)
5. exp Chronic Pain/ (79)
6. (chronic adj2 pain).mp. (2585)
7. Opioid-Related Disorders/ (571)
8. (opioid adj2 (abuse or addict* or misuse or diversion)).mp. (116)
9. 4 and (5 or 6) (523)
10. 7 or 8 (630)
11. 9 or 10 (1139)
12. Patient Compliance/
13. Health Services Misuse/
14. Substance Abuse Detection/
15. Drug Monitoring/
16. (urine adj7 (screen$ or test$ or detect$)).mp.
17. (abus$ or misus$ or diversion$ or divert$).mp.
18. (opioid$ adj7 (contract$ or agree$)).mp.
19. Contracts/
20. Patient Education as Topic/
21. Drug Overdose/
22. or/12-21
23. ((risk$ adj7 mitigat$) or reduc$).mp.
24. ("risk evaluation and mitigation" or "rems").mp.

25. Risk Reduction Behavior/ or Risk/
26. or/23-25
27. 11 and 22 and 26
28. limit 27 to yr="2008 - 2013"

KQ 4d: Treatment Strategies
1. exp Analgesics, Opioid/
2. opioid*.mp.
3. (alfentanil or alphaprodine or beta-casomorphins or buprenorphine or carfentanil or codeine or deltorphin or dextromethorphan or dezocine or dihydrocodeine or dihydromorphine or enkephalin$ or ethylketocyclazocine or ethylmorphine or etorphine or fentanyl or heroin or hydrocodone or hydromorphone or ketobemidone or levorphanol or lofentanil or meperidine or meptazinol or methadone or methadyl acetate or morphine or nalbuphine or opium or oxycodone or oxymorphone or pentazocine or phenazocine or phenoperidine or pirinitramide or promedol or propoxyphene or remifentanil or sufentanil or tilidine or tapentadol).mp.
4. or/1-3
5. Opioid-Related Disorders/
6. (opioid adj2 (abuse or addict* or misuse or diversion)).mp.
7. Patient Compliance/
8. Health Services Misuse/
9. Substance Abuse Detection/
10. Drug Monitoring/
11. (urine adj7 (screen$ or test$ or detect$)).mp.
12. (abus$ or misus$ or diversion$ or divert$).mp.
13. (opioid$ adj7 (contract$ or agree$)).mp.
14. Contracts/
15. Patient Education as Topic/
16. Drug Overdose/
17. or/7-16
18. Substance Abuse Detection/
19. Opiate Substitution Treatment/
20. Risk Management/
21. or/18-20
22. or/4-6
23. 17 and 21 and 22
24. treatment outcome.mp. or Treatment Outcome/
25. (treatment and (strateg$ or plan$)).mp.
26. 23 and (24 or 25)

Database: PsycINFO

KQ 1 and 2: Comparative Effectiveness and Harms
1. opioid*.mp.
2. (alfentanil or alphaprodine or beta-casomorphins or buprenorphine or carfentanil or codeine or deltorphin or dextromethorphan or dezocine or dihydrocodeine or

dihydromorphine or enkephalin$ or ethylketocyclazocine or ethylmorphine or etorphine or fentanyl or heroin or hydrocodone or hydromorphone or ketobemidone or levorphanol or lofentanil or meperidine or meptazinol or methadone or methadyl acetate or morphine or nalbuphine or opium or oxycodone or oxymorphone or pentazocine or phenazocine or phenoperidine or pirinitramide or promedol or propoxyphene or remifentanil or sufentanil or tilidine or tapentadol).mp.
3. (chronic and pain).mp.
4. (1 or 2) and 3
5. (random$ or control$ or trial or cohort or prospective or retrospective).mp.
6. 4 and 5
7. limit 6 to yr="2008 - 2014"
8. limit 7 to human

KQ 3a-3g, 3i: Dosing Strategies
1. opioid*.mp.
2. (alfentanil or alphaprodine or beta-casomorphins or buprenorphine or carfentanil or codeine or deltorphin or dextromethorphan or dezocine or dihydrocodeine or dihydromorphine or enkephalin$ or ethylketocyclazocine or ethylmorphine or etorphine or fentanyl or heroin or hydrocodone or hydromorphone or ketobemidone or levorphanol or lofentanil or meperidine or meptazinol or methadone or methadyl acetate or morphine or nalbuphine or opium or oxycodone or oxymorphone or pentazocine or phenazocine or phenoperidine or pirinitramide or promedol or propoxyphene or remifentanil or sufentanil or tilidine or tapentadol).mp.
3. (chronic and pain).mp.
4. (1 or 2) and 3
5. 4 and (dose or dosing or dosage).mp.
6. limit 5 to human
7. limit 6 to yr="2008 - 2014"

KQ 3h: Tapered Dosing
1. opioid*.mp.
2. (alfentanil or alphaprodine or beta-casomorphins or buprenorphine or carfentanil or codeine or deltorphin or dextromethorphan or dezocine or dihydrocodeine or dihydromorphine or enkephalin$ or ethylketocyclazocine or ethylmorphine or etorphine or fentanyl or heroin or hydrocodone or hydromorphone or ketobemidone or levorphanol or lofentanil or meperidine or meptazinol or methadone or methadyl acetate or morphine or nalbuphine or opium or oxycodone or oxymorphone or pentazocine or phenazocine or phenoperidine or pirinitramide or promedol or propoxyphene or remifentanil or sufentanil or tilidine or tapentadol).mp.
3. (chronic and pain).mp.
4. (1 or 2) and 3
5. 4 and (taper$ or decreas$).mp.
6. limit 5 to human

KQ 4a-4c: Risk Prediction and Mitigation
1. opioid*.mp.
2. (alfentanil or alphaprodine or beta-casomorphins or buprenorphine or carfentanil or codeine or deltorphin or dextromethorphan or dezocine or dihydrocodeine or dihydromorphine or enkephalin$ or ethylketocyclazocine or ethylmorphine or etorphine or fentanyl or heroin or hydrocodone or hydromorphone or ketobemidone or levorphanol or lofentanil or meperidine or meptazinol or methadone or methadyl acetate or morphine or nalbuphine or opium or oxycodone or oxymorphone or pentazocine or phenazocine or phenoperidine or pirinitramide or promedol or propoxyphene or remifentanil or sufentanil or tilidine or tapentadol).mp.
3. (chronic and pain).mp.
4. (1 or 2) and 3
5. risk.mp.
6. 4 and
7. limit 6 to human
8. limit 7 to yr="2008 - 2014"

KQ 4d: Treatment Strategies
1. opioid*.mp
2. (alfentanil or alphaprodine or beta-casomorphins or buprenorphine or carfentanil or codeine or deltorphin or dextromethorphan or dezocine or dihydrocodeine or dihydromorphine or enkephalin$ or ethylketocyclazocine or ethylmorphine or etorphine or fentanyl or heroin or hydrocodone or hydromorphone or ketobemidone or levorphanol or lofentanil or meperidine or meptazinol or methadone or methadyl acetate or morphine or nalbuphine or opium or oxycodone or oxymorphone or pentazocine or phenazocine or phenoperidine or pirinitramide or promedol or propoxyphene or remifentanil or sufentanil or tilidine or tapentadol).mp
3. (chronic and pain).mp
4. (1 or 2) and 3
5. 4 and ((treatment and (strateg$ or plan$).mp
6. 5 and (overdose or abuse or misuse or pain or function or "quality of life" or "qol").mp
7. limit 6 to human

Database: EBSCO CINAHL Plus with Full Text

All Key Questions (except 3h, 4d)
1. (MH "Analgesics, Opioid") OR (MH "Narcotics") OR (MH "Alfentanil") OR "alfentanil" (MH "Alphaprodine") OR "alphaprodine" OR "beta-casomorphins" (MH "Buprenorphine") OR "buprenorphine" OR "carfentanil" (MH "Codeine") OR "codeine" OR (MH "Oxycodone") OR "deltorphin" OR (MH "Dextromethorphan") OR "dextromethorphan" OR "dezocine" OR "dihydrocodeine" OR "dihydromorphine" OR (MH "Enkephalins") OR "enkephalin" OR "ethylketocyclazocine" OR "ethylmorphine" "etorphine" OR (MH "Fentanyl") OR "fentanyl" (MH "Heroin") OR "heroin" "hydrocodone" OR (MH "Dihydromorphinone") OR "hydromorphone" OR "ketobemidone" OR "levorphanol" OR "lofentanil" OR (MH "Meperidine") OR

"meperidine" OR "meptazinol" OR (MH "Methadone") OR "methadone" OR "methadyl acetate" OR (MH "Morphine") OR "morphine" OR (MH "Nalbuphine") OR (MH "Opium") OR "oxycodone" OR "oxymorphone" OR (MH "Pentazocine") OR "pentazocine" OR "phenazocine" OR "phenoperidine" OR "pirinitramide" OR "promedol" OR (MH "Propoxyphene") OR "propoxyphene" OR "remifentanil" OR (MH "Sufentanil") OR "sufentanil" OR "tilidine" OR (MH "Tapentadol") OR "tapentadol"
2. (MH "Chronic Pain") OR "chronic pain"
3. 1 and 2
4. "random*" OR "control*" OR "trial" OR "cohort" OR "prospective" OR "retrospective"
5. 3 and 4
6. Limit 4 to published date 20080101-20131015

KQ 3h: Tapered Dosing

1. (MH "Analgesics, Opioid") OR (MH "Narcotics") OR (MH "Alfentanil") OR "alfentanil" (MH "Alphaprodine") OR "alphaprodine" OR "beta-casomorphins" (MH "Buprenorphine") OR "buprenorphine" OR "carfentanil" (MH "Codeine") OR "codeine" OR (MH "Oxycodone") OR "deltorphin" OR (MH "Dextromethorphan") OR "dextromethorphan" OR "dezocine" OR "dihydrocodeine" OR "dihydromorphine" OR (MH "Enkephalins") OR "enkephalin" OR "ethylketocyclazocine" OR "ethylmorphine" "etorphine" OR (MH "Fentanyl") OR "fentanyl" (MH "Heroin") OR "heroin" "hydrocodone" OR (MH "Dihydromorphinone") OR "hydromorphone" OR "ketobemidone" OR "levorphanol" OR "lofentanil" OR (MH "Meperidine") OR "meperidine" OR "meptazinol" OR (MH "Methadone") OR "methadone" OR "methadyl acetate" OR (MH "Morphine") OR "morphine" OR (MH "Nalbuphine") OR (MH "Opium") OR "oxycodone" OR "oxymorphone" OR (MH "Pentazocine") OR "pentazocine" OR "phenazocine" OR "phenoperidine" OR "pirinitramide" OR "promedol" OR (MH "Propoxyphene") OR "propoxyphene" OR "remifentanil" OR (MH "Sufentanil") OR "sufentanil" OR "tilidine" OR (MH "Tapentadol") OR "tapentadol"
2. (MH "Chronic Pain") OR "chronic pain"
3. 1 and 2
4. "random*" OR "control*" OR "trial" OR "cohort" OR "prospective" OR "retrospective"
5. 3 and 4
6. "taper*" OR "decreas*"
7. 5 and 6
8. Limit 6 to published date 19920101-20071231

KQ 4d: Treatment Strategies

1. (MH "Analgesics, Opioid") OR (MH "Narcotics") OR (MH "Alfentanil") OR "alfentanil" (MH "Alphaprodine") OR "alphaprodine" OR "beta-casomorphins" (MH "Buprenorphine") OR "buprenorphine" OR "carfentanil" (MH "Codeine") OR "codeine" OR (MH "Oxycodone") OR "deltorphin" OR (MH "Dextromethorphan") OR "dextromethorphan" OR "dezocine" OR "dihydrocodeine" OR "dihydromorphine" OR (MH "Enkephalins") OR "enkephalin" OR "ethylketocyclazocine" OR "ethylmorphine" "etorphine" OR (MH "Fentanyl") OR "fentanyl" (MH "Heroin") OR "heroin" "hydrocodone" OR (MH "Dihydromorphinone") OR "hydromorphone" OR "ketobemidone" OR "levorphanol" OR "lofentanil" OR (MH "Meperidine") OR

"meperidine" OR "meptazinol" OR (MH "Methadone") OR "methadone" OR "methadyl acetate" OR (MH "Morphine") OR "morphine" OR (MH "Nalbuphine") OR (MH "Opium") OR "oxycodone" OR "oxymorphone" OR (MH "Pentazocine") OR "pentazocine" OR "phenazocine" OR "phenoperidine" OR "pirinitramide" OR "promedol" OR (MH "Propoxyphene") OR "propoxyphene" OR "remifentanil" OR (MH "Sufentanil") OR "sufentanil" OR "tilidine" OR (MH "Tapentadol") OR "tapentadol"
2. (MH "Chronic Pain") OR "chronic pain"
3. 1 and 2
4. "random*" OR "control*" OR "trial" OR "cohort" OR "prospective" OR "retrospective"
5. 3 and 4
6. "treatment" AND ("strateg*" OR "plan*")
7. 5 and 6
8. Limit 7 to published date 19920101-20071231

Database: EBM Reviews – Cochrane Database of Systematic Reviews

All KQs: Systematic Reviews

1. (opioid$ or alfentanil or alphaprodine or beta-casomorphin$ or buprenorphine or carfentanil or codeine or deltorphin or dextromethorphan or dezocine or dihydrocodeine or dihydromorphine or enkephalin$ or ethylketocyclazocine or ethylmorphine or etorphine or fentanyl or heroin or hydrocodone or hydromorphone or ketobemidone or levorphanol or lofentanil or meperidine or meptazinol or methadone or methadyl acetate or morphine or nalbuphine or opium or oxycodone or oxymorphone or pentazocine or phenazocine or phenoperidine or pirinitramide or promedol or propoxyphene or remifentanil or sufentanil or tilidine or tapentadol).ti.
2. 1 and (chronic and pain).mp.
3. limit 2 to full systematic reviews

Appendix B. PICOTS

PICOT	Include	Exclude
Population and Conditions of Interest	<ul><li>For all KQs: Adults (age >18 years) with various types of chronic pain (defined as pain lasting >3 months), including patients with acute exacerbations of chronic pain (KQ Ig)</li><li>For KQs 1b, 2b: Subgroups as defined by specific pain condition, patient demographics (e.g., age, race, ethnicity, sex), comorbidities (including medical comorbidities and mental health disorders, including past or current alcohol or substance abuse and related disorders, and those at high risk for addiction);</li><li>For KQ 2b: Subgroups also defined by the dose of opioids used</li></ul>	<ul><li>Patients with pain at end of life, acute pain, pregnant or breastfeeding, patients treated with opioids for addiction</li></ul>
Interventions	<ul><li>For KQs 1, 2, 3: Long- or short-acting opioids (including tapentadol) used as long-term therapy (defined as use of opioids on most days for >3months)</li><li>For KQ 1d: Also include combination of opioid plus nonopioid therapy (pharmacological or nonpharmacological)</li><li>For KQ 1Va, b: Risk prediction instruments</li><li>For KQ 1Vc: Opioid management plans, patient education, urine drug screening, use of prescription drug monitoring program data, use of monitoring instruments, more frequent monitoring intervals, pill counts, use of abuse deterrent formulations</li><li>For KQ 1Vd: Opioid management strategies</li></ul>	<ul><li>Intravenous or intramuscular administration of opioids</li><li>Tramadol</li></ul>
Comparators	<ul><li>For KQs 1a, 1b, 2a, 2b: Opioid vs. placebo or nonopioid therapy (including usual care)</li><li>For KQ 1c: Opioid vs. nonopioid therapy (pharmacological or nonpharmacological [e.g., exercise therapy, cognitive behavioral therapy, interdisciplinary rehabilitation])</li><li>For KQ 1d: Opioid plus nonopioid therapy (pharmacological or nonpharmacological) vs. opioid or nonopioid therapy alone</li><li>For KQ 3a: Comparisons of different dose initiation and titration strategies</li><li>For KQ 3b: Short- vs. long-acting opioids</li><li>For KQ 3c: One long-acting opioid vs. another long-acting opioid</li><li>For KQ 3d: Short- plus long-acting opioid vs. long-acting opioid</li><li>For KQ 3e: Scheduled, continuous vs. as-needed dosing of opioid</li><li>For KQ 3f: Dose escalation vs. dose maintenance or use of maximum dosing thresholds</li><li>For KQ 3g: Opioid rotation vs. continuation of current opioid</li><li>For KQ 3h: Comparisons of different methods for treating acute exacerbations of chronic pain</li><li>For KQ 3i: Decreasing or tapering opioid doses vs. continuation of opioids</li><li>For KQ 3j: Comparisons of different tapering protocols and strategies</li><li>For KQ 4a: Risk prediction instruments vs. reference standard for overdose or opioid addiction, abuse or misuse</li><li>For KQ 4b: Risk prediction instruments vs. nonuse of risk prediction instruments</li><li>For KQ 4c: Risk mitigation strategies (see Interventions above) vs. nonuse of risk mitigation strategies</li><li>For KQ 4d: Comparisons of treatment strategies for managing patients with addiction to prescription opioids</li></ul>	

PICOT	Include	Exclude
Outcomes	- For KQs 1, 3, 4: Pain (intensity, severity, bothersomeness), function (physical disability, activity limitations, activity interference, work function), and quality of life (including depression), doses of opioids used - Also for KQs 2, 3, 4: Overdose, opioid use disorder, addiction, abuse, and misuse; other opioid-related harms (including gastrointestinal, falls, fractures, motor vehicle accidents, endocrinological harms, infections, cardiovascular events, cognitive harms, and psychological harms (e.g., depression)	- Intermediate outcomes (e.g., pharmacokinetics/pharmacodynamics, drug-drug interactions, dose conversions)
Timing	- Any duration for outcomes related to overdose and injuries (falls, fractures, motor vehicle accidents), studies on treatment of acute exacerbations of chronic pain, studies on dose initiation and titration, and studies on discontinuation of opioid therapy - For other outcomes: >1 year	
Setting	- Outpatient settings (e.g., primary care, pain clinics, other specialty clinics)	- Addiction treatment settings, inpatient settings
Study Design	- For all KQs, randomized controlled trials, controlled cohort studies, and case-control studies (controlled observational studies must have performed adjustment on potential confounders) - For all KQs, we excluded uncontrolled observational studies, case series, and case reports, with the exception of KQ 2a for which we included uncontrolled observational studies of patients with chronic pain prescribed long-term opioid therapy for at least one year that used predefined methods to assess rates of abuse, misuse, or addiction - For KQ 4a, we included studies that evaluated the predictive ability of risk prediction instruments, and excluded studies that did not evaluate the performance of a risk prediction instrument against a reference standard.	

KQ, key question; PICOT=populations, interventions, comparators, outcomes, timing, setting.

Appendix C. Included Studies*

Akbik H, Butler SF, Budman SH, et al. Validation and clinical application of the screener and opioid assessment for patients with pain (SOAPP). J Pain Symptom Manage. 2006;32(3):287-93. PMID: 16939853.

Allan L, Richarz U, Simpson K, et al. Transdermal fentanyl versus sustained release oral morphine in strong-opioid naive patients with chronic low back pain. Spine. 2005;30(22):2484-90. PMID: 16284584.

Ashburn MA, Slevin KA, Messina J, et al. The efficacy and safety of fentanyl buccal tablet compared with immediate-release oxycodone for the management of breakthrough pain in opioid-tolerant patients with chronic pain. Anesth Analg. 2011;112(3):693-702. PMID: 21304148.

Banta-Green CJ, Merrill JO, Doyle SR, et al. Opioid use behaviors, mental health and pain--development of a typology of chronic pain patients. Drug Alcohol Depend. 2009;104(1-2):34-42. PMID: 19473786.

Boscarino JA, Rukstalis M, Hoffman SN, et al. Risk factors for drug dependence among out-patients on opioid therapy in a large us health-care system. Addiction. 2010;105(10):1776-82. PMID: 20712819.

Carman WJ, Su S, Cook SF, et al. Coron0ary heart disease outcomes among chronic opioid and cyclooxygenase-2 users compared with a general population cohort. Pharmacoepidemiol Drug Saf. 2011;20(7):754-62. PMID: 21567652.

Compton PA, Wu SM, Schieffer B, et al. Introduction of a self-report version of the prescription drug use questionnaire and relationship to medication agreement noncompliance. J Pain Symptom Manage. 2008;36(4):383-95. PMID: 18508231.

Cowan DT, Wilson-Barnett J, Griffiths P, et al. A survey of chronic noncancer pain patients prescribed opioid analgesics. Pain Med. 2003;4(4):340-51. PMID: 14750910.

Cowan DT, Wilson-Barnett J, Griffiths P, et al. A randomized, double-blind, placebo-controlled, cross-over pilot study to assess the effects of long-term opioid drug consumption and subsequent abstinence in chronic noncancer pain patients receiving controlled-release morphine. Pain Med. 2005;6(2):113-21. PMID: 15773875.

Davies A, Sitte T, Elsner F, et al. Consistency of efficacy, patient acceptability, and nasal tolerability of fentanyl pectin nasal spray compared with immediate-release morphine sulfate in breakthrough cancer pain. J Pain Symptom Manage. 2011;41(2):358-66. PMID: 21334555.

Deyo RA, Smith DH, Johnson ES, et al. Prescription opioids for back pain and use of medications for erectile dysfunction. Spine. 2013;38(11):909-15. PMID: 23459134.

Dunn KM, Saunders KW, Rutter CM, et al. Opioid prescriptions for chronic pain and overdose: a cohort study.[summary for patients in Ann Intern Med.

2010;152(2):I-42]. Ann Intern Med. 2010;152(2):85-92. PMID: 20083827.

Edlund MJ, Martin BC, Russo JE, et al. The role of opioid prescription in incident opioid abuse and dependence among individuals with chronic noncancer pain. Clin J Pain. 2014;30(7):557-64. PMID: 24281273.

Fleming MF, Balousek SL, Klessig CL, et al. Substance use disorders in a primary care sample receiving daily opioid therapy. J Pain. 2007;8(7):573-82. PMID: 17499555.

Gomes T, Mamdani MM, Dhalla IA, et al. Opioid dose and drug-related mortality in patients with nonmalignant pain. Arch Intern Med. 2011;171(7):686-91. PMID: 21482846.

Gomes T, Redelmeier DA, Juurlink DN, et al. Opioid dose and risk of road trauma in Canada: a population-based study. JAMA Intern Med. 2013;173(3):196-201. PMID: 23318919.

Hartung DM, Middleton L, Haxby DG, et al. Rates of adverse events of long-acting opioids in a state Medicaid program. Ann Pharmacother. 2007;41(6):921-8. PMID: 17504834.

Hojsted J, Nielsen PR, Guldstrand SK, et al. Classification and identification of opioid addiction in chronic pain patients. Eur J Pain. 2010;14(10):1014-20. PMID: 20494598.

Jamison RN, Raymond SA, Slawsby EA, et al. Opioid therapy for chronic noncancer back pain. a randomized prospective study. Spine. 1998;23(23):2591-600. PMID: 9854758.

Jones T, Moore T. Preliminary data on a new opioid risk assessment measure: the Brief Risk Interview. J Opioid Manag. 2013;9(1):19-27. PMID: 23709300.

Krebs EE, Becker WC, Zerzan J, et al. Comparative mortality among Department of Veterans Affairs patients prescribed methadone or long-acting morphine for chronic pain. Pain. 2011;152(8):1789-95. PMID: 21524850.

Li L, Setoguchi S, Cabral H, et al. Opioid use for noncancer pain and risk of myocardial infarction amongst adults. J Intern Med. 2013;273(5):511-26. PMID: 23331508.

Li L, Setoguchi S, Cabral H, et al. Opioid use for noncancer pain and risk of fracture in adults: a nested case- control study using the general practice research database. Am J Epidemiol. 2013;178(4):559-69. PMID: 23639937.

Mitra F, Chowdhury S, Shelley M, et al. A feasibility study of transdermal buprenorphine versus transdermal fentanyl in the long-term management of persistent non-cancer pain. Pain Med. 2013;14(1):75-83. PMID: 23320402.

Moore TM, Jones T, Browder JH, et al. A comparison of common screening methods for predicting aberrant drug-related behavior among patients receiving opioids for chronic pain management. Pain Med. 2009;10(8):1426-33. PMID: 20021601.

Naliboff BD, Wu SM, Schieffer B, et al. A randomized trial of 2 prescription strategies for opioid treatment of chronic nonmalignant pain. J Pain. 2011;12(2):288-96. PMID: 21111684.

Portenoy RK, Farrar JT, Backonja MM, et al. Long-term use of controlled-release oxycodone for noncancer pain: results of a 3-year registry study. Clin J Pain. 2007;23(4):287-99. PMID: 17449988.

Portenoy RK, Messina J, Xie F, et al. Fentanyl buccal tablet (FBT) for relief of breakthrough pain in opioid-treated patients with chronic low back pain: a randomized, placebo-controlled study. Curr Med Res Opin. 2007;23(1):223-33. PMID: 17207304.

Ralphs JA, Williams AC, Richardson PH, et al. Opiate reduction in chronic pain patients: a comparison of patient-controlled reduction and staff controlled cocktail methods. Pain. 1994;56(3):279-88. PMID: 8022621.

Reid MC, Engles-Horton LL, Weber MB, et al. Use of opioid medications for chronic noncancer pain syndromes in primary care. J Gen Intern Med. 2002;17(3):173-9. PMID: 11929502.

Saffier K, Colombo C, Brown D, et al. Addiction severity index in a chronic pain sample receiving opioid therapy. J Subst Abuse Treat. 2007;33(3):303-11. PMID: 17376639.

Salzman RT, Roberts MS, Wild J, et al. Can a controlled-release oral dose form of oxycodone be used as readily as an immediate-release form for the purpose of titrating to stable pain control? J Pain Symptom Manage. 1999;18(4):271-9. PMID: 10534967.

Saunders KW, Dunn KM, Merrill JO, et al. Relationship of opioid use and dosage levels to fractures in older chronic pain patients. J Gen Intern Med. 2010;25(4):310-5. PMID: 20049546.

Schneider JP, Kirsh KL. Defining clinical issues around tolerance, hyperalgesia, and addiction: a quantitative and qualitative outcome study of long-term opioid dosing in a chronic pain practice. J Opioid Manag. 2010;6(6):385-95. PMID: 21268999.

Simpson DM, Messina J, Xie F, et al. Fentanyl buccal tablet for the relief of breakthrough pain in opioid-tolerant adult patients with chronic neuropathic pain: a multicenter, randomized, double-blind, placebo-controlled study. Clin Ther. 2007;29(4):588-601. PMID: 17617282.

Tennant FS, Jr., Rawson RA. Outpatient treatment of prescription opioid dependence: comparison of two methods. Arch Intern Med. 1982;142(10):1845-7. PMID: 6181749.

Wasan AD, Butler SF, Budman SH, et al. Does report of craving opioid medication predict aberrant drug behavior among chronic pain patients? Clin J Pain. 2009;25(3):193-8. PMID: 19333168.

Webster LR, Slevin KA, Narayana A, et al. Fentanyl buccal tablet compared with immediate-release oxycodone for the management of breakthrough pain in opioid-tolerant patients with chronic cancer and noncancer pain: a randomized, double-blind, crossover study followed by a 12-week open-label phase to evaluate patient outcomes. Pain Med. 2013;14(9):1332-45. PMID: 23855816.

Webster LR, Webster RM. Predicting aberrant behaviors in opioid-treated patients: preliminary validation of the Opioid Risk Tool. Pain Med. 2005;6(6):432-42. PMID: 16336480.

Wild JE, Grond S, Kuperwasser B, et al. Long-term safety and tolerability of tapentadol extended release for the management of chronic low back pain or osteoarthritis pain. Pain Pract. 2010;10(5):416-27. PMID: 20602712.

*Appendix C is the reference list for all appendixes.

Appendix D. Excluded Studies

No Author. Use of opioids to control arthritis pain under scrutiny. Increase in falls, fractures in older adults attributed to narcotic painkillers, such as oxycodone, Vicodin or Percocet. Duke Med Health News. 2013;19(5):7. PMID: 23802330. *Excluded: wrong study design*

Abrahamsen B, Brixen K. Mapping the prescriptiome to fractures in men--a national analysis of prescription history and fracture risk. Osteoporos Int. 2009;20(4):585-97. PMID: 18690484. *Excluded: wrong population.*

Adams EH, Breiner S, Cicero TJ, et al. A comparison of the abuse liability of tramadol, NSAIDs, and hydrocodone in patients with chronic pain. J Pain Symptom Manage. 2006;31(5):465-76. PMID: 16716877. *Excluded: wrong study design.*

Afilalo M, Etropolski MS, Kuperwasser B, et al. Efficacy and safety of Tapentadol extended release compared with oxycodone controlled release for the management of moderate to severe chronic pain related to osteoarthritis of the knee: a randomized, double-blind, placebo- and active-controlled phase III study. Clin Drug Investig. 2010;30(8):489-505. PMID: 20586515. *Excluded: inadequate duration.*

Agarwal S, Polydefkis M, Block B, et al. Transdermal fentanyl reduces pain and improves functional activity in neuropathic pain states. Pain Med. 2007;8(7):554-62. PMID: 17883740. *Excluded: inadequate duration.*

Albert S, Brason FW, 2nd, Sanford CK, et al. Project Lazarus: community-based overdose prevention in rural North Carolina. Pain Med. 2011;12 Suppl 2:S77-85. PMID: 21668761. *Excluded: wrong population.*

Amass L, Bickel WK, Higgins ST, et al. A preliminary investigation of outcome following gradual or rapid buprenorphine detoxification. J Addict Dis. 1994;13(3):33-45. PMID: 7734458. *Excluded: wrong population.*

Amass L, Ling W, Freese TE, et al. Bringing buprenorphine-naloxone detoxification to community treatment providers: the NIDA Clinical Trials Network field experience. American Journal on Addictions. 2004;13 Suppl 1:S42-66. PMID: 15204675. *Excluded: wrong population.*

Amato J-N, Marie S, Lelong-Boulouard V, et al. Effects of three therapeutic doses of codeine/paracetamol on driving performance, a psychomotor vigilance test, and subjective feelings. Psychopharmacology. 2013;228(2):309-20. PMID: 23474890. *Excluded: wrong comparator.*

Amato P. Clinical experience with fortnightly buprenorphine/naloxone versus buprenorphine in Italy: preliminary observational data in an office-based setting. Clin Drug Investig. 2010;30 Suppl 1:33-9. PMID: 20450244. *Excluded: wrong population.*

Anderson VC, Burchiel KJ. A prospective study of long-term intrathecal morphine in the management of chronic nonmalignant pain. Neurosurgery. 1999;44(2):289-300. PMID: 9932882. *Excluded: wrong intervention.*

Annemans L. Pharmacoeconomic impact of adverse events of long-term opioid treatment for the management of persistent pain. Clin Drug Investig. 2011;31(2):73-86. PMID: 21067250. *Excluded: wrong publication type.*

Anonymous. Tapentadol. Acute or chronic pain: No therapeutic advance. Prescrire Int. 2014: 121-4. PMID: 24926510. *Excluded: wrong publication type*

Aoki T, Kuroki Y, Kageyama T, et al. Multicentre double-blind comparison of piroxicam and indomethacin in the treatment of lumbar diseases. Eur J Rheumatol Inflamm. 1983;6(3):247-52. PMID: 6239779. *Excluded: wrong intervention.*

Apolone G, Deandrea S, Montanari M, et al. Evaluation of the comparative analgesic effectiveness of transdermal and oral opioids in cancer patients: a propensity score analysis. Eur J Pain. 2012;16(2):229-38. PMID: 22323375. *Excluded: wrong population.*

Arner S, Meyerson BA. Lack of analgesic effect of opioids on neuropathic and idiopathic forms of pain. Pain. 1988;33(1):11-23. PMID: 2454440. *Excluded: wrong intervention.*

Ashworth J, Green DJ, Dunn KM, et al. Opioid use among low back pain patients in primary care: Is opioid prescription associated with disability at 6-month follow-up? Pain. 2013: 1038-44. PMID: 23688575. *Excluded: inadequate duration*

Assadi SM, Hafezi M, Mokri A, et al. Opioid detoxification using high doses of buprenorphine in 24 hours: a randomized, double blind, controlled clinical trial. J Subst Abuse Treat. 2004;27(1):75-82. PMID: 15223097. *Excluded: wrong population.*

Attal N, Guirimand F, Brasseur L, et al. Effects of IV morphine in central pain: a randomized placebo-controlled study. Neurology. 2002;58(4):554-63. PMID: 11865132. *Excluded: wrong intervention.*

Babul N, Noveck R, Chipman H, et al. Efficacy and safety of extended-release, once-daily tramadol in chronic pain: a randomized 12-week clinical trial in osteoarthritis of the knee. J Pain Symptom Manage. 2004;28(1):59-71. PMID: 15223085. *Excluded: inadequate duration.*

Ballantyne JC. Treating pain in patients with drug-dependence problems. BMJ. 2013;347:f3213. PMID: 24324214. *Excluded: wrong publication type.*

Banning A, Sjogren P. Cerebral effects of long-term oral opioids in cancer patients measured by continuous reaction time. Clin J Pain. 1990;6(2):91-5. PMID: 2135009. *Excluded: inadequate duration.*

Banning A, Sjogren P, Kaiser F. Reaction time in cancer patients receiving peripherally acting analgesics alone or in combination with opioids. Acta Anaesthesiol Scand. 1992;36(5):480-2. PMID: 1378679. *Excluded: wrong population.*

Barrera-Chacon JM, Mendez-Suarez JL, Jáuregui-Abrisqueta ML, et al. Oxycodone improves pain control and quality of life in anticonvulsant-pretreated spinal cord-injured patients with neuropathic pain. Spinal Cord. 2011;49(1):36-42. PMID: 20820176. *Excluded: wrong comparator.*

Baumblatt JAG, Wiedeman C, Dunn JR, et al. High-risk use by patients prescribed opioids for pain and its role in overdose deaths. JAMA Intern Med. 2014;174(5):796-801. PMID: 24589873. *Excluded: wrong comparator.*

Becker WC, O'Connor PG. The safety of opioid analgesics in the elderly: new data raise new concerns: comment on "the comparative safety of opioids for nonmalignant pain in older adults". Arch Intern Med. 2010;170(22):1986-8. PMID: 21149755. *Excluded: wrong publication type.*

Becker WC, Sullivan LE, Tetrault JM, et al. Non-medical use, abuse and dependence on prescription opioids among U.S. adults: psychiatric, medical and substance use correlates. Drug Alcohol Depend. 2008;94(1-3):38-47. PMID: 18063321. *Excluded: wrong study design.*

Benavidez DC, Flores AM, Fierro I, et al. Road rage among drug dependent patients. Accid Anal Prev. 2013;50:848-53. PMID: 22840213. *Excluded: wrong population.*

Benitez-Rosario MA, Feria M, Salinas-Martin A, et al. Opioid switching from transdermal fentanyl to oral methadone in patients with cancer pain. Cancer. 2004;101(12):2866-73. PMID: 15529307. *Excluded: wrong study design.*

Benitez-Rosario MA, Salinas-Martin A, Aguirre-Jaime A, et al. Morphine-methadone opioid rotation in cancer patients: analysis of dose ratio predicting factors. J Pain Symptom Manage. 2009;37(6):1061-8. PMID: 19171458. *Excluded: wrong study design.*

Bickel WK, Stitzer ML, Bigelow GE, et al. A clinical trial of buprenorphine: comparison with methadone in the detoxification of heroin addicts. Clin Pharmacol Ther. 1988;43(1):72-8. PMID: 3275523. *Excluded: wrong population.*

Binsfeld H, Szczepanski L, Waechter S, et al. A randomized study to demonstrate noninferiority of once-daily OROS((R)) hydromorphone with twice-daily sustained-release oxycodone for moderate to severe chronic noncancer pain. Pain Pract. 2010;10(5):404-15. PMID: 20384968. *Excluded: wrong comparator.*

Binswanger IA, Blatchford PJ, Mueller SR, et al. Mortality after prison release: opioid overdose and other causes of death, risk factors, and time trends from 1999 to 2009. Ann Intern Med. 2013;159(9):592-600. PMID: 24189594. *Excluded: wrong population.*

Biondi D, Xiang J, Benson C, et al. Tapentadol immediate release versus oxycodone immediate release for treatment of acute low back pain. Pain Physician. 2013;16(3):E237-46. PMID: 23703422. *Excluded: inadequate duration.*

Biondi D, Xiang J, Etropolski M, et al. A post hoc pooled data analysis to evaluate blood pressure (bp) and heart rate (hr) measurements in patients with a current or prior history of hypertension who received tapentadol er, oxycodone cr, or placebo in chronic pain studies. J Pain. Conference: 30th Annual Scientific Meeting of the American Pain Society Austin, TX United States. 2011;12(4 SUPPL. 1):55. PMID: N/A. *Excluded: wrong publication type.*

Bjorkman R, Ullman A, Hedner J. Morphine-sparing effect of diclofenac in cancer pain. Eur J Clin Pharmacol. 1993;44(1):1-5. PMID: 8436146. *Excluded: inadequate duration.*

Blalock SJ, Casteel C, Roth MT, et al. Impact of enhanced pharmacologic care on the prevention of falls: a randomized controlled trial. Am J Geriatr Pharmacother. 2010;8(5):428-40. PMID: 21335296. *Excluded: wrong population.*

Block C, Cianfrini L. Neuropsychological and neuroanatomical sequelae of chronic non-malignant pain and opioid analgesia. Neurorehabilitation. 2013: 343-66. PMID: 2013-35225-021. *Excluded: wrong publication type*

Blondell RD, Ashrafioun L, Dambra CM, et al. A clinical trial comparing tapering doses of buprenorphine with steady doses for chronic pain and co-existent opioid addiction. J Addict Med. 2010;4(3):140-6. PMID: 20959867. *Excluded: inadequate duration.*

Bohnert ASB, Valenstein M, Bair MJ, et al. Association between opioid prescribing patterns and opioid overdose-related deaths. JAMA. 2011;305(13):1315-21. PMID: 21467284. *Excluded: wrong population.*

Boscarino JA, Rukstalis MR, Hoffman SN, et al. Prevalence of prescription opioid-use disorder among chronic pain patients: comparison of the DSM-5 vs. DSM-4 diagnostic criteria. J Addict Dis. 2011;30(3):185-94. PMID: 21745041. *Excluded: wrong outcome.*

Bosek V, Miguel R. Comparison of morphine and ketorolac for intravenous patient-controlled analgesia in postoperative cancer patients. Clin J Pain. 1994;10(4):314-8. PMID: 7858362. *Excluded: inadequate duration.*

Braden JB, Russo J, Fan MY, et al. Emergency department visits among recipients of chronic opioid therapy. Arch Intern Med. 2010;170(16):1425-32. PMID: 20837827. *Excluded: wrong comparator.*

Bramness JG, Skurtveit S, Morland J, et al. An increased risk of motor vehicle accidents after prescription of methadone. Addiction. 2012;107(5):967-72. PMID: 22151376. *Excluded: wrong population.*

Breckenridge J, Clark JD. Patient characteristics associated with opioid versus nonsteroidal anti-inflammatory drug management of chronic low back pain. J Pain. 2003;4(6):344-50. PMID: 14622692. *Excluded: wrong study design.*

Breivik H, Ljosaa TM, Stengaard-Pedersen K, et al. A 6-months, randomised, placebo-controlled evaluation of efficacy and tolerability of a low-dose 7-day buprenorphine transdermal patch in osteoarthritis patients naive to potent opioids. Scand J Pain. 2010;1(3):122-41. PMID: N/A. *Excluded: inadequate duration.*

Brookoff D, Polomano R. Treating sickle cell pain like cancer pain. Ann Intern Med. 1992;116(5):364-8. PMID: 1736768. *Excluded: wrong intervention.*

Brown J, Setnik B, Lee K, et al. Assessment, stratification, and monitoring of the risk for prescription opioid misuse and abuse in the primary care setting. J Opioid Manag. 2011;7(6):467-83. PMID: 22320029. *Excluded: wrong population.*

Brown RT, Zuelsdorff M, Fleming M. Adverse effects and cognitive function among primary care patients taking opioids for chronic nonmalignant pain. J Opioid Manag. 2006;2(3):137-46. PMID: 17319447. *Excluded: wrong population.*

Bruera E, Belzile M, Pituskin E, et al. Randomized, double-blind, cross-over trail comparing safety and efficacy or oral controlled-release oxycodone with controlled-release morphine in patients with cancer pain. J Clin Oncol. 1998;16(10):3222-9. PMID: 9779695. *Excluded: wrong population.*

Bruera E, Macmillan K, Hanson J, et al. The cognitive effects of the administration of narcotic analgesics in patients with cancer pain. Pain. 1989;39(1):13-6. PMID: 2812850. *Excluded: inadequate duration.*

Buckeridge D, Huang A, Hanley J, et al. Risk of injury associated with opioid use in older adults. J Am Geriatr Soc. 2010;58(9):1664-70. PMID: 20863326. *Excluded: wrong population.*

Buelow AK, Haggard R, Gatchel RJ. Additional validation of the pain medication questionnaire in a heterogeneous sample of chronic pain patients. Pain Pract. 2009;9(6):428-34. PMID: 19735363. *Excluded: wrong outcome.*

Butler SF, Budman SH, Fanciullo GJ, et al. Cross validation of the current opioid misuse measure to monitor chronic pain patients on opioid therapy. Clin J Pain. 2010;26(9):770-6. PMID: 20842012. *Excluded: wrong population.*

Butler SF, Budman SH, Fernandez K, et al. Validation of a screener and opioid assessment measure for patients with chronic pain. Pain. 2004;112(1-2):65-75. PMID: 15494186. *Excluded: wrong population.*

Butler SF, Budman SH, Fernandez KC, et al. Cross-validation of a screener to predict opioid misuse in chronic pain patients (SOAPP-R). J Addict Med. 2009;3(2):66-73. PMID: 20161199. *Excluded: wrong population.*

Butler SF, Budman SH, Fernandez KC, et al. Development and validation of the current opioid misuse measure. Pain. 2007;130(1-2):144-56. PMID: 17493754. *Excluded: wrong population.*

Butler SF, Fernandez K, Benoit C, et al. Validation of the revised screener and opioid assessment for patients with pain (soapp-r). J Pain. 2008;9(4):360-72. PMID: 18203666. *Excluded: wrong population.*

Buynak R, Shapiro D, Okamoto A, et al. Efficacy, safety, and gastrointestinal tolerability of tapentadol er in a randomized, double-blind, placebo- and active-controlled phase III study of patients with chronic low back pain. J Pain. 2009;10(4, Supplement 1):S48. PMID: 20578811. *Excluded: wrong publication type.*

Buynak R, Shapiro DY, Okamoto A, et al. Efficacy and safety of tapentadol extended release for the management of chronic low back pain: results of a prospective, randomized, double-blind, placebo- and active-controlled Phase III study. Expert Opin Pharmacother. 2010;11(11):1787-804. PMID: 20578811. *Excluded: inadequate duration.*

Byas-Smith MG, Chapman SL, Reed B, et al. The effect of opioids on driving and psychomotor performance in patients with chronic pain. Clin J Pain. 2005;21(4):345-52. PMID: 15951653. *Excluded: inadequate duration.*

Caldwell JR, Rapoport RJ, Davis JC, et al. Efficacy and safety of a once-daily morphine formulation in chronic, moderate-to-severe osteoarthritis pain: results from a randomized, placebo-controlled, double-blind trial and an open-label extension trial. J Pain Symptom Manage. 2002;23(4):278-91. PMID: 11997197. *Excluded: inadequate duration.*

Callaghan RC, Gatley JM, Veldhuizen S, et al. Alcohol- or drug-use disorders and motor vehicle accident mortality: a retrospective cohort study. Accid Anal Prev. 2013;53:149-55. PMID: 23434842. *Excluded: wrong population.*

Carlson RW, Borrison RA, Sher HB, et al. A multiinstitutional evaluation of the analgesic efficacy and safety of ketorolac tromethamine, acetaminophen plus codeine, and placebo in cancer pain. Pharmacotherapy. 1990;10(3):211-6. PMID: 2196536. *Excluded: inadequate duration.*

Carr DB, Goudas LC, Denman WT, et al. Safety and efficacy of intranasal ketamine for the treatment of breakthrough pain in patients with chronic pain: a randomized, double-blind, placebo-controlled, crossover study. Pain. 2004;108(1-2):17-27. PMID: 15109503. *Excluded: wrong intervention.*

Cepeda M, Fife D, Ma Q, et al. Comparison of the risks of opioid abuse or dependence between tapentadol and oxycodone: Results from a cohort study. J Pain. 2013;14(10):1227-41. PMID: 24370606. *Excluded: wrong comparator.*

Chabal C, Erjavec MK, Jacobson L, et al. Prescription opiate abuse in chronic pain patients: clinical criteria, incidence, and predictors. Clin J Pain. 1997;13(2):150-5. PMID: 9186022. *Excluded: wrong study design.*
Chaparro EL, Furlan AD, Deshpande A, et al. Opioids compared to placebo or other treatments for chronic low-back pain. Cochrane Database Syst Rev. 2013;(8)PMID: 17636781. *Excluded: systematic review or meta-analysis used only as a source document.*

Chaparro LEMD, Furlan ADMDP, Deshpande AMD, et al. Opioids compared with placebo or other treatments for chronic low back pain: an update of the cochrane review. Spine. 2014;39(7):556-63. PMID: 24480962. *Excluded: systematic review or meta-analysis used only as a source document.*

Chary S, Goughnour BR, Moulin DE, et al. The dose-response relationship of controlled-release codeine (codeine contin) in chronic cancer pain. J Pain Symptom Manage. 1994;9(6):363-71. PMID: 7963789. *Excluded: inadequate duration.*

Chelminski PR, Ives TJ, Felix KM, et al. A primary care, multi-disciplinary disease management program for opioid-treated patients with chronic non-cancer pain and a high burden of psychiatric comorbidity. BMC Health Serv Res. 2005;5(1):3. PMID: 15649331. *Excluded: wrong population.*

Chen L, Vo T, Seefeld L, et al. Lack of correlation between opioid dose adjustment and pain score change in a group of chronic pain patients. J Pain. 2013;14(4):384-92. PMID: 23452826. *Excluded: inadequate duration.*

Cheskin LJ, Fudala PJ, Johnson RE. A controlled comparison of buprenorphine and clonidine for acute detoxification from opioids. Drug Alcohol Depend. 1994;36(2):115-21. PMID: 7851278. *Excluded: inadequate duration.*

Chu LF, D'Arcy N, Brady C, et al. Analgesic tolerance without demonstrable opioid-induced hyperalgesia: a double-blinded, randomized, placebo-controlled trial of sustained-release morphine for treatment of chronic nonradicular low-back pain. Pain. 2012;153(8):1583-92. PMID: 22704854. *Excluded: inadequate duration.*

Cicero TJ, Lynskey M, Todorov A, et al. Co-morbid pain and psychopathology in males and females admitted to treatment for opioid analgesic abuse. Pain. 2008;139(1):127-35. PMID: 18455314. *Excluded: wrong study design.*

Clemons M, Regnard C, Appleton T. Alertness, cognition and morphine in patients with advanced cancer. Cancer Treat Rev. 1996;22(6):451-68. PMID: 9134005. *Excluded: inadequate duration.*

Coffey RJ, Owens ML, Broste SK, et al. Mortality associated with implantation and management of intrathecal opioid drug infusion systems to treat noncancer pain. Anesthesiology. 2009;111(4):881-91. PMID: 20029253. *Excluded: wrong study design.*

Collins ED, Kleber HD, Whittington RA, et al. Anesthesia-assisted vs buprenorphine- or clonidine-assisted heroin detoxification and naltrexone induction: a randomized trial. JAMA. 2005;294(8):903-13. PMID: 16118380. *Excluded: wrong population.*

Collins ED, Whittington RA, Heitler NE, et al. A randomised comparison of anaesthesia-assisted heroin detoxification with buprenorphine- and clonidine-assisted detoxifications. . 2002;PMID: N/A. *Excluded: wrong population.*

Corli O, Cozzolino A, Scaricabarozzi I. Nimesulide and diclofenac in the control of cancer-related pain. comparison between oral and rectal administration. Drugs. 1993;46 Suppl 1:152-5. PMID: 7506158. *Excluded: wrong intervention.*

Couto JE, Romney MC, Leider HL, et al. High rates of inappropriate drug use in the chronic pain population. Popul Health Manag. 2009;12(4):185-90. PMID: 19663620. *Excluded: wrong population.*

Crisostomo RA, Schmidt JE, Hooten WM, et al. Withdrawal of analgesic medication for chronic low-back pain patients: improvement in outcomes of multidisciplinary rehabilitation regardless of surgical history. Am J Phys Med Rehabil 2008;87(7):527-36. PMID: 18574345. *Excluded: inadequate duration.*

Currie SR, Hodgins DC, Crabtree A, et al. Outcome from integrated pain management treatment for recovering substance abusers. J Pain. 2003;4(2):91-100. PMID: 14622720. *Excluded: wrong population.*

Dagtekin O, Gerbershagen HJ, Wagner W, et al. Assessing cognitive and psychomotor performance under long-term treatment with transdermal buprenorphine in chronic noncancer pain patients. Anesth Analg. 2007;105(5):1442-8, table of contents. PMID: 17959980. *Excluded: inadequate duration.*

Daitch J, Frey ME, Silver D, et al. Conversion of chronic pain patients from full-opioid agonists to sublingual buprenorphine. Pain Physician. 2012;15(3 Suppl):ES59-66. PMID: 22786462. *Excluded: inadequate duration.*

D'Amore A, Romano F, Biancolillo V, et al. Evaluation of buprenorphine dosage adequacy in opioid receptor agonist substitution therapy for heroin dependence: first use of the buprenorphine-naloxone dosage adequacy evaluation (buava) questionnaire. Clin Drug Investig. 2012;32(7):427-32. PMID: 22559256. *Excluded: wrong population.*

Daniell HW. Hypogonadism in men consuming sustained-action oral opioids. J Pain. 2002;3:377-84. PMID: 14622741. *Excluded: wrong population.*

Daniell HW. DHEAS deficiency during consumption of sustained-action prescribed opioids: evidence for opioid-induced inhibition of adrenal androgen production. J Pain. 2006;7(12):901-7. PMID: 17157776. *Excluded: wrong population.*

Daniell HW. Opioid endocrinopathy in women consuming prescribed sustained-action opioids for control of nonmalignant pain. J Pain. 2008;9:28-36. PMID: 14622741. *Excluded: wrong population.*

Daniels S, Casson E, Stegmann JU, et al. A randomized, double-blind, placebo-controlled phase 3 study of the relative efficacy and tolerability of tapentadol IR and oxycodone IR for acute pain. Curr Med Res Opin. 2009;25(6):1551-61. PMID: 19445652. *Excluded: inadequate duration.*

Daniels SE, Upmalis D, Okamoto A, et al. A randomized, double-blind, phase III study comparing multiple doses of tapentadol IR, oxycodone IR, and placebo for postoperative (bunionectomy) pain. Curr Med Res Opin. 2009;25(3):765-76. PMID: 19203298. *Excluded: inadequate duration.*

Danninger R, Jaske R, Beubler E. Randomized crossovercomparison of 2g- and 4g- doses of paracetamol per day in the case of mild to moderate pain caused by head and neck cancers.1993;PMID: N/A. *Excluded: wrong intervention.*

Dassanayake T, Michie P, Carter G, et al. Effects of benzodiazepines, antidepressants and opioids on driving: a systematic review and meta-analysis of epidemiological and experimental evidence. Drug Saf. 2011;34(2):125-56. PMID: 21247221. *Excluded: systematic review or meta-analysis used only as a source document.*

Davis MP. Fentanyl for breakthrough pain: a systematic review. Expert Rev Neurother. 2011;11(8):1197-216. PMID: 21797660. *Excluded: systematic review or meta-analysis used only as a source document.*

De Conno F, Groff L, Brunelli C, et al. Clinical experience with oral methadone administration in the treatment of pain in 196 advanced cancer patients. J Clin Oncol. 1996;14(10):2836-42. PMID: 8874346. *Excluded: inadequate duration.*

Dellemijn PL, Vanneste JA. Randomised double-blind active-placebo-controlled crossover trial of intravenous fentanyl in neuropathic pain. Lancet. 1997;349(9054):753-8. PMID: 9074573. *Excluded: wrong intervention.*

Dellemijn PL, Verbiest HB, van Vliet JJ, et al. Medical therapy of malignant nerve pain. A randomised double-blind explanatory trial with naproxen versus slow-release morphine. Eur J Cancer. 1994;30A(9):1244-50. PMID: 7999406. *Excluded: wrong population.*

Dersh J, Mayer TG, Gatchel RJ, et al. Prescription opioid dependence is associated with poorer outcomes in disabling spinal disorders. Spine. 2008;33(20):2219-27. PMID: 18725868. *Excluded: wrong study design.*

Devulder J, Jacobs A, Richarz U, et al. Impact of opioid rescue medication for breakthrough pain on the efficacy and tolerability of long-acting opioids in patients with chronic non-malignant pain. Br J Anaesth. 2009;103(4):576-85. PMID: 19736216. *Excluded: systematic review or meta-analysis used only as a source document.*

Doyon S. Opioid overdose-related deaths. JAMA. 2011;306(4):379-80; author reply 80-1. PMID: 21791680. *Excluded: wrong publication type.*

Dubois S, Bedard M, Weaver B. The association between opioid analgesics and unsafe driving actions preceding fatal crashes. Accid Anal Prev. 2010;42(1):30-7. PMID: 19887141. *Excluded: wrong population.*

Duehmke MR, Hollingshead J, Cornblath DR. Tramadol for neuropathic pain. Cochrane Database Syst Rev. 2009;(2)PMID: 15106216. *Excluded: wrong intervention.*

Dunbar SA, Katz NP. Chronic opioid therapy for nonmalignant pain in patients with a history of substance abuse: report of 20 cases. J Pain Symptom Manage. 1996;11(3):163-71. PMID: 8851374. *Excluded: wrong study design.*

Dunn KM, Hay EM. Opioids for chronic musculoskeletal pain. BMJ. 2010;341:c3533. PMID: 20605881. *Excluded: wrong publication type.*

DuPont RL, Graham NA, Gold MS. Opioid treatment for chronic back pain and its association with addiction. Ann Intern Med. 2007;147(5):349; author reply -50. PMID: 17785497. *Excluded: wrong publication type.*

Dupouy J, Dassieu L, Bourrel R, et al. Effectiveness of drug tests in outpatients starting opioid substitution therapy. J Subst Abuse Treat. 2013;44(5):515-21. PMID: 23337248. *Excluded: wrong outcome.*

Edlund MJ, Martin BC, Fan M-Y, et al. Risks for opioid abuse and dependence among recipients of chronic opioid therapy: results from the TROUP study. Drug Alcohol Depend. 2010;112(1-2):90-8. PMID: 20634006. *Excluded: wrong population.*

Edlund MJ, Steffick D, Hudson T, et al. Risk factors for clinically recognized opioid abuse and dependence among veterans using opioids for chronic non-cancer pain. Pain. 2007;129(3):355-62. PMID: 17449178. *Excluded: wrong study design.*

Edlund MJ, Sullivan M, Steffick D, et al. Do users of regularly prescribed opioids have higher rates of substance use problems than nonusers? Pain Med. 2007;8(8):647-56. PMID: 18028043. *Excluded: wrong population.*

Eide PK, Jorum E, Stubhaug A, et al. Relief of post-herpetic neuralgia with the N-methyl-D-aspartic acid receptor antagonist ketamine: a double-blind, cross-over comparison with morphine and placebo. Pain. 1994;58(3):347-54. PMID: 7838584. *Excluded: wrong intervention.*

Eide PK, Stubhaug A, Stenehjem AE. Central dysesthesia pain after traumatic spinal cord injury is dependent on N-methyl-D-aspartate receptor activation. Neurosurgery. 1995;37(6):1080-7. PMID: 8584148. *Excluded: wrong intervention.*

Elander J, Lusher J, Bevan D, et al. Pain management and symptoms of substance dependence among patients with sickle cell disease. Soc Sci Med. 2003;57(9):1683-96. PMID: 12948577. *Excluded: wrong study design.*

Ensrud KE, Blackwell T, Mangione CM, et al. Central nervous system active medications and risk for fractures in older women. Arch Intern Med. 2003;163(8):949-57. PMID: 12719205. *Excluded: wrong population.*

Estape J, Vinolas N, Gonzalez B, et al. Ketorolac, a new non-opioid analgesic: a double-blind trial versus pentazocine in cancer pain. J Int Med Res1990;18(4):298-304. PMID: 2227077. *Excluded: wrong intervention.*

Etropolski M, Kelly K, Okamoto A, et al. Comparable efficacy and superior gastrointestinal tolerability (nausea, vomiting, constipation) of tapentadol compared with oxycodone hydrochloride. Adv Ther. 2011;28(5):401-17. PMID: 21494892. *Excluded: inadequate duration.*

Etropolski M, Lange B, Goldberg J, et al. A pooled analysis of patient-specific factors and efficacy and tolerability of tapentadol extended release treatment for moderate to severe chronic pain. J Opioid Manag. 2013;9(5):343-56. PMID: 24353047. *Excluded: inadequate duration.*

Etropolski M, Kuperwasser B, Flügel M, et al. Safety and tolerability of tapentadol extended release in moderate to severe chronic osteoarthritis or low back pain management: Pooled analysis of randomized controlled trials. Adv Ther. 2014: 604-20. PMID: 2012636416. Excluded: *systematic review or meta-analysis used only as a source document.*

Evans DP, Burke MS, Newcombe RG. Medicines of choice in low back pain. Curr Med Res Opin. 1980;6(8):540-7. PMID: 6446445. *Excluded: inadequate duration.*

Farrar JT, Messina J, Xie F, et al. A novel 12-week study, with three randomized, double-blind placebo-controlled periods to evaluate fentanyl buccal tablets for the relief of breakthrough pain in opioid-tolerant patients with noncancer-related chronic pain. Pain Med. 2010;11(9):1313-27. PMID: 20807345. *Excluded: wrong study design.*

Ferrer-Brechner T, Ganz P. Combination therapy with ibuprofen and methadone for chronic cancer pain. Am J Med. 1984;77(1A):78-83. PMID: 6380281. *Excluded: inadequate duration.*

Fine PG. Overdose risk with opioids for chronic noncancer pain. J Pain Palliat Care Pharmacother. 2010;24(3):287-8. PMID: N/A. *Excluded: wrong population.*

Fine PG, Fishman SM. Reducing opioid abuse and diversion. JAMA. 2011;306(4):382; author reply -3. PMID: 21791685. *Excluded: wrong publication type.*

Fine PG, Narayana A, Passik SD. Treatment of breakthrough pain with fentanyl buccal tablet in opioid-tolerant patients with chronic pain: appropriate patient selection and management. Pain Med. 2010;11(7):1024-36. PMID: 20642730. *Excluded: wrong publication type.*

Fishbain DA, Cutler RB, Rosomoff HL, et al. Can patients taking opioids drive safely? A structured evidence-based review. J Pain Palliat Care Pharmacother. 2002;16(1):9-28. PMID: 14650448. *Excluded: inadequate duration.*

Fishbain DA, Cutler RB, Rosomoff HL, et al. Are opioid-dependent/tolerant patients impaired in driving-related skills? a structured evidence-based review. J Pain Symptom Manage. 2003;25(6):559-77. PMID: 12782437. *Excluded: inadequate duration.*

Fishman SM. Strategies for selecting treatment and mitigating risk in patients with chronic pain. J Clin Psychiatry. 2011;72(1):e02. PMID: 21272509. *Excluded: wrong publication type.*

Fishman SM, Mahajan G, Jung S, et al. The trilateral opioid contract: bridging the pain clinic and the primary care physician through the opioid contract. J Pain Symptom Manage. 2002;24(3):335-44. PMID: 12458115. *Excluded: inadequate duration.*

Frank B, Serpell MG, Hughes J, et al. Comparison of analgesic effects and patient tolerability of nabilone and dihydrocodeine for chronic neuropathic pain: randomised, crossover, double blind study. BMJ. 2008;336(7637):199-201. PMID: 18182416. *Excluded: inadequate duration.*

Franklin GM, Stover BD, Turner JA, et al. Early opioid prescription and subsequent disability among workers with back injuries: The disability risk identification study cohort. Spine. 2008; 33(2):199-204. PMID: 18197107. *Excluded: wrong population*

Fraser LA, Morrison D, Morley-Forster P, et al. Oral opioids for chronic non-cancer pain: higher prevalence of hypogonadism in men than in women. Exp Clin Endocrinol Diabetes. 2009;117(1):38-43. PMID: 18523930. *Excluded: wrong study design.*

Fredheim OM, Kaasa S, Dale O, et al. Opioid switching from oral slow release morphine to oral methadone may improve pain control in chronic non-malignant pain: a nine-month follow-up study. Palliat Med. 2006;20(1):35-41. PMID: 16482756. *Excluded: inadequate duration.*

French DD, Campbell R, Spehar A, et al. National outpatient medication profiling: medications associated with outpatient fractures in community-dwelling elderly veterans. Br J Clin Pharmacol. 2007;63(2):238-44. PMID: 17096682. *Excluded: wrong population.*

Frich LM, Sorensen J, Jacobsen S, et al. Outcomes of follow-up visits to chronic nonmalignant pain patients. Pain Manag Nurs. 2012;13(4):223-35. PMID: 23158704. *Excluded: wrong intervention.*

Friedmann N, Klutzaritz V, Webster L. Efficacy and safety of an extended-release oxycodone (remoxy) formulation in patients with moderate to severe osteoarthritic pain. J Opioid Manag. 2011;7(3):193-202. PMID: 21823550. *Excluded: wrong outcome.*

Friedmann N, Klutzaritz V, Webster L. Long-term safety of Remoxy (extended-release oxycodone) in patients with moderate to severe chronic osteoarthritis or low back pain. Pain Med. 2011;12(5):755-60. PMID: 21481168. *Excluded: inadequate duration.*

Furlan A, Chaparro LE, Irvin E, et al. A comparison between enriched and nonenriched enrollment randomized withdrawal trials of opioids for chronic noncancer pain. Pain Res Manag. 2011;16(5):337-51. PMID: 22059206. *Excluded: inadequate duration.*

Furlan AD, Sandoval JA, Mailis-Gagnon A, et al. Opioids for chronic noncancer pain: a meta-analysis of effectiveness and side effects. CMAJ. 2006;174(11):1589-94. PMID: 16717269. *Excluded: systematic review or meta-analysis used only as a source document.*

Gabrail NY, Dvergsten C, Ahdieh H. Establishing the dosage equivalency of oxymorphone extended release and oxycodone controlled release in patients with cancer pain: a randomized controlled study. Curr Med Res Opin. 2004;20(6):911-8. PMID: 15200750. *Excluded: inadequate duration.*

Gaertner J, Frank M, Bosse B, et al. [Oral controlled-release oxycodone for the treatment of chronic pain. data from 4196 patients]. Schmerz. 2006;20(1):61-8. PMID: 15926076. *Excluded: inadequate duration.*

Gaertner J, Radbruch L, Giesecke T, et al. Assessing cognition and psychomotor function under long-term treatment with controlled release oxycodone in non-cancer pain patients. Acta Anaesthesiol Scand. 2006;50(6):664-72. PMID: 16987359. *Excluded: inadequate duration.*

Gajria K, Kosinski M, Schein J, et al. Health-related quality-of-life outcomes in patients treated with push-pull OROS hydromorphone versus extended-release oxycodone for chronic hip or knee osteoarthritis pain: a randomized, open-label, parallel-group, multicenter study. Patient. 2008;1(3):223-38. PMID: 22272928. *Excluded: inadequate duration.*

Galer BS, Lee D, Ma T, et al. MorphiDex (morphine sulfate/dextromethorphan hydrobromide combination) in the treatment of chronic pain: three multicenter, randomized, double-blind, controlled clinical trials fail to demonstrate enhanced opioid analgesia or reduction in tolerance. Pain. 2005;115(3):284-95. PMID: 15911155. *Excluded: inadequate duration.*

Gallucci M, Toscani F, Mapelli A, et al. Nimesulide in the treatment of advanced cancer pain. double-blind comparison with naproxen. Arzneimittelforschung. 1992;42(8):1028-30. PMID: 1418076. *Excluded: wrong population.*

Galski T, Williams JB, Ehle HT. Effects of opioids on driving ability. J Pain Symptom Manage. 2000;19(3):200-8. PMID: 10760625. *Excluded: inadequate duration.*

Gana TJ, Pascual ML, Fleming RR, et al. Extended-release tramadol in the treatment of osteoarthritis: a multicenter, randomized, double-blind, placebo-controlled clinical trial. Curr Med Res Opin. 2006;22(7):1391-401. PMID: 16834838. *Excluded: inadequate duration.*

Gatti A, Longo G, Sabato E, et al. Long-term controlled-release oxycodone and pregabalin in the treatment of non-cancer pain: an observational study. Eur Neurol. 2011;65(6):317-22. PMID: 21576968. *Excluded: wrong study design.*

Gatti A, Reale C, Luzi M, et al. Effects of opioid rotation in chronic pain patients: ORTIBARN study. Clin Drug Investig. 2010;30 Suppl 2:39-47. PMID: 20670048. *Excluded: inadequate duration.*

Gatti A, Reale C, Occhioni R, et al. Standard therapy with opioids in chronic pain management: ORTIBER study. Clin Drug Investig. 2009;29 Suppl 1:17-23. PMID: 19445551. *Excluded: inadequate duration.*

Garland EL, Manusov EG, Froeliger B, et al. Mindfulness-oriented recovery enhancement for chronic pain and prescription opioid misuse: Results from an early-stage randomized controlled trial. J Consult Clin Psychol. 2014: 448-59. PMID: 24491075. *Excluded: inadequate duration*

Gerra G, Fantoma A, Zaimovic A. Naltrexone and buprenorphine combination in the treatment of opioid dependence. J Psychopharmacol. 2006;20(6):806-14. PMID: 16401652. *Excluded: wrong population.*

Gerra G, Saenz E, Busse A, et al. Supervised daily consumption, contingent take-home incentive and non-contingent take-home in methadone maintenance. Prog Neuropsychopharmacol Biol Psychiatry. 2011;35(2):483-9. PMID: 21147192. *Excluded: wrong population.*

Gianutsos L, Safrenek S. Is there a well-tested tool to detect drug-seeking behaviors in chronic pain patients? J Fam Pract. 2008;57(9):609-10. PMID: 18786335. *Excluded: wrong publication type.*

Gimbel JS, Richards P, Portenoy RK. Controlled-release oxycodone for pain in diabetic neuropathy: a randomized controlled trial. Neurology. 2003;60(6):927-34. PMID: 12654955. *Excluded: inadequate duration.*

Gordon A, Callaghan D, Spink D, et al. Buprenorphine transdermal system in adults with chronic low back pain: a randomized, double-blind, placebo-controlled crossover study, followed by an open-label extension phase. Clin Ther. 2010;32(5):844-60. PMID: 20685494. *Excluded: inadequate duration.*

Gordon A, Rashiq S, Moulin DE, et al. Buprenorphine transdermal system for opioid therapy in patients with chronic low back pain. Pain Res Manag. 2010;15(3):169-78. PMID: 20577660. *Excluded: inadequate duration.*

Gourlay GK, Plummer JL, Cherry DA, et al. Comparison of intermittent bolus with continuous infusion of epidural morphine in the treatment of severe cancer pain. Pain. 1991;47(2):135-40. PMID: 1762806. *Excluded: wrong intervention.*

Gowing L, Ali R, White JM. Buprenorphine for the management of opioid withdrawal. Cochrane Database Syst Rev. 2009;(4)PMID: 16625553. *Excluded: wrong population.*

Grattan A, Sullivan MD, Saunders KW, et al. Depression and prescription opioid misuse among chronic opioid therapy recipients with no history of substance abuse. Ann Fam Med. 2012;10(4):304-11. PMID: 22778118. *Excluded: wrong study design.*

Gravolin M, Rowell K, de Groot J. Interventions to support the decision-making process for older people facing the possibility of long-term residential care. Cochrane Database Syst Rev. 2007;(3):CD005213. PMID: 17636790. *Excluded: wrong intervention.*

Gregory TB. Chronic pain perspectives: How to safely prescribe long-acting opioids. J Fam Pract. 2013: S12-8. PMID: 2012429988. *Excluded: wrong publication type*

Grellner W, Rettig-Sturmer A, Kuhn-Becker H, et al. Daytime sleepiness and traffic-relevant psychophysical capability of patients with chronic pain under long-term therapy with opioids. 16th international conference on alcohol, drugs and traffic safety; 2002; Montreal, Canada. Societe de l'Assurance Automobile du Quebec; Volume 1. xviii [89]+349 pp. *Excluded: wrong outcomes*

Grider JS, Harned ME, Etscheidt MA. Patient selection and outcomes using a low-dose intrathecal opioid trialing method for chronic nonmalignant pain. Pain Physician. 2011;14(4):343-51. PMID: 21785477. *Excluded: inadequate duration.*

Guo Z, Wills P, Viitanen M, et al. Cognitive impairment, drug use, and the risk of hip fracture in persons over 75 years old: a community-based prospective study. Am J Epidemiol. 1998;148(9):887-92. PMID: 9801019. *Excluded: wrong population.*

Hagen NA, Babul N. Comparative clinical efficacy and safety of a novel controlled-release oxycodone formulation and controlled-release hydromorphone in the treatment of cancer pain. Cancer. 1997;79(7):1428-37. PMID: 9083166. *Excluded: inadequate duration.*

Hale M, Khan A, Kutch M, et al. Once-daily OROS hydromorphone ER compared with placebo in opioid-tolerant patients with chronic low back pain. Curr Med Res Opin. 2010;26(6):1505-18. PMID: 20429852. *Excluded: inadequate duration.*

Hale M, Speight K, Harsanyi Z, et al. Efficacy of 12 hourly controlled-release codeine compared with as required dosing of acetaminophen plus codeine in patients with chronic low back pain. Pain Res Manag. 1997;2(1):33 - 8. PMID: N/A. *Excluded: inadequate duration.*

Hale M, Upmalis D, Okamoto A, et al. Tolerability of tapentadol immediate release in patients with lower back pain or osteoarthritis of the hip or knee over 90 days: a randomized, double-blind study. Curr Med Res Opin. 2009;25(5):1095-104. PMID: 19301989. *Excluded: inadequate duration.*

Hale ME, Fleischmann R, Salzman R, et al. Efficacy and safety of controlled-release versus immediate-release oxycodone: randomized, double-blind evaluation in patients with chronic back pain. Clin J Pain. 1999;15(3):179-83. PMID: 10524470. *Excluded: inadequate duration.*

Hale ME, Wallace MS, Taylor DR, et al. Safety and tolerability of OROS hydromorphone er in adults with chronic noncancer and cancer pain: pooled analysis of 13 studies. J Opioid Manag. 2012;8(5):299-314. PMID: 23247907. *Excluded: systematic review or meta-analysis used only as a source document.*

Hamann S, Sloan P. Oral naltrexone to enhance analgesia in patients receiving continuous intrathecal morphine for chronic pain: a randomized, double-blind, prospective pilot study. J Opioid Manag. 2007;3(3):137-44. PMID: 18027539. *Excluded: inadequate duration.*

Hambleton S. Opioids for chronic noncancer pain: are they safe and effective? J Miss State Med Assoc. 2013;54(1):4-7. PMID: 23550383. *Excluded: wrong publication type.*

Hanlon JT, Boudreau RM, Roumani YF, et al. Number and dosage of central nervous system medications on recurrent falls in community elders: the Health, Aging and Body Composition study. J Gerontol A Biol Sci Med Sci. 2009;64(4):492-8. PMID: 19196642. *Excluded: wrong population.*

Hanna M, Thipphawong J. A randomized, double-blind comparison of OROS hydromorphone and controlled-release morphine for the control of chronic cancer pain. BMC Palliat Care. 2008;7(1):17. PMID: 18976472. *Excluded: inadequate duration.*

Harke H, Gretenkort P, Ladleif HU, et al. The response of neuropathic pain and pain in complex regional pain syndrome I to carbamazepine and sustained-release morphine in patients pretreated with spinal cord stimulation: a double-blinded randomized study. Anesth Analg. 2001;92(2):488-95. PMID: 11159256. *Excluded: inadequate duration.*

Haroutiunian S, McNicol ED, Lipman AG. Methadone for chronic non-cancer pain in adults. Cochrane Database Syst Rev. 2012;(11)PMID: 23152251. *Excluded: inadequate duration.*

Hartrick C, Van Hove I, Stegmann JU, et al. Efficacy and tolerability of tapentadol immediate release and oxycodone HCl immediate release in patients awaiting primary joint replacement surgery for end-stage joint disease: a 10-day, phase III, randomized, double-blind, active- and placebo-controlled study. Clin Ther. 2009;31(2):260-71. PMID: 19302899. *Excluded: inadequate duration.*

Hausmann LR, Gao S, Lee ES, et al. Racial disparities in the monitoring of patients on chronic opioid therapy. Pain. 2013: 46-52. PMID: 23273103. *Excluded: wrong intervention*

Havens JR, Walker R, Leukefeld CG. Prescription opioid use in the rural Appalachia: a community-based study. J Opioid Manag. 2008;4(2):63-71. PMID: 18557162. *Excluded: wrong population.*

Havens JR, Leukefeld CG, DeVeaugh-Geiss AM, et al. The impact of a reformulation of extended-release oxycodone designed to deter abuse in a sample of prescription opioid abusers. Drug Alcohol Depend. 2014. 139: 9-17. PMID: 24721614. *Excluded: wrong population*

Haythornthwaite JA, Menefee LA, Quatrano-Piacentini AL, et al. Outcome of chronic opioid therapy for non-cancer pain. J Pain Symptom Manage. 1998;15(3):185-94. PMID: 9564120. *Excluded: inadequate duration.*

Heiskanen T, Kalso E. Controlled-release oxycodone and morphine in cancer related pain. Pain. 1997;73(1):37-45. PMID: 9414055. *Excluded: inadequate duration.*

Hendler N, Cimini C, Ma T, et al. A comparison of cognitive impairment due to benzodiazepines and to narcotics. Am J Psychiatry. 1980;137(7):828-30. PMID: 6104445. *Excluded: wrong study design.*

Hermos JA, Lawler EV. Opioid overdose-related deaths. JAMA. 2011;306(4):380; author reply -1. PMID: 21791682. *Excluded: wrong publication type.*

Hermos JA, Young MM, Gagnon DR, et al. Characterizations of long-term oxycodone/acetaminophen prescriptions in veteran patients. Arch Intern Med. 2004;164(21):2361-6. PMID: 15557416. *Excluded: wrong study design.*

Hetland A, Carr DB. Medications and Impaired Driving. Ann Pharmacother. 2014;48(4):494-506. PMID: 24473486. *Excluded: systematic review or meta-analysis used only as a source document.*

Hirsch A, Proescholdbell SK, Bronson W, et al. Prescription histories and dose strengths associated with overdose deaths. Pain Med. 2014. 15(7): 1187-95. PMID: 25202775. *Excluded: wrong population*

Hochman JS, Pergolizzi J. Cohort study finds nine times increased overdose risk (fatal plus non-fatal) in patients receiving 100 mg/day for 90 days compared with 1-20 mg/day opioids for chronic non-cancer pain, but wide CI and possibility of unmeasured confounders. Evid Based Nurs. 2010;13(2):55-6. PMID: 20436154. *Excluded: wrong publication type.*

Hojsted J, Nielsen PR, Kendall S, et al. Validation and usefulness of the Danish version of the pain medication questionnaire in opioid-treated chronic pain patients. Acta Anaesthesiol Scand. 2011;55(10):1231-8. PMID: 22092128. *Excluded: wrong study design.*

Hojsted J, Ekholm O, Kurita GP, et al. Addictive behaviors related to opioid use for chronic pain: A population-based study. Pain. 2013; 154(12): 2677-83. PMID: 23906554. *Excluded: wrong study design*

Holmes CP. An opioid screening instrument: Long-term evaluation of the utility of the ain medication questionnaire: Holmes, Cara Pearson: U Texas Southwestern Medical Center At Dallas, US; 2004. *Excluded: wrong population.*

Holmes CP, Gatchel RJ, Adams LL, et al. An opioid screening instrument: long-term evaluation of the utility of the pain medication questionnaire. Pain Pract. 2006;6(2):74-88. PMID: 17309714. *Excluded: wrong population.*

Hopper JA, Wu J, Martus W, et al. A randomized trial of one-day vs. three-day buprenorphine inpatient detoxification protocols for heroin dependence. J Opioid Manag. 2005;1(1):31-5. PMID: 17315409. *Excluded: wrong population.*

Howe CQ, Sullivan MD. The missing 'p' in pain management: How the current opioid epidemic highlights the need for psychiatric services in chronic pain care. Gen Hosp Psychiatry. 2014; 36(1): 99-104. PMID: 24211157. *Exclude: wrong publication type*

Hser YI, Li J, Jiang H, et al. Effects of a randomized contingency management intervention on opiate abstinence and retention in methadone maintenance treatment in

China. Addiction. 2011;106(10):1801-9. PMID: 21793958. *Excluded: wrong population.*

Huffman KL, Sweis GW, Gase A, et al. Opioid use 12 months following interdisciplinary pain rehabilitation with weaning. Pain Med. 2013; 14(12): 1908-17. PMID: 2012396855. *Excluded: wrong comparator*

Humeniuk R, Ali R, Babor T, et al. A randomized controlled trial of a brief intervention for illicit drugs linked to the alcohol, smoking and substance involvement screening test (ASSIST) in clients recruited from primary health-care settings in four countries. Addiction. 2012;107(5):957-66. PMID: 22126102. *Excluded: wrong intervention.*

Huse E, Larbig W, Flor H, et al. The effect of opioids on phantom limb pain and cortical reorganization. Pain. 2001;90(1-2):47-55. PMID: 11166969. *Excluded: inadequate duration.*

Iraurgi Castillo I, Gonzalez Saiz F, Lozano Rojas O, et al. Estimation of cutoff for the severity of dependence scale (SDS) for opiate dependence by ROC analysis. Actas Esp Psiquiatr. 2010;38(5):270-7. PMID: 21117001. *Excluded: wrong outcome.*

Ivanova JI, Birnbaum HG, Yushkina Y, et al. The prevalence and economic impact of prescription opioid-related side effects among patients with chronic noncancer pain. J Opioid Manage. 2013; 9(4): 239-54. PMID: 24353017. *Excluded: inadequate duration*

Ives TJ, Chelminski PR, Hammett-Stabler CA, et al. Predictors of opioid misuse in patients with chronic pain: a prospective cohort study. BMC Health Serv Res. 2006;6:46. PMID: 16595013. *Excluded: wrong population.*

Jacobson J. Controlling chronic noncancer pain in an era of opioid misuse. Am J Nurs. 2012;112(9):19-21. PMID: 22932046. *Excluded: wrong publication type.*

Jadad AR, Carroll D, Glynn CJ, et al. Morphine responsiveness of chronic pain: double-blind randomised crossover study with patient-controlled analgesia. Lancet. 1992;339(8806):1367-71. PMID: 1350803. *Excluded: inadequate duration.*

James IG, O'Brien CM, McDonald CJ. A randomized, double-blind, double-dummy comparison of the efficacy and tolerability of low-dose transdermal buprenorphine (BuTrans seven-day patches) with buprenorphine sublingual tablets (Temgesic) in patients with osteoarthritis pain. J Pain Symptom Manage. 2010;40(2):266-78. PMID: 20541900. *Excluded: inadequate duration.*

Jamison RN, Butler SF, Budman SH, et al. Gender differences in risk factors for aberrant prescription opioid use. J Pain. 2010;11(4):312-20. PMID: 19944648. *Excluded: wrong study design.*

Jamison RN, Edwards RR. Risk factor assessment for problematic use of opioids for chronic pain. Clinical Neuropsychologist. 2013;27(1):60-80. PMID: 22935011. *Excluded: wrong publication type.*

Jamison RN, Edwards RR, Liu X, et al. Relationship of negative affect and outcome of an opioid therapy trial among low back pain patients. Pain Pract. 2013;13(3):173-81. PMID: 22681407. *Excluded: wrong outcome.*
Jamison RN, Link CL, Marceau LD. Do pain patients at high risk for substance misuse experience more pain? A longitudinal outcomes study. Pain Med. 2009;10(6):1084-94. PMID: 19671087. *Excluded: wrong population.*

Jamison RN, Ross EL, Michna E, et al. Substance misuse treatment for high-risk chronic pain patients on opioid therapy: a randomized trial. Pain. 2010;150(3):390-400. PMID: 20334973. *Excluded: inadequate duration.*

Jamison RN, Schein JR, Vallow S, et al. Neuropsychological effects of long-term opioid use in chronic pain patients. J Pain Symptom Manage. 2003;26(4):913-21. PMID: 14527760. *Excluded: inadequate duration.*

Janiri L, Mannelli P, Persico AM, et al. Opiate detoxification of methadone maintenance patients using lefetamine, clonidine and buprenorphine. Drug Alcohol Depend. 1994;36(2):139-45. PMID: 7851281. *Excluded: wrong population.*

Janiri L, Mannelli P, Serretti A, et al. Low-dose buprenorphine detoxification in long term methadone addicts. . 1994;PMID: N/A. *Excluded: wrong population.*

Jawahar R, Oh U, Yang S, et al. A systematic review of pharmacological pain management in multiple sclerosis. Drugs. 2013; 73(15): 1711-22. PMID: 24085618. *Excluded: wrong population*

Jenkins DG, Ebbutt AF, Evans CD. Tofranil in the treatment of low back pain. J Int Med Res1976;4(2 Suppl):28-40. PMID: 140827. *Excluded: inadequate duration.*

Jensen E, Ginsberg F. Tramadol versus dextropropoxyphene in the treatment of osteoarthritis. Drug Investigation. 1994;8(4):211-8. PMID: N/A. *Excluded: wrong intervention.*

Johnson, Johnson Pharmaceutical R, GrA'Anenthal G. A Study to evaluate the effectiveness and safety of tapentadol (CG5503) extended release (ER) in patients with moderate to severe chronic low back pain. 2010 PMID: N/A. *Excluded: inadequate duration.*

Johnson JR, Miller AJ. The efficacy of choline magnesium trisalicylate (CMT) in the management of metastatic bone pain: a pilot study. Palliat Med. 1994;8(2):129-35. PMID: 7521713. *Excluded: wrong intervention.*

Jones T, Moore T. Preliminary data on a new opioid risk assessment measure: the Brief Risk Interview. J Opioid Manag. 2013;9(1):19-27. PMID: 23709300. *Excluded: wrong population.*

Jones T, Passik SD. A comparison of methods of administering the Opioid Risk Tool. J Opioid Manag. 2011;7(5):347-51. PMID: 22165033. *Excluded: wrong outcome.*

Jorum E, Warncke T, Stubhaug A. Cold allodynia and hyperalgesia in neuropathic pain: the effect of N-methyl-D-aspartate (NMDA) receptor antagonist ketamine--a double-blind, cross-over comparison with alfentanil and placebo. Pain. 2003;101(3):229-35. PMID: 12583865. *Excluded: inadequate duration.*

Juárez Pichardo JS, Kassian Rank AA, Hernández Pérez AL, et al. Comparación de la eficacia en el alivio de dolor neuropático crónico agudizado con oxicodona más lidocaína intravenosas frente a tramadol más lidocaína intravenosas. Revista de la Sociedad Española del Dolor. 2009;16:307-13. PMID: N/A. *Excluded: wrong intervention.*

Jungquist CR. The relationship among chronic pain, opiates, and sleep: Jungquist, Carla R : U Rochester School of Nursing, US; 2009. *Excluded: wrong study design.*

Jungquist CR, Flannery M, Perlis ML, et al. Relationship of chronic pain and opioid use with respiratory disturbance during sleep. Pain Management Nursing. 2012;13(2):70-9. PMID: 22652280. *Excluded: wrong study design.*

Kalso E, Edwards JE, Moore RA, et al. Opioids in chronic non-cancer pain: systematic review of efficacy and safety. Pain. 2004;112(3):372-80. PMID: 15561393. *Excluded: inadequate duration.*

Kalso E, Vainio A. Morphine and oxycodone hydrochloride in the management of cancer pain. Clin Pharmacol Ther. 1990;47(5):639-46. PMID: 2188774. *Excluded: wrong population.*

Kamal-Bahl SJ, Stuart BC, Beers MH. Propoxyphene use and risk for hip fractures in older adults. Am J Geriatr Pharmacother. 2006;4(3):219-26. PMID: 17062322. *Excluded: wrong population.*

Kapil RP, Cipriano A, Friedman K, et al. Once-weekly transdermal buprenorphine application results in sustained and consistent steady-state plasma levels. J Pain Symptom Manage. 2013;46(1):65-75. PMID: 23026548. *Excluded: wrong population.*

Kaplan R, Slywka J, Slagle S, et al. A titrated morphine analgesic regimen comparing substance users and non-users with AIDS-related pain. J Pain Symptom Manage. 2000;19(4):265-73. PMID: 10799793. *Excluded: wrong study design.*

Kapural L, Kapural M, Bensitel T, et al. Opioid-sparing effect of intravenous outpatient ketamine infusions appears short-lived in chronic-pain patients with high opioid requirements. Pain Physician. 2010;13(4):389-94. PMID: 20648208. *Excluded: wrong intervention.*

Karlsson M, Berggren AC. Efficacy and safety of low-dose transdermal buprenorphine patches (5, 10, and 20 microg/h) versus prolonged-release tramadol tablets (75, 100, 150, and 200 mg) in patients with chronic osteoarthritis pain: a 12-week, randomized, open-label, controlled, parallel-group noninferiority study. Clin Ther. 2009;31(3):503-13. PMID: 19393841. *Excluded: wrong comparator.*

Katz N, Hale M, Morris D, et al. Morphine sulfate and naltrexone hydrochloride extended release capsules in patients with chronic osteoarthritis pain. Postgrad Med. 2010;122(4):112-28. PMID: 20675975. *Excluded: inadequate duration.*

Katz N, Sun S, Johnson F, et al. ALO-01 (morphine sulfate and naltrexone hydrochloride) extended-release capsules in the treatment of chronic pain of osteoarthritis of the hip or knee: pharmacokinetics, efficacy, and safety. J Pain. 2010;11(4):303-11. PMID: 19944650. *Excluded: inadequate duration.*

Katz NP, Birnbaum HG, Castor A. Volume of prescription opioids used nonmedically in the United States. J Pain Palliat Care Pharmacother. 2010;24(2):141-4. PMID: 20504136. *Excluded: inadequate duration.*

Katz NP, Sherburne S, Beach M, et al. Behavioral monitoring and urine toxicology testing in patients receiving long-term opioid therapy. Anesth Analg. 2003;97(4):1097-102, table of contents. PMID: 14500164. *Excluded: wrong population.*

Kendall SE, Sjogren P, Pimenta CAdM, et al. The cognitive effects of opioids in chronic non-cancer pain. Pain. 2010;150(2):225-30. PMID: 20554115. *Excluded: systematic review or meta-analysis used only as a source document.*

Kennedy JA, Crowley TJ. Chronic pain and substance abuse: a pilot study of opioid maintenance. J Subst Abuse Treat. 1990;7(4):233-8. PMID: 1981244. *Excluded: wrong population.*

Keskinbora K, Aydinli I. Perineural morphine in patients with chronic ischemic lower extremity pain: efficacy and long-term results. J Anesth. 2009;23(1):11-8. PMID: 19234816. *Excluded: wrong intervention.*

Khan BA, James K, Stickevers S. Retrospective review of opiate abuse in a veterans administration pain clinic. Am J Phys Med Rehabil. 2014: a75. PMID: 2012576996. *Excluded: wrong publication type*

Khatami M, Woody G, O'Brien C. Chronic pain and narcotic addiction: a multitherapeutic approach--a pilot study. Compr Psychiatry. 1979;20(1):55-60. PMID: 365441. *Excluded: wrong study design.*

Kinney MA, Hooten WM, Cassivi SD, et al. Chronic postthoracotomy pain and health-related quality of life. Ann Thorac Surg. 2012;93(4):1242-7. PMID: 22397986. *Excluded: wrong study design.*

Kleinert R, Lange C, Steup A, et al. Single dose analgesic efficacy of tapentadol in postsurgical dental pain: the results of a randomized, double-blind, placebo-controlled study. Anesth Analg. 2008;107(6):2048-55. PMID: 19020157. *Excluded: inadequate duration.*

Koeppe J, Lyda K, Armon C. Association between opioid use and health care utilization as measured by emergency room visits and hospitalizations among persons living with HIV. Clin J Pain. 2013; 29(11): 957-61. PMID: 2012337041. *Excluded: wrong study design*

Korkmazsky M, Ghandehari J, Sanchez A, et al. Feasibility study of rapid opioid rotation and titration.[Erratum appears in Pain Physician. 2011 Mar-Apr;14(2):217 Note: Lin, Huong-Mo [corrected to Lin, Hung-Mo]]. Pain Physician. 2011;14(1):71-82. PMID: 21267044. *Excluded: inadequate duration.*

Kragh A, Elmstahl S, Atroshi I. Older adults' medication use 6 months before and after hip fracture: a population-based cohort study. J Am Geriatr Soc. 2011;59(5):863-8. PMID: 21517788. *Excluded: wrong comparator.*

Krebs EE, Ramsey DC, Miloshoff JM, et al. Primary care monitoring of long-term opioid therapy among veterans with chronic pain. Pain Med. 2011;12(5):740-6. PMID: 21481167. *Excluded: wrong study design.*

Kress HG, Orońska A, Kaczmarek Z, et al. Efficacy and tolerability of intranasal fentanyl spray 50 to 200 μg for breakthrough pain in patients with cancer: a phase III, multinational, randomized, double-blind, placebo-controlled, crossover trial with a 10-month, open-label extension treatment period. Clin Ther. 2009;31(6):1177-91. PMID: N/A. *Excluded: wrong population.*

Kroenke K, Krebs E, Wu J, et al. Stepped care to optimize pain care rffectiveness (SCOPE) trial study design and sample characteristics. Contemp Clin Trials. 2013;34(2):270-81. PMID: 23228858. *Excluded: wrong publication type.*

Kroenke K, Krebs EE, Wu J, et al. Telecare collaborative management of chronic pain in primary care: A randomized clinical trial. JAMA. 2014; 312(3): 240-8. PMID: 25027139. *Excluded: wrong population*

Krumova EK, Bennemann P, Kindler D, et al. Low pain intensity after opioid withdrawal as a first step of a comprehensive pain rehabilitation program predicts long-term nonuse of opioids in chronic noncancer pain. Clin J Pain. 2013; 29(9): 760-9. PMID: 23567163. *Excluded: wrong study design*

Krymchantowski A, Moreira P. Out-patient detoxification in chronic migraine: comparison of strategies. Cephalalgia. 2003;23(10):982-93. PMID: 14984232. *Excluded: inadequate duration.*

Kuijpers T, van Middelkoop M, Rubinstein SM, et al. A systematic review on the effectiveness of pharmacological interventions for chronic non-specific low-back pain. Eur Spine J. 2011;20(1):40-50. PMID: 20680369. *Excluded: inadequate duration.*

Kupers RC, Konings H, Adriaensen H, et al. Morphine differentially affects the sensory and affective pain ratings in neurogenic and idiopathic forms of pain. Pain. 1991;47(1):5-12. PMID: 1663226. *Excluded: inadequate duration.*

Kurita GP, de Mattos Pimenta CA. Cognitive impairment in cancer pain patients receiving opioids: a pilot study. Cancer Nurs. 2008;31(1):49-57. PMID: 18176132. *Excluded: inadequate duration.*

Lake AE, III, Saper JR, Hamel RL. Comprehensive inpatient treatment of refractory chronic daily headache. Headache. 2009;49(4):555-62. PMID: 15613222. *Excluded: wrong study design.*

Landro NI, Fors EA, Vapenstad LL, et al. The extent of neurocognitive dysfunction in a multidisciplinary pain centre population. Is there a relation between reported and tested neuropsychological functioning? Pain. 2013; 154(7): 972-7. PMID: 23473784. *Excluded: inadequate duration*

Lange B, Kuperwasser B, Okamoto A, et al. Efficacy and safety of tapentadol prolonged release for chronic osteoarthritis pain and low back pain.[Erratum appears in Adv Ther. 2010 Dec;27(12):981]. Adv Ther. 2010;27(6):381-99. PMID: 20556560. *Excluded: inadequate duration.*

Langley PC, Patkar AD, Boswell KA, et al. Adverse event profile of tramadol in recent clinical studies of chronic osteoarthritis pain. Curr Med Res Opin. 2010;26(1):239-51. PMID: 19929615. *Excluded: wrong intervention.*

Lara NA, Teixeira MJ, Fonoff ET. Long term intrathecal infusion of opiates for treatment of failed back surgery syndrome. Acta Neurochir Suppl. 2011;108:41-7. PMID: 21107937. *Excluded: wrong intervention.*

Lauretti GR, Oliveira GM, Pereira NL. Comparison of sustained-release morphine with sustained-release oxycodone in advanced cancer patients. Br J Cancer. 2003;89(11):2027-30. PMID: 14647133. *Excluded: inadequate duration.*

Layne RD, Pellegrino RJ, Lerfald NM. Prescription opioids and overdose deaths. JAMA. 2009;301(17):1766-7; author reply 7-9. PMID: 19417188. *Excluded: wrong publication type.*

LeFort SM. Review: intravenous and oral opioids reduce chronic non-cancer pain but are associated with high rates of constipation, nausea, and sleepiness. Evid Based Nurs. 2005;8(3):88-. PMID: 16021719. *Excluded: systematic review or meta-analysis used only as a source document.*

Lemberg KK, Heiskanen TE, Neuvonen M, et al. Does co-administration of paroxetine change oxycodone analgesia: an interaction study in chronic pain patients. Scand J Pain. 2010;1(1):24-33. PMID: N/A. *Excluded: inadequate duration.*

Lemming D, Sorensen J, Graven-Nielsen T, et al. Managing chronic whiplash associated pain with a combination of low-dose opioid (remifentanil) and NMDA-antagonist (ketamine). Eur J Pain. 2007;11(7):719-32. PMID: 17197214. *Excluded: wrong intervention.*

Lennernäs B, Frank-Lissbrant I, Lennernäs H, et al. Sublingual administration of fentanyl to cancer patients is an effective treatment for breakthrough pain: results from a randomized phase II study. Palliat Med. 2010;24(3):286-93. PMID: 20015921. *Excluded: wrong population.*

Leonard R, Kourlas H. Too much of a good thing? treating the emerging syndrome of opioid-induced hyperalgesia. J Pharm Pract. 2008;21(2):165-8. PMID: N/A. *Excluded: wrong publication type.*

Leppert W. The role of methadone in opioid rotation-a Polish experience. Support Care Cancer. 2009;17(5):607-12. PMID: 19043743. *Excluded: wrong study design.*

Leslie H, Shapiro DY, Okamoto A, et al. Tapentadol ER for chronic low back pain: brief pain inventory (BPI) results. Ann Neurol. 2009;66(3, Supplement 13):S5. PMID: N/A. *Excluded: wrong publication type.*

Leung A, Wallace MS, Ridgeway B, et al. Concentration-effect relationship of intravenous alfentanil and ketamine on peripheral neurosensory thresholds, allodynia and hyperalgesia of neuropathic pain. Pain. 2001;91(1-2):177-87. PMID: 11240090. *Excluded: wrong intervention.*

Levick S, Jacobs C, Loukas DF, et al. Naproxen sodium in treatment of bone pain due to metastatic cancer. Pain. 1988;35(3):253-8. PMID: 3226754. *Excluded: inadequate duration.*

Li L. Safety of opioids for non-cancer pain: Li, Lin: Boston U , US; 2012. *Excluded: wrong study design.*

Lieb JG, Shuster JJ, Theriaque D, et al. A pilot study of octreotide lar vs. octreotide tid for pain and quality of life in chronic pancreatitis. JOP. 2009;10(5):518-22. PMID: 19734628. *Excluded: wrong intervention.*

Liguori S, Gottardi M, Micheletto G, et al. Pharmacological approach to chronic visceral pain. Focus on oxycodone controlled release: an open multicentric study. Eur Rev Med Pharmacol Sci. 2010;14(3):185-90. PMID: 20391956. *Excluded: inadequate duration.*

Likar R, Vadlau E-M, Breschan C, et al. Comparable analgesic efficacy of transdermal buprenorphine in patients over and under 65 years of age. Clin J Pain. 2008;24(6):536-43. PMID: 18574363. *Excluded: inadequate duration.*

Lin TC, Hsu CH, Lu CC, et al. Chronic opioid therapy in patients with chronic noncancer pain in Taiwan. J Anesth. 2010;24(6):882-7. PMID: 20886242. *Excluded: wrong study design.*

Ling W, Amass L, Shoptaw S, et al. A multi-center randomized trial of buprenorphine-naloxone versus clonidine for opioid detoxification: findings from the National Institute on Drug Abuse Clinical Trials Network. Addiction. 2005;100(8):1090-100. PMID: 16042639. *Excluded: wrong population.*

Ling W, Hillhouse M, Jenkins J, et al. Comparisons of analgesic potency and side effects of buprenorphine and buprenorphine with ultra-low-dose naloxone. J Addict Med. 2012;6(2):118-23. PMID: 22475985. *Excluded: wrong intervention.*

Lintzeris N, Bell J, Bammer G, et al. A randomized controlled trial of buprenorphine in the management of short-term ambulatory heroin withdrawal. Addiction. 2002;97(11):1395-404. PMID: 12410780. *Excluded: wrong population.*

Littlejohn C, Baldacchino A, Bannister J. Chronic non-cancer pain and opioid dependence. J R Soc Med. 2004;97(2):62-5. PMID: 14749399. *Excluded: wrong study design.*

Lo Presti C, Roscetti A, Muriess D, et al. Time to pain relief after immediate-release morphine in episodic pain: the TIME study. Clin Drug Investig. 2010;30 Suppl 2:49-55. PMID: 20670049. *Excluded: wrong study design.*

Loeber S, Nakovics H, Kniest A, et al. Factors affecting cognitive function of opiate-dependent patients. Drug Alcohol Depend. 2012;120(1-3):81-7. PMID: 21802223. *Excluded: wrong population.*

Lomen PL, Samal BA, Lamborn KR, et al. Flurbiprofen for the treatment of bone pain in patients with metastatic breast cancer. Am J Med. 1986;80(3A):83-7. PMID: 3515928. *Excluded: inadequate duration.*

Lotsch J, Freynhagen R, von Hentig N, et al. Higher pain scores, similar opioid doses and side effects associated with antipyretic analgesics in specialised tertiary pain care. Inflamm Res. 2010;59(11):989-95. PMID: 20490889. *Excluded: wrong study design.*

Lowenstein O, Leyendecker P, Hopp M, et al. Combined prolonged-release oxycodone and naloxone improves bowel function in patients receiving opioids for moderate-to-severe non-malignant chronic pain: a randomised controlled trial. Expert Opin Pharmacother.

2009;10(4):531-43. PMID: 19243306. *Excluded: inadequate duration.*

Madadi P, Hildebrandt D, Lauwers AE, et al. Characteristics of opioid-users whose death was related to opioid-toxicity: a population-based study in Ontario, Canada. PLoS ONE. 2013;8(4):e60600. PMID: 23577131. *Excluded: wrong population.*

Magnelli F, Biondi L, Calabria R, et al. Safety and efficacy of buprenorphine/naloxone in opioid-dependent patients: an Italian observational study. Clin Drug Investig. 2010;30 Suppl 1:21-6. PMID: 20450242. *Excluded: wrong comparator.*

Mailis-Gagnon A, Lakha SF, Furlan A, et al. Systematic review of the quality and generalizability of studies on the effects of opioids on driving and cognitive/psychomotor performance. Clin J Pain. 2012;28(6):542-55. PMID: 22673489. *Excluded: systematic review or meta-analysis used only as a source document.*

Maltoni M, Scarpi E, Modonesi C, et al. A validation study of the WHO analgesic ladder: a two-step vs three-step strategy. Support Care Cancer. 2005;13(11):888-94. PMID: 15818486. *Excluded: wrong population.*

Manchikanti L, Ailinani H, Koyyalagunta D, et al. A systematic review of randomized trials of long-term opioid management for chronic non-cancer pain. Pain Physician. 2011;14(2):91-121. PMID: 21412367. *Excluded: systematic review or meta-analysis used only as a source document.*

Manchikanti L, Cash KA, Damron KS, et al. Controlled substance abuse and illicit drug use in chronic pain patients: An evaluation of multiple variables. Pain Physician. 2006;9(3):215-25. PMID: 16886030. *Excluded: wrong population.*

Manchikanti L, Fellows B, Ailinani H, et al. Therapeutic use, abuse, and nonmedical use of opioids: a ten-year perspective. Pain Physician. 2010;13(5):401-35. PMID: 20859312. *Excluded: wrong publication type.*

Manchikanti L, Giordano J, Boswell MV, et al. Psychological factors as predictors of opioid abuse and illicit drug use in chronic pain patients. J Opioid Manag. 2007;3(2):89-100. PMID: 17520988. *Excluded: wrong population.*

Manchikanti L, Helm S, 2nd, Fellows B, et al. Opioid epidemic in the United States. Pain Physician. 2012;15(3 Suppl):ES9-38. PMID: 22786464. *Excluded: wrong publication type.*

Manchikanti L, Manchikanti KN, Pampati V, et al. Prevalence of side effects of prolonged low or moderate dose opioid therapy with concomitant benzodiazepine and/or antidepressant therapy in chronic non-cancer pain. Pain Physician. 2009;12(1):259-67. PMID: 19165308. *Excluded: wrong intervention.*

Manchikanti L, Manchukonda R, Damron KS, et al. Does adherence monitoring reduce controlled substance abuse in chronic pain patients? Pain Physician. 2006;9(1):57-60. PMID: 16700282. *Excluded: wrong population.*

Manchikanti L, Manchukonda R, Pampati V, et al. Evaluation of abuse of prescription and illicit drugs in chronic pain patients receiving short-acting (hydrocodone) or long-acting (methadone) opioids. Pain Physician. 2005;8(3):257-61. PMID: 16850081. *Excluded: wrong population.*

Manchikanti L, Pampati V, Damron KS, et al. Prevalence of prescription drug abuse and dependency in patients with chronic pain in western Kentucky. J Ky Med Assoc. 2003;101(11):511-7. PMID: 14635580. *Excluded: wrong population.*

Manchikanti L, Pampati V, Damron KS, et al. Prevalence of opioid abuse in interventional pain medicine practice settings: a randomized clinical evaluation. Pain Physician. 2001;4(4):358-65. PMID: 16902682. *Excluded: wrong population.*

Manchikanti L, Vallejo R, Manchikanti KN, et al. Effectiveness of long-term opioid therapy for chronic non-cancer pain. Pain Physician. 2011;14(2):E133-56. PMID: 21412378. *Excluded: systematic review or meta-analysis used only as a source document.*

Manterola C, Vial M, Moraga J, et al. Analgesia in patients with acute abdominal pain. Cochrane Database Syst Rev. 2011;(1):CD005660. PMID: 21249672. *Excluded: inadequate duration.*

Mariconti P, Collini R. Tramadol SR in arthrosic and neuropathic pain. Minerva Anestesiol. 2008;74(3):63-8. PMID: 18288068. *Excluded: wrong intervention.*

Marino EN, Rosen KD, Gutierrez A, et al. Impulsivity but not sensation seeking is associated with opioid analgesic misuse risk in patients with chronic pain. Addict Behav. 2013;38(5):2154-7. PMID: 23454878. *Excluded: wrong study design.*

Marsch LA, Bickel WK, Badger GJ, et al. Comparison of pharmacological treatments for opioid-dependent adolescents: a randomized controlled trial. Arch Gen Psychiatry. 2005;62(10):1157-64. PMID: 16203961. *Excluded: wrong population.*

Martel M, Wasan A, Jamison R, et al. Catastrophic thinking and increased risk for prescription opioid misuse in patients with chronic pain. Drug Alcohol Depend. 2013; 132(1-2): 335-41. PMID: 23618767. *Excluded: wrong study design*

Martel MO, Dolman AJ, Edwards RR, et al. The association between negative affect and prescription opioid misuse in patients with chronic pain: The mediating role of opioid craving. J Pain. 2014; 15(1): 90-100. PMID: 24295876. *Excluded: wrong study design*

Martell BA, O'Connor PG, Kerns RD, et al. Systematic review: opioid treatment for chronic back pain: prevalence, efficacy, and association with addiction. Ann Intern Med. 2007;146(2):116-27. PMID: 17227935. *Excluded: systematic review or meta-analysis used only as a source document.*

Martin BC, Fan MY, Edlund MJ, et al. Long-term chronic opioid therapy discontinuation rates from the troup study. J Gen Intern Med. 2011; 26(12): 1450-7. PMID: 21751058. *Excluded: wrong population*

Martino G, Ventafridda V, Parini J, et al. A controlled study on the analgesic activity of indoprofen in patients with cancer pain. Adv Pain Res Ther. 1976;1:573-8. PMID: 383108. *Excluded: wrong intervention.*

Matthews ML, Lufkin R. Tapentadol: a novel, centrally acting analgesic for moderate-to-severe acute pain. J Pharm Technol. 2011;27(1):27-34. PMID: N/A. *Excluded: wrong population.*

Max MB, Byas-Smith MG, Gracely RH, et al. Intravenous infusion of the NMDA antagonist, ketamine, in chronic posttraumatic pain with allodynia: a double-blind comparison to alfentanil and placebo. Clin Neuropharmacol. 1995;18(4):360-8. PMID: 8665549. *Excluded: wrong intervention.*

Max MB, Schafer SC, Culnane M, et al. Association of pain relief with drug side effects in postherpetic neuralgia: a single-dose study of clonidine, codeine, ibuprofen, and placebo. Clin Pharmacol Ther. 1988;43(4):363-71. PMID: 3281774. *Excluded: inadequate duration.*

Mayyas F, Fayers P, Kaasa S, et al. A systematic review of oxymorphone in the management of chronic pain. J Pain Symptom Manage. 2010;39(2):296-308. PMID: 20152592. *Excluded: inadequate duration.*

McCann B, Lange R, Wagner B, et al. Patient global impression of change results from a 1-year open-label extension study of tapentadol extended release in patients with chronic osteoarthritis or low back pain. [abstract]. *Excluded: wrong publication type.*

Arthritis Rheum. 2010; Conference: American College of Rheumatology/Association of Rheumatology Health Professionals Annual Scientific Meeting, ACR/ARHP Atlanta, Georgia, Nov. 6-11, 2010(62 Suppl 10):950. PMID: N/A. *Excluded: wrong publication type.*

McKay L, Pritham UA, Radzyminski S, et al. Safe use of opioid analgesics for chronic pain in pregnancy. J Obstet Gynecol Neonatal Nurs2013;42:S74-S. PMID: N/A. *Excluded: wrong population.*

McNamara P. Opioid switching from morphine to transdermal fentanyl for toxicity reduction in palliative care. Palliat Med. 2002;16(5):425-34. PMID: 12380661. *Excluded: wrong population.*

McNicol ED, Midbari A, Eisenberg E. Opioids for neuropathic pain. Cochrane Database Syst Rev. 2013;(9)PMID: 16856116. *Excluded: systematic review or meta-analysis used only as a source document.*

McNicol ED, Strassels S, Goudas L, et al. NSAIDS or paracetamol, alone or combined with opioids, for cancer pain. Cochrane Database Syst Rev. 2011;(6)PMID: 15654708. *Excluded: systematic review or meta-analysis used only as a source document.*

Meghani SH, Wiedemer NL, Becker WC, et al. Predictors of resolution of aberrant drug behavior in chronic pain patients treated in a structured opioid risk management program. Pain Med. 2009;10(5):858-65. PMID: 19523029. *Excluded: wrong study design.*

Meissner W, Leyendecker P, Mueller-Lissner S, et al. A randomised controlled trial with prolonged-release oral oxycodone and naloxone to prevent and reverse opioid-induced constipation. Eur J Pain. 2009;13(1):56-64. PMID: 18762438. *Excluded: wrong outcome.*

Meissner W, Schmidt U, Hartmann M, et al. Oral naloxone reverses opioid-associated constipation. Pain. 2000;84(1):105-9. PMID: 10601678. *Excluded: wrong comparator.*

Meltzer EC, Rybin D, Meshesha LZ, et al. Aberrant drug-related behaviors: unsystematic documentation does not identify prescription drug use disorder. Pain Med. 2012;13(11):1436-43. PMID: 23057631. *Excluded: wrong population.*

Meltzer EC, Rybin D, Saitz R, et al. Identifying prescription opioid use disorder in primary care: diagnostic characteristics of the current opioid misuse measure (COMM). Pain. 2011;152(2):397-402. PMID: 21177035. *Excluded: wrong population.*

Menefee LA, Frank ED, Crerand C, et al. The effects of transdermal fentanyl on driving, cognitive performance, and balance in patients with chronic nonmalignant pain conditions. Pain Med. 2004;5(1):42-9. PMID: 14996236. *Excluded: inadequate duration.*

Mercadante S, Caraceni A. Conversion ratios for opioid switching in the treatment of cancer pain: a systematic review. Palliat Med. 2011;25(5):504-15. PMID: 21708857. *Excluded: systematic review or meta-analysis used only as a source document.*

Mercadante S, Casuccio A, Calderone L. Rapid switching from morphine to methadone in cancer patients with poor response to morphine. J Clin Oncol. 1999;17(10):3307-12. PMID: 10506634. *Excluded: inadequate duration.*

Mercadante S, Casuccio A, Fulfaro F, et al. Switching from morphine to methadone to improve analgesia and tolerability in cancer patients: a prospective study. J Clin Oncol. 2001;19(11):2898-904. PMID: 11387363. *Excluded: inadequate duration.*

Mercadante S, Casuccio A, Tirelli W, et al. Equipotent doses to switch from high doses of opioids to transdermal buprenorphine. Support Care Cancer. 2009;17(6):715-8. PMID: 19104845. *Excluded: wrong study design.*

Mercadante S, Ferrera P, Villari P, et al. Rapid switching between transdermal fentanyl and methadone in cancer patients. J Clin Oncol. 2005;23(22):5229-34. PMID: 16051965. *Excluded: wrong population.*

Mercadante S, Ferrera P, Villari P, et al. Frequency, indications, outcomes, and predictive factors of opioid switching in an acute palliative care unit. J Pain Symptom Manage. 2009;37(4):632-41. PMID: 19345298. *Excluded: wrong study design.*

Mercadante S, Porzio G, Ferrera P, et al. Sustained-release oral morphine versus transdermal fentanyl and oral methadone in cancer pain management. Eur J Pain. 2008;12(8):1040-6. PMID: 18353696. *Excluded: inadequate duration.*

Mercadante S, Porzio G, Fulfaro F, et al. Switching from transdermal drugs: an observational "N of 1" study of fentanyl and buprenorphine. J Pain Symptom Manage. 2007;34(5):532-8. PMID: 17629666. *Excluded: wrong study design.*

Mercadante S, Radbruch L, Davies A, et al. A comparison of intranasal fentanyl spray with oral transmucosal fentanyl citrate for the treatment of breakthrough cancer pain: an open-label, randomised, crossover trial. Curr Med Res Opin 2009;25(11):2805-15. PMID: 19792837. *Excluded: wrong population.*

Mercadante S, Villari P, Ferrera P, et al. Opioid plasma concentrations during a switch from transdermal fentanyl to methadone. J Palliat Med. 2007;10(2):338-44. PMID: 17472504. *Excluded: wrong outcome.*

Merchant S, Provenzano D, Mody S, et al. Composite measure to assess efficacy/gastrointestinal tolerability of tapentadol er versus oxycodone cr for chronic pain: pooled analysis of randomized studies. J Opioid Manag. 2013;9(1):51-61. PMID: 23709304. *Excluded: inadequate duration.*

Merrill JO, Von Korff M, Banta-Green CJ, et al. Prescribed opioid difficulties, depression and opioid dose among chronic opioid therapy patients. Gen Hosp Psychiatry.2012;34(6):581-7. PMID: 22959422. *Excluded: wrong comparator.*

Merza Z, Edwards N, Walters S, et al. Patients with chronic pain and abnormal pituitary function require investigation. Lancet. 2003;361(9376):2203-4. PMID: 12842375. *Excluded: wrong study design.*

Messina J, Darwish M, Fine PG. Fentanyl buccal tablet. Drugs Today. 2008;44(1):41-54. PMID: 18301803. *Excluded: wrong publication type.*

Meuleners LB, Duke J, Lee AH, et al. Psychoactive medications and crash involvement requiring hospitalization for older drivers: a population-based study. J Am Geriatr Soc. 2011;59(9):1575-80. PMID: 21883110. *Excluded: wrong population.*

Miller M, Sturmer T, Azrael D, et al. Opioid analgesics and the risk of fractures in older adults with arthritis. J Am Geriatr Soc. 2011;59(3):430-8. PMID: 21391934. *Excluded: wrong population.*

Milligan K, Lanteri-Minet M, Borchert K, et al. Evaluation of long-term efficacy and safety of transdermal fentanyl in the treatment of chronic noncancer pain. J Pain. 2001;2(4):197-204. PMID: 14622817. *Excluded: wrong study design.*

Minotti V, Betti M, Ciccarese G, et al. A double-blind study comparing two single-dose regimens of ketorolac with diclofenac in pain due to cancer. Pharmacotherapy. 1998;18(3):504-8. PMID: 9620101. *Excluded: inadequate duration.*

Minotti V, De Angelis V, Righetti E, et al. Double-blind evaluation of short-term analgesic efficacy of orally administered diclofenac, diclofenac plus codeine, and diclofenac plus imipramine in chronic cancer pain. Pain. 1998;74(2-3):133-7. PMID: 9520227. *Excluded: inadequate duration.*

Minotti V, Patoia L, Roila F, et al. Double-blind evaluation of analgesic efficacy of orally administered diclofenac, nefopam, and acetylsalicylic acid (asa) plus codeine in chronic cancer pain. Pain. 1989;36(2):177-83. PMID: 2645561. *Excluded: inadequate duration.*

Minozzi S, Amato L, Davoli M. Development of dependence following treatment with opioid analgesics for pain relief: A systematic review. Addiction. 2013;108(4):688-98. PMID: 22775332. *Excluded: systematic review or meta-analysis used only as a source document.*

Moden B, Merlo J, Ohlsson H, et al. Psychotropic drugs and falling accidents among the elderly: a nested case control study in the whole population of Scania, Sweden. J Epidemiol Community Health. 2010;64(5):440-6. PMID: 20445213. *Excluded: wrong population.*

Moertel CG, Ahmann DL, Taylor WF, et al. Aspirin and pancreatic cancer pain. Gastroenterology. 1971;60(4):552-3. PMID: 5573227. *Excluded: inadequate duration.*

Moertel CG, Ahmann DL, Taylor WF, et al. Relief of pain by oral medications. A controlled evaluation of analgesic combinations. JAMA. 1974;229(1):55-9. PMID: 4599149. *Excluded: inadequate duration.*

Monterubbianesi MC, Capuccini J, Ferioli I, et al. High opioid dosage rapid detoxification of cancer patient in palliative care with the Raffaeli model. J Opioid Manag.

2012;8(5):292-8. PMID: 23247906. *Excluded: wrong intervention.*

Moore AR, Edwards J, Derry S, et al. Single dose oral dihydrocodeine for acute postoperative pain. Cochrane Database Syst Rev. 2011;(3)PMID: 11034754. *Excluded: wrong population.*

Moore KT, Adams HD, Natarajan J, et al. Bioequivalence and safety of a novel fentanyl transdermal matrix system compared with a transdermal reservoir system. J Opioid Manag. 2011;7(2):99-107. PMID: 21561033. *Excluded: inadequate duration.*

Moore RA, McQuay HJ. Prevalence of opioid adverse events in chronic non-malignant pain: systematic review of randomised trials of oral opioids. Arthritis Res Ther. 2005;7(5):R1046-51. PMID: 16207320. *Excluded: inadequate duration.*

Morasco BJ, Dobscha SK. Prescription medication misuse and substance use disorder in VA primary care patients with chronic pain. Gen Hosp Psychiatry.2008;30(2):93-9. PMID: 18291290. *Excluded: wrong population.*

Morasco BJ, Duckart JP, Dobscha SK. Adherence to clinical guidelines for opioid therapy for chronic pain in patients with substance use disorder. J Gen Intern Med. 2011;26(9):965-71. PMID: 21562923. *Excluded: wrong outcome.*

Morasco BJ, Gritzner S, Lewis L, et al. Systematic review of prevalence, correlates, and treatment outcomes for chronic non-cancer pain in patients with comorbid substance use disorder. Pain. 2011;152(3):488-97. PMID: 21185119. *Excluded: systematic review or meta-analysis used only as a source document.*

Morasco BJ, Turk DC, Donovan DM, et al. Risk for prescription opioid misuse among patients with a history of substance use disorder. Drug Alcohol Depend. 2013;127(1-3):193-9. PMID: 22818513. *Excluded: wrong study design.*

Morasco BJ, Cavanagh R, Gritzner S, et al. Care management practices for chronic pain in veterans prescribed high doses of opioid medications. Fam Pract. 2013; 30(6): 671-8. PMID: 23901065. *Excluded: wrong study design*

Moriarty M, McDonald CJ, Miller AJ. A randomized crossover comparison of controlled release hydromorphone tablets with controlled release morphine tablets in patients with cancer pain. J Drug Assessment. 1999;2:41-8. PMID: N/A. *Excluded: inadequate duration.*

Morley JS, Bridson J, Nash TP, et al. Low-dose methadone has an analgesic effect in neuropathic pain: a double-blind randomized controlled crossover trial. Palliat Med. 2003;17(7):576-87. PMID: 14594148. *Excluded: inadequate duration.*

Morrison RA. Update on sickle cell disease: incidence of addiction and choice of opioid in pain management. Pediatr Nurs. 1991;17(5):503. PMID: 1923659. *Excluded: wrong publication type.*

Moryl N, Pope J, Obbens E. Hypoglycemia during rapid methadone dose escalation. J Opioid Manag. 2013;9(1):29-34. PMID: 23709301. *Excluded: wrong comparator.*

Moser HR, Giesler GJ, Jr. Itch and analgesia resulting from intrathecal application of morphine: Contrasting effects on different populations of trigeminothalamic tract neurons. J Neurosci. 2013; 33(14): 6093-101. PMID: 23554490. *Excluded: wrong intervention*

Mosher HJ, Jiang L, Vaughan Sarrazin MS, et al. Prevalence and characteristics of hospitalized adults on chronic opioid therapy. J Hosp Med. 2014;9(2):82-7. PMID: 24311455. *Excluded: wrong population.*

Moulin DE, Iezzi A, Amireh R, et al. Randomised trial of oral morphine for chronic non-cancer pain. Lancet. 1996;347(8995):143-7. PMID: 8544547. *Excluded: inadequate duration.*

Moulin DE, Johnson NG, Murray-Parsons N, et al. Subcutaneous narcotic infusions for cancer pain: treatment outcome and guidelines for use. CMAJ. 1992;146(6):891-7. PMID: 1371946. *Excluded: wrong intervention.*

Moulin DE, Richarz U, Wallace M, et al. Efficacy of the sustained-release hydromorphone in neuropathic pain management: pooled analysis of three open-label studies. J Pain Palliat Care Pharmacother. 2010;24(3):200-12. PMID: 20718640. *Excluded: inadequate duration.*

Mowatt G, Glazener C, Jarrett M. Sacral nerve stimulation for faecal incontinence and constipation in adults. Cochrane Database Syst Rev. 2007;(3):CD004464. PMID: 17636759. *Excluded: wrong intervention.*

Mucci-LoRusso P, Berman BS, Silberstein PT, et al. Controlled-release oxycodone compared with controlled-release morphine in the treatment of cancer pain: A randomized, double-blind, parallel-group study. Eur J Pain. 1998;2(3):239-49. PMID: 15102384. *Excluded: inadequate duration.*

Murphy JL, Clark ME, Banou E. Opioid cessation and multidimensional outcomes after interdisciplinary chronic pain treatment. Clin J Pain. 2013;29(2):109-17. PMID: 22751033. *Excluded: wrong population.*

Mystakidou K, Parpa E, Tsilika E, et al. Long-term management of noncancer pain with transdermal therapeutic system-fentanyl. J Pain. 2003;4(6):298-306. PMID: 14622686. *Excluded: wrong study design.*

Mystakidou K, Tsilika E, Parpa E, et al. Long-term cancer pain management in morphine pre-treated and opioid naive patients with transdermal fentanyl. Int J Cancer.

2003;107(3):486-92. PMID: 14506751. *Excluded: wrong study design.*

Nalamachu SR, Kutch M, Hale ME. Safety and tolerability of once-daily OROS hydromorphone extended-release in opioid-tolerant adults with moderate-to-severe chronic cancer and noncancer pain: pooled analysis of 11 clinical studies. J Pain Symptom Manage. 2012;44(6):852-65. PMID: 22795050. *Excluded: systematic review or meta-analysis used only as a source document.*

Nalamachu SR, Narayana A, Janka L. Long-term dosing, safety, and tolerability of fentanyl buccal tablet in the management of noncancer-related breakthrough pain in opioid-tolerant patients. Curr Med Res Opin. 2011;27(4):751-60. PMID: 21288055. *Excluded: systematic review or meta-analysis used only as a source document.*

Narabayashi M, Saijo Y, Takenoshita S, et al. Opioid rotation from oral morphine to oral oxycodone in cancer patients with intolerable adverse effects: an open-label trial. Jpn J Clin Oncol. 2008;38(4):296-304. PMID: 18326541. *Excluded: inadequate duration.*

Neumann AM, Blondell RD, Jaanimagi U, et al. A preliminary study comparing methadone and buprenorphine in patients with chronic pain and coexistent opioid addiction. J Addict Dis. 2013;32(1):68-78. PMID: 23480249. *Excluded: inadequate duration.*

Newshan G, Lefkowitz M. Transdermal fentanyl for chronic pain in AIDS: A pilot study. J Pain Symptom Manage. 2001;21(1):69-77. PMID: 11223316. *Excluded: inadequate duration.*

Nicholson B, Ross E, Sasaki J, et al. Randomized trial comparing polymer-coated extended-release morphine sulfate to controlled-release oxycodone HCl in moderate to severe nonmalignant pain. Curr Med Res Opin. 2006;22(8):1503-14. PMID: 16870075. *Excluded: inadequate duration.*

Nielsen S, Larance B, Lintzeris N, et al. Correlates of pain in an in-treatment sample of opioid-dependent people. Drug Alcohol Rev. 2013; 32(5): 489-94. PMID: 23594352. *Excluded: wrong population*

Nigam AK, Ray R, Tripathi BM. Buprenorphine in opiate withdrawal: a comparison with clonidine. J Subst Abuse Treat. 1993;10(4):391-4. PMID: 8257551. *Excluded: wrong population.*

Njee TB, Irthum B, Roussel P, et al. Intrathecal morphine infusion for chronic non-malignant pain: a multiple center retrospective survey. Neuromodulation. 2004;7(4):249-59. PMID: 22151334. *Excluded: wrong intervention.*

Noble M, Schoelles K. Opioid treatment for chronic back pain and its association with addiction. Ann Intern Med. 2007;147(5):348-9; author reply 9-50. PMID: 17785496. *Excluded: wrong publication type.*

Noble M, Tregear SJ, Treadwell JR, et al. Long-term opioid therapy for chronic noncancer pain: a systematic review and meta-analysis of efficacy and safety. J Pain Symptom Manage. 2008;35(2):214-28. PMID: 18178367. *Excluded: systematic review or meta-analysis used only as a source document.*

Notley C, Blyth A, Maskrey V, et al. The experience of long-term opiate maintenance treatment and reported barriers to recovery: A qualitative systematic review. Eur Addict Res. 2013; 19(6): 287-98. PMID: 23652159. *Excluded: wrong outcome*

Oberleitner LMS. Emotional risk factors for substance abuse in a chronic pain population: developing a predictive model and testing methods for assessing stigmatized behaviors: Oberleitner, Lindsay M S : Wayne State U , US; 2012. *Excluded: wrong study design.*

O'Connor PG, Carroll KM, Shi JM, et al. Three methods of opioid detoxification in a primary care setting. a randomized trial. Ann Intern Med. 1997;127(7):526-30. PMID: 9313020. *Excluded: wrong population.*

O'Donnell JB, Ekman EF, Spalding WM, et al. The effectiveness of a weak opioid medication versus a cyclo-oxygenase-2 (COX-2) selective non-steroidal anti-inflammatory drug in treating flare-up of chronic low-back pain: results from two randomized, double-blind, 6-week studies. J Int Med Res2009;37(6):1789-802. PMID: 20146877. *Excluded: inadequate duration.*

Oosterman JM, Derksen LC, van Wijck AJ, et al. Executive and attentional functions in chronic pain: Does performance decrease with increasing task load? Pain Res Manag. 2012;17(3):159-65. PMID: 22606680. *Excluded: wrong study design.*

Oreskovich MR, Saxon AJ, Ellis ML, et al. A double-blind, double-dummy, randomized, prospective pilot study of the partial mu opiate agonist, buprenorphine, for acute detoxification from heroin. Drug Alcohol Depend. 2005;77(1):71-9. PMID: 15607843. *Excluded: wrong population.*

Palangio M, Northfelt DW, Portenoy RK, et al. Dose conversion and titration with a novel, once-daily, OROS osmotic technology, extended-release hydromorphone formulation in the treatment of chronic malignant or nonmalignant pain. J Pain Symptom Manage. 2002;23(5):355-68. PMID: 12007754. *Excluded: inadequate duration.*

Pani PP, Trogu E, Maremmani I, et al. Qtc interval screening for cardiac risk in methadone treatment of opioid dependence. Cochrane Database Syst Rev. 2013; 6: CD008939. PMID: 23787716. *Excluded: wrong population*

Pannuti F, Robustelli della Cuna G, Ventaffrida V, et al. A double-blind evaluation of the analgesic efficacy and toxicity of oral ketorolac and diclofenac in cancer pain. the TD/10 recordati protocol study group. Tumori.

1999;85(2):96-100. PMID: 10363074. *Excluded: wrong intervention.*

Park J, Clement R, Lavin R. Factor structure of pain medication questionnaire in community-dwelling older adults with chronic pain. Pain Pract. 2011;11(4):314-24. PMID: 21143370. *Excluded: wrong study design.*

Passik SD, Kirsh KL, Donaghy KB, et al. Pain and aberrant drug-related behaviors in medically ill patients with and without histories of substance abuse. Clin J Pain. 2006;22(2):173-81. PMID: 16428952. *Excluded: wrong study design.*

Passik SD, Messina J, Golsorkhi A, et al. Aberrant drug-related behavior observed during clinical studies involving patients taking chronic opioid therapy for persistent pain and fentanyl buccal tablet for breakthrough pain. J Pain Symptom Manage. 2011;41(1):116-25. PMID: 20580202. *Excluded: wrong population.*

Paulozzi LJ, Kilbourne EM, Shah NG, et al. A history of being prescribed controlled substances and risk of drug overdose death. Pain Med. 2012;13(1):87-95. PMID: 22026451. *Excluded: wrong population.*

Pedersen L, Borchgrevink PC, Breivik HP, et al. A randomized, double-blind, double-dummy comparison of short- and long-acting dihydrocodeine in chronic non-malignant pain. Pain. 2014; 155(5): 881-8. PMID: 24345428. *Excluded: inadequate duration*

Peloso PM, Fortin L, Beaulieu A, et al. Analgesic efficacy and safety of tramadol/ acetaminophen combination tablets (ultracet) in treatment of chronic low back pain: a multicenter, outpatient, randomized, double blind, placebo controlled trial. J Rheumatol. 2004;31(12):2454-63. PMID: 15570651. *Excluded: inadequate duration.*

Pergolizzi JV, Jr., Labhsetwar SA, Puenpatom RA, et al. Exposure to potential CYP450 pharmacokinetic drug-drug interactions among osteoarthritis patients: incremental risk of multiple prescriptions. Pain Pract. 2011;11(4):325-36. PMID: 21199317. *Excluded: wrong comparator.*

Phifer J, Skelton K, Weiss T, et al. Pain symptomatology and pain medication use in civilian PTSD. Pain. 2011;152(10):2233-40. PMID: 21665366. *Excluded: wrong population.*

Pink LR, Smith AJ, Peng PWH, et al. Intake assessment of problematic use of medications in a chronic noncancer pain clinic. Pain Res Manag. 2012;17(4):276-80. PMID: 22891193. *Excluded: wrong study design.*

Pinn S. Fewer opioid-related side effects with tapentadol. Br J Hosp Med. 2009;70(10):558-. PMID: N/A. *Excluded: wrong publication type.*

Ponizovsky AM, Grinshpoon A, Margolis A, et al. Well-being, psychosocial factors, and side-effects among heroin-dependent inpatients after detoxification using buprenorphine versus clonidine. Addict Behav. 2006;31(11):2002-13. PMID: 16524668. *Excluded: wrong population.*

Portenoy RK, Bruns D, Shoemaker B, et al. Breakthrough pain in community-dwelling patients with cancer pain and noncancer pain, part 2: impact on function, mood, and quality of life. J Opioid Manag. 2010;6(2):109-16. PMID: 20481175. *Excluded: wrong comparator.*

Portenoy RK, Burton AW, Gabrail N, et al. A multicenter, placebo-controlled, double-blind, multiple-crossover study of fentanyl pectin nasal spray (fpsn) in the treatment of breakthrough cancer pain. Pain. 2010;151(3):617-24. PMID: 20800358. *Excluded: wrong study design.*

Portenoy RK, Foley KM. Chronic use of opioid analgesics in non-malignant pain: report of 38 cases. Pain. 1986;25(2):171-86. PMID: 2873550. *Excluded: wrong study design.*

Portenoy RK, Ganae-Motan ED, Allende S, et al. Nabiximols for opioid-treated cancer patients with poorly-controlled chronic pain: a randomized, placebo-controlled, graded-dose trial. J Pain. 2012;13(5):438-49. PMID: 22483680. *Excluded: inadequate duration.*

Portenoy RK, Raffaeli W, Torres LM, et al. Long-term safety, tolerability, and consistency of effect of fentanyl pectin nasal spray for breakthrough cancer pain in opioid-tolerant patients.[Erratum appears in J Opioid Manag. 2011 Jan-Feb;7(1):26], [Erratum appears in J Opioid Manag. 2010 Nov-Dec;6(6):407]. J Opioid Manag. 2010;6(5):319-28. PMID: 21046929. *Excluded: wrong comparator.*

Proctor SL, Estroff TW, Empting LD, et al. Prevalence of substance use and psychiatric disorders in a highly select chronic pain population. J Addict Med. 2013;7(1):17-24. PMID: 23131838. *Excluded: wrong study design.*

Przeklasa-Muszynska A, Dobrogowski J. Transdermal buprenorphine for the treatment of moderate to severe chronic pain: results from a large multicenter, non-interventional post-marketing study in Poland. Curr Med Res Opin. 2011;27(6):1109-17. PMID: 21456888. *Excluded: wrong comparator.*

Pycha C, Resnick RB, Galanter M, et al. Buprenorphine: rapid and slow dose-reductions for heroin detoxification in: NIDA, ed 55th annual scientific meeting, Problems of drug dependence. 1994. p. 453. *Excluded: wrong population.*

Quang-Cantagrel ND, Wallace MS, Magnuson SK. Opioid substitution to improve the effectiveness of chronic noncancer pain control: a chart review. Anesth Analg. 2000;90(4):933-7. PMID: 10735802. *Excluded: inadequate duration.*

Quigley C. Hydromorphone for acute and chronic pain. Cochrane Database Syst Rev. 2002;(1)PMID: 11869661. *Excluded: systematic review or meta-analysis used only as a source document.*

Quigley C. Hydromorphone for acute and chronic pain. Cochrane Database Syst Rev. 2009;(4)PMID: 11869661. *Excluded: systematic review or meta-analysis used only as a source document.*

Quigley C. Opioid switching to improve pain relief and drug tolerability. Cochrane Database Syst Rev. 2010;(11)PMID: 15266542. *Excluded: systematic review or meta-analysis used only as a source document.*

Rabben T, Skjelbred P, Oye I. Prolonged analgesic effect of ketamine, an N-methyl-D-aspartate receptor inhibitor, in patients with chronic pain. J Pharmacol Exp Ther. 1999;289(2):1060-6. PMID: 10215688. *Excluded: wrong intervention.*

Radat F, Creac'h C, Guegan-Massardier E, et al. Behavioral dependence in patients with medication overuse headache: a cross-sectional study in consulting patients using the DSM-IV criteria. Headache. 2008;48(7):1026-36. PMID: 18081820. *Excluded: wrong study design.*

Radner H, Ramiro S, Buchbinder R, et al. Pain management for inflammatory arthritis (rheumatoid arthritis, psoriatic arthritis, ankylosing spondylitis and other spondyloarthritis) and gastrointestinal or liver comorbidity. Cochrane Database Syst Rev. 2012;(1)PMID: 22258995. *Excluded: wrong outcome.*

Raffaeli W, Pari C, Corvetta A, et al. Oxycodone/acetaminophen at low dosage: an alternative pain treatment for patients with rheumatoid arthritis. J Opioid Manag. 2010;6(1):40-6. PMID: 20297613. *Excluded: wrong comparator.*

Raistrick D, West D, Finnegan O, et al. A comparison of buprenorphine and lofexidine for community opiate detoxification: results from a randomized controlled trial. Addiction. 2005;100(12):1860-7. PMID: 16367987. *Excluded: wrong population.*

Raja SN, Haythornthwaite JA, Pappagallo M, et al. Opioids versus antidepressants in postherpetic neuralgia: a randomized, placebo-controlled trial. Neurology. 2002;59(7):1015-21. PMID: 12370455. *Excluded: inadequate duration.*

Rauck R, Deer T, Rosen S, et al. Long-term follow-up of a novel implantable programmable infusion pump. Neuromodulation. 2013;16(2):163-7. PMID: 23057877. *Excluded: inadequate duration.*

Rauck R, Ma T, Kerwin R, et al. Titration with oxymorphone extended release to achieve effective long-term pain relief and improve tolerability in opioid-naive patients with moderate to severe pain. Pain Med. 2008;9(7):777-85. PMID: 18950436. *Excluded: wrong comparator.*

Rauck R, North J, Gever LN, et al. Fentanyl buccal soluble film (fbsf) for breakthrough pain in patients with cancer: a randomized, double-blind, placebo-controlled study. Ann Oncol. 2010;21(6):1308-14. PMID: 19940014. *Excluded: wrong population.*

Rauck R, Rapoport R, Thipphawong J. Results of a double-blind, placebo-controlled, fixed-dose assessment of once-daily OROS® hydromorphone ER in Patients with moderate to severe pain associated with chronic osteoarthritis. Pain Pract. 2013;13(1):18-29. PMID: 22537100. *Excluded: inadequate duration.*

Rauck RL, Bookbinder SA, Bunker TR, et al. A randomized, open-label,multicenter trial comparing once-a-dayAvinza (morphine sulfate extended-release capsules) versus twice-a-day oxy- Contin (oxycodone hydrochloride controlled release tablets) for the treatment of chronic, moderate to severe low back pain: Improved physical functioning in the ACTION trial. J Opioid Manag. 2007;3(1):35-46. PMID: 17367093. *Excluded: inadequate duration.*

Rauck RL, Tark M, Reyes E, et al. Efficacy and long-term tolerability of sublingual fentanyl orally disintegrating tablet in the treatment of breakthrough cancer pain. Curr Med Res Opin 2009;25(12):2877-85. PMID: 19814586. *Excluded: wrong study design.*

Rawool V, Dluhy C. Auditory sensitivity in opiate addicts with and without a history of noise exposure. Noise Health. 2011;13(54):356-63. PMID: 21959116. *Excluded: wrong study design.*

Reguly P, Dubois S, Bédard M. Examining the impact of opioid analgesics on crash responsibility in truck drivers involved in fatal crashes. Forensic Sci Int. 2014;234(0):154-61. PMID: 24378316. *Excluded: wrong population.*

Reid M, Henderson CR, Jr., Papaleontiou M, et al. Characteristics of older adults receiving opioids in primary care: treatment duration and outcomes. Pain Med. 2010;11(7):1063-71. PMID: 20642732. *Excluded: wrong study design.*

Rhodin A, Gronbladh A, Ginya H, et al. Combined analysis of circulating -endorphin with gene polymorphisms in OPRM1, CACNAD2 and ABCB1 reveals correlation with pain, opioid sensitivity and opioid-related side effects. Mol Brain. 2013;6:8. PMID: 23402298. *Excluded: wrong study design.*

Rhodin A, Gronbladh L, Nilsson LH, et al. Methadone treatment of chronic non-malignant pain and opioid dependence--a long-term follow-up. Eur J Pain. 2006;10(3):271-8. PMID: 15972261. *Excluded: wrong study design.*

Rhodin A, Stridsberg M, Gordh T. Opioid endocrinopathy: a clinical problem in patients with chronic pain and long-term oral opioid treatment. Clin J Pain. 2010;26(5):374-80. PMID: 20473043. *Excluded: wrong study design.*

Rice JB, White AG, Birnbaum HG, et al. A model to identify patients at risk for prescription opioid abuse, dependence, and misuse. Pain Med. 2012;13(9):1162-73. PMID: 22845054. *Excluded: wrong study design.*

Richardson LP, Russo JE, Katon W, et al. Mental health disorders and long-term opioid use among adolescents and young adults with chronic pain. J Adolesc Health. 2012;50(6):553-8. PMID: 22626480. *Excluded: wrong study design.*

Richarz U, Waechter S, Sabatowski R, et al. Sustained safety and efficacy of once-daily hydromorphone extended-release (OROS hydromorphone ER) compared with twice-daily oxycodone controlled-release over 52 weeks in patients with moderate to severe chronic noncancer pain. Pain Pract. 2013;13(1):30-40. PMID: 22510252. *Excluded: wrong comparator.*

Riemsma R, Forbes C, Harker J, et al. Systematic review of tapentadol in chronic severe pain. Curr Med Res Opin. 2011;27(10):1907-30. PMID: 21905968. *Excluded: wrong population.*

Riley J, Ross JR, Rutter D, et al. No pain relief from morphine? individual variation in sensitivity to morphine and the need to switch to an alternative opioid in cancer patients. Support Care Cancer. 2006;14(1):56-64. PMID: 15952009. *Excluded: inadequate duration.*

Riley JL, Hastie BA, Glover TL, et al. Cognitive-affective and somatic side effects of morphine and pentazocine: side-effect profiles in healthy adults. Pain Med. 2010;11(2):195-206. PMID: 19671086. *Excluded: wrong intervention.*

Ringe JD, Schafer S, Wimmer AM, et al. Use of OROS hydromorphone in the treatment of osteoarthritis and osteoporosis: a pooled analysis of three non-interventional studies focusing on different starting doses. Wien Klin Wochenschr. 2012;124(1-2):25-31. PMID: 22045112. *Excluded: inadequate duration.*

Ripamonti C, Groff L, Brunelli C, et al. Switching from morphine to oral methadone in treating cancer pain: what is the equianalgesic dose ratio? J Clin Oncol. 1998;16(10):3216-21. PMID: 9779694. *Excluded: wrong study design.*

Robbins L. Long-acting opioids for severe chronic daily headache. Headache Q-curr Trea. 1999;10(2):135-9. PMID: N/A. *Excluded: wrong comparator.*

Robinson RC, Gatchel RJ, Polatin P, et al. Screening for problematic prescription opioid use. Clin J Pain. 2001;17(3):220-8. PMID: 11587112. *Excluded: wrong publication type.*

Robinson-Papp J, Elliott K, Simpson DM, et al. Problematic prescription opioid use in an HIV-infected cohort: the importance of universal toxicology testing. J Acquir Immune Defic Syndr. 2012;61(2):187-93. PMID: 22820804. *Excluded: wrong study design.*

Rodriguez M, Barutell C, Rull M, et al. Efficacy and tolerance of oral dipyrone versus oral morphine for cancer pain. Eur J Cancer. 1994;30A(5):584-7. PMID: 8080670. *Excluded: inadequate duration.*

Rodriguez RF, Castillo JM, Castillo MP, et al. Hydrocodone/acetaminophen and tramadol chlorhydrate combination tablets for the management of chronic cancer pain: a double-blind comparative trial.[Erratum appears in Clin J Pain. 2008 Sep;24(7):649]. Clin J Pain. 2008;24(1):1-4. PMID: 18180628. *Excluded: inadequate duration.*

Rodriguez RF, Castillo JM, Castillo MP, et al. "Hydrocodone/acetaminophen and tramadol chlorhydrate combination tablets for the management of chronic cancer pain: a double-blind comparative trial": Correction. Clin J Pain. 2008;24(7):649. PMID: 18180628. *Excluded: wrong population.*

Rodriguez RF, Castillo JM, del Pilar Castillo M, et al. Codeine/acetaminophen and hydrocodone/acetaminophen combination tablets for the management of chronic cancer pain in adults: a 23-day, prospective, double-blind, randomized, parallel-group study. Clin Ther. 2007;29(4):581-7. PMID: 17617281. *Excluded: inadequate duration.*

Roelofs PD, Deyo RA, Koes BW, et al. Nonsteroidal anti-inflammatory drugs for low back pain: an updated Cochrane review. Spine. 2008;33(16):1766-74. PMID: 18580547. *Excluded: systematic review or meta-analysis used only as a source document.*

Roland CL, Setnik B, Cleveland JM, et al. Clinical outcomes during opioid titration following initiation with or conversion to Remoxy(R), an extended-release formulation of oxycodone. Postgrad Med. 2011;123(4):148-59. PMID: 21680999. *Excluded: wrong study design.*

Rosenblum A, Cruciani RA, Strain EC, et al. Sublingual buprenorphine/naloxone for chronic pain in at-risk patients: development and pilot test of a clinical protocol. J Opioid Manag. 2012;8(6):369-82. PMID: 23264315. *Excluded: wrong study design.*

Rosenthal M, Moore P, Groves E, et al. Sleep improves when patients with chronic OA pain are managed with morning dosing of once a day extended-release morphine sulfate (AVINZA): findings from a pilot study. J Opioid Manag. 2007;3(3):145-54. PMID: 18027540. *Excluded: wrong comparator.*

Rosti G, Gatti A, Costantini A, et al. Opioid-related bowel dysfunction: prevalence and identification of predictive factors in a large sample of Italian patients on chronic treatment. Eur Rev Med Pharmacol Sci 2010;14(12):1045-50. PMID: 21375137. *Excluded: wrong comparator.*

Roth SH, Fleischmann RM, Burch FX, et al. Around-the-clock, controlled-release oxycodone therapy for osteoarthritis-related pain: placebo-controlled trial and long-term evaluation. Arch Intern Med. 2000;160(6):853-60. PMID: 10737286. *Excluded: inadequate duration.*

Rowbotham MC, Reisner-Keller LA, Fields HL. Both intravenous lidocaine and morphine reduce the pain of postherpetic neuralgia. Neurology. 1991;41(7):1024-8. PMID: 1712433. *Excluded: inadequate duration.*

Rowbotham MC, Twilling L, Davies PS, et al. Oral opioid therapy for chronic peripheral and central neuropathic pain. N Engl J Med. 2003;348(13):1223-32. PMID: 12660386. *Excluded: inadequate duration.*

Rubinstein AL, Carpenter DM, Minkoff JR. Hypogonadism in men with chronic pain linked to the use of long-acting rather than short-acting opioids. Clin J Pain. 2013; 29(10): 840-5. PMID: 2012423819. *Excluded: wrong comparator*

Ruoff GE, Rosenthal N, Jordan D, et al. Tramadol/acetaminophen combination tablets for the treatment of chronic lower back pain: a multicenter, randomized, double-blind, placebo-controlled outpatient study. Clin Ther. 2003;25(4):1123-41. PMID: 12809961. *Excluded: inadequate duration.*

Saadat H, Ziai SA, Ghanemnia M, et al. Opium addiction increases interleukin 1 receptor antagonist (IL-1Ra) in the coronary artery disease patients. PLoS ONE. 2012;7(9):e44939. PMID: 23028694. *Excluded: wrong population.*

Saarialho-Kere U, Julkunen H, Mattila MJ, et al. Psychomotor performance of patients with rheumatoid arthritis: cross-over comparison of dextropropoxyphene, dextropropoxyphene plus amitriptyline, indomethacin, and placebo. Pharmacol Toxicol. 1988;63(4):286-92. PMID: 3057482. *Excluded: wrong intervention.*

Sabatowski R, Schwalen S, Rettig K, et al. Driving ability under long-term treatment with transdermal fentanyl. J Pain Symptom Manage. 2003;25(1):38-47. PMID: 12565187. *Excluded: inadequate duration.*

Sacchetti G, Camera P, Rossi AP, et al. Injectable ketoprofen vs. acetylsalicylic acid for the relief of severe cancer pain: a double-blind, crossover trial. Drug Intell Clin Pharm. 1984;18(5):403-6. PMID: 6373214. *Excluded: wrong intervention.*

Salengros JC, Huybrechts I, Ducart A, et al. Different anesthetic techniques associated with different incidences of chronic post-thoracotomy pain: low-dose remifentanil plus presurgical epidural analgesia is preferable to high-dose remifentanil with postsurgical epidural analgesia. J Cardiothorac Vasc Anesth. 2010;24(4):608-16. PMID: 20005744. *Excluded: wrong intervention.*

Sanders JC, Gerstein N, Torgeson E, et al. Intrathecal baclofen for postoperative analgesia after total knee arthroplasty. J Clin Anesth. 2009;21(7):486-92. PMID: 20006256. *Excluded: wrong intervention.*

Sandner-Kiesling A, Leyendecker P, Hopp M, et al. Long-term efficacy and safety of combined prolonged-release oxycodone and naloxone in the management of non-cancer chronic pain. Int J Clin Pract. 2010;64(6):763-74. PMID: 20370845. *Excluded: wrong comparator.*

Santiago-Palma J, Khojainova N, Kornick C, et al. Intravenous methadone in the management of chronic cancer pain: safe and effective starting doses when substituting methadone for fentanyl. Cancer. 2001;92(7):1919-25. PMID: 11745266. *Excluded: wrong comparator.*

Saper JR, Lake AE, 3rd, Bain PA, et al. A practice guide for continuous opioid therapy for refractory daily headache: patient selection, physician requirements, and treatment monitoring. Headache. 2010;50(7):1175-93. PMID: 20649650. *Excluded: wrong publication type.*

Sator-Katzenschlager SM, Schiesser AW, Kozek-Langenecker SA, et al. Does pain relief improve pain behavior and mood in chronic pain patients? Anesth Analg. 2003;97(3):791-7. PMID: 12933404. *Excluded: wrong comparator.*

Saunders KW, Von Korff M, Campbell CI, et al. Concurrent use of alcohol and sedatives among persons prescribed chronic opioid therapy: prevalence and risk factors. J Pain. 2012;13(3):266-75. PMID: 22285611. *Excluded: wrong study design.*

Sawe J, Hansen J, Ginman C, et al. Patient-controlled dose regimen of methadone for chronic cancer pain. Br Med J. 1981;282(6266):771-3. PMID: 6163497. *Excluded: inadequate duration.*

Saxon AJ, Wells EA, Fleming C, et al. Pre-treatment characteristics, program philosophy and level of ancillary services as predictors of methadone maintenance treatment outcome. Addiction. 1996;91(8):1197-209. PMID: 8828247. *Excluded: wrong population.*

Saxon AJ, Ling W, Hillhouse M, et al. Buprenorphine/naloxone and methadone effects on laboratory indices of liver health: A randomized trial. Drug Alcohol Depend. 2013; 128(1-2): 71-6. PMID: 22921476. *Excluded: wrong population*

Schackman BR, Leff JA, Polsky D, et al. Cost-effectiveness of long-term outpatient buprenorphine-naloxone treatment for opioid dependence in primary care. J Gen Intern Med. 2012;27(6):669-76. PMID: 22215271. *Excluded: wrong study design.*

Schein JR, Kosinski MR, Janagap-Benson C, et al. Functionality and health-status benefits associated with reduction of osteoarthritis pain. Curr Med Res Opin 2008;24(5):1255-65. PMID: 18358082. *Excluded: wrong intervention.*

Scher A, Lipton R, Stewart W, et al. Patterns of medication use by chronic and episodic headache sufferers in the general population: Results from the frequent headache epidemiology study. Cephalalgia. 2010;30(3):321-8. PMID: 19614708. *Excluded: wrong outcome.*

Scherbaum N, Specka M. Factors influencing the course of opiate addiction. Int J Methods Psychiatr Res 2008;17 Suppl 1:S39-44. PMID: 18543361. *Excluded: wrong population.*

Schmader K. Treatment and prevention strategies for herpes zoster and postherpetic neuralgia in older adults. Clin Geriatr. 2006;14(1):26-33. PMID: N/A. *Excluded: wrong publication type.*

Schmittner J, Schroeder JR, Epstein DH, et al. Electrocardiographic effects of lofexidine and methadone coadministration: secondary findings from a safety study. Pharmacotherapy. 2009;29(5):495-502. PMID: 19397459. *Excluded: wrong population.*

Schneider U, Paetzold W, Eronat V, et al. Buprenorphine and carbamazepine as a treatment for detoxification of opiate addicts with multiple drug misuse: a pilot study. Addiction Biology. 2000;5(1):65-9. PMID: 20575820. *Excluded: wrong population.*

Schnitzer TJ, Gray WL, Paster RZ, et al. Efficacy of tramadol in treatment of chronic low back pain. J Rheumatol. 2000;27(3):772-8. PMID: 10743823. *Excluded: wrong intervention.*

Schoedel KA, McMorn S, Chakraborty B, et al. Positive and negative subjective effects of extended-release oxymorphone versus controlled-release oxycodone in recreational opioid users. J Opioid Manag. 2011;7(3):179-92. PMID: 21823549. *Excluded: wrong population.*

Scholes CF, Gonty N, Trotman IF. Methadone titration in opioid-resistant cancer pain. Eur J Cancer Care (Engl). 1999;8(1):26-9. PMID: 10362950. *Excluded: wrong study design.*

Schottenfeld RS, Chawarski MC, Pakes JR, et al. Methadone versus buprenorphine with contingency management or performance feedback for cocaine and opioid dependence. Am J Psychiatry. 2005;162(2):340-9. PMID: 15677600. *Excluded: wrong population.*

Schottenfeld RS, Pakes JR, Kosten TR. Prognostic factors in buprenorphine- versus methadone-maintained patients. J Nerv Ment Dis. 1998;186(1):35-43. PMID: 9457145. *Excluded: wrong population.*

Schutter U, Grunert S, Meyer C, et al. Innovative pain therapy with a fixed combination of prolonged-release oxycodone/naloxone: a large observational study under conditions of daily practice. Curr Med Res Opin. 2010;26(6):1377-87. PMID: 20380506. *Excluded: wrong population.*

Schwartz RP, Kelly SM, O'Grady KE, et al. Antecedents and correlates of methadone treatment entry: a comparison of out-of-treatment and in-treatment cohorts. Drug Alcohol Depend. 2011;115(1-2):23-9. PMID: 21126830. *Excluded: wrong population.*

Schwittay A, Schumann C, Litzenburger BC, et al. Tapentadol Prolonged Release for Severe Chronic Pain: Results of a Noninterventional study involving general practitioners and internists. J Pain Palliat Care Pharmacother. 2013;27(3):225-34. PMID: 23957433. *Excluded: wrong comparator.*

Seal K, Krebs E, Neylan T. "Posttraumatic stress disorder and opioid use among US veterans": In reply. JAMA. 2012;307(23):2485-6. PMID: 22797438. *Excluded: wrong publication type.*

Seal KH, Shi Y, Cohen G, et al. Association of mental health disorders with prescription opioids and high-risk opioid use in US veterans of Iraq and Afghanistan.[Erratum appears in JAMA. 2012 Jun 20;307(23):2489]. JAMA. 2012;307(9):940-7. PMID: 22396516. *Excluded: wrong study design.*

Seidel S, Aigner M, Ossege M, et al. Antipsychotics for acute and chronic pain in adults. Cochrane Database Syst Rev. 2008;(4):CD004844. PMID: 18843669. *Excluded: wrong intervention.*

Seifert J, Metzner C, Paetzold W, et al. Mood and affect during detoxification of opiate addicts: a comparison of buprenorphine versus methadone. Addict Biol. 2005;10(2):157-64. PMID: 16191668. *Excluded: wrong population.*

Seifert J, Metzner C, Paetzold W, et al. Detoxification of opiate addicts with multiple drug abuse: a comparison of buprenorphine vs. methadone. Pharmacopsychiatry. 2002;35(5):159-64. PMID: 12237786. *Excluded: wrong population.*

Sekhon R, Aminjavahery N, Davis CN, Jr., et al. Compliance with opioid treatment guidelines for chronic non-cancer pain (CNCP) in primary care at a Veterans Affairs Medical Center (VAMC). Pain Med. 2013;14(10):1548-56. PMID: 23746149. *Excluded: wrong population.*

Senay EC, Barthwell A, Marks R, et al. Medical maintenance: an interim report. J Addict Dis. 1994;13(3):65-9. PMID: 7734460. *Excluded: wrong population.*

Setnik B, Roland CL, Cleveland JM, et al. The abuse potential of remoxy((r)), an extended-release formulation of oxycodone, compared with immediate- and extended-release oxycodone. Pain Med. 2011;12(4):618-31. PMID: 21463474. *Excluded: wrong population.*

Shapiro BJ, Lynch KL, Toochinda T, et al. Promethazine misuse among methadone maintenance patients and community-based injection drug users. J Addict Med.

2013;7(2):96-101. PMID: 23385449. *Excluded: wrong population.*

Shapiro D, Buynak R, Okamoto A, et al. Results of a randomized, double-blind, placebo- and active-controlled trial of tapentadol extended release for chronic low back pain. Rheumatology Conference Proceedings. 2010. British Society for Rheumatology, BSR and British Health Professionals in Rheumatology, BHPR Annual Meeting 2010, Birmingham United Kingdom.. Conference Publication: i78-9. PMID: N/A. *Excluded: inadequate duration.*

Sharek PJ, McClead RE, Jr., Taketomo C, et al. An intervention to decrease narcotic-related adverse drug events in children's hospitals. Pediatrics. 2008;122(4):e861-6. PMID: 18829784. *Excluded: wrong population.*

Sharkey KM, Kurth ME, Corso RP, et al. Home polysomnography in methadone maintenance patients with subjective sleep complaints. Am J Drug Alcohol Abuse. 2009;35(3):178-82. PMID: 19462301. *Excluded: wrong population.*

Sheard L, Wright NM, El-Sayeh HG, et al. The leeds evaluation of efficacy of detoxification Study (LEEDS) prisons project: a randomised controlled trial comparing dihydrocodeine and buprenorphine for opiate detoxification. Subst Abuse Treat Prev Policy. 2009;4(1). PMID: 19196468. *Excluded: wrong population.*

Shi L, Liu J, Zhao Y. Comparative effectiveness in pain-related outcomes and health care utilizations between veterans with major depressive disorder treated with duloxetine and other antidepressants: a retrospective propensity score-matched comparison. Pain Pract. 2012;12(5):374-81. PMID: 21951787. *Excluded: wrong intervention.*

Shorr RI, Griffin MR, Daugherty JR, et al. Opioid analgesics and the risk of hip fracture in the elderly: codeine and propoxyphene. J Gerontol. 1992;47(4):M111-5. PMID: 1624693. *Excluded: wrong population.*

Shram MJ, Sathyan G, Khanna S, et al. Evaluation of the abuse potential of extended release hydromorphone versus immediate release hydromorphone. J Clin Psychopharmacol. 2010;30(1):25-33. PMID: 20075644. *Excluded: inadequate duration.*

Sia AT, Sng BL, Lim EC, et al. The influence of ATP-binding cassette sub-family B member -1 (ABCB1) genetic polymorphisms on acute and chronic pain after intrathecal morphine for caesarean section: a prospective cohort study. Int J Obstet Anesth. 2010;19(3):254-60. PMID: 20627697. *Excluded: wrong intervention.*

Siddall PJ, Gray M, Rutkowski S, et al. Intrathecal morphine and clonidine in the management of spinal cord injury pain: A case report. Pain. 1994;59(1):147-8. PMID: 7854795. *Excluded: wrong study design.*

Singh K, Phillips FM, Kuo E, et al. A prospective, randomized, double-blind study of the efficacy of postoperative continuous local anesthetic infusion at the iliac crest bone graft site after posterior spinal arthrodesis: a minimum of 4-year follow-up. Spine. 2007;32(25):2790-6. PMID: 18245999. *Excluded: wrong intervention.*

Sittl R, Griessinger N, Likar R. Analgesic efficacy and tolerability of transdermal buprenorphine in patients with inadequately controlled chronic pain related to cancer and other disorders: a multicenter, randomized, double-blind, placebo-controlled trial. Clin Ther. 2003;25(1):150-68. PMID: 12637117. *Excluded: inadequate duration.*

Sjogren P, Banning A. Pain, sedation and reaction time during long-term treatment of cancer patients with oral and epidural opioids. Pain. 1989;39(1):5-11. PMID: 2812854. *Excluded: wrong population.*

Sjogren P, Banning AM, Christensen CB, et al. Continuous reaction time after single dose, long-term oral and epidural opioid administration. Eur J Anaesthesiol. 1994;11(2):95-100. PMID: 8174541. *Excluded: inadequate duration.*

Sjogren P, Christrup LL, Petersen MA, et al. Neuropsychological assessment of chronic non-malignant pain patients treated in a multidisciplinary pain centre. Eur J Pain. 2005;9(4):453-62. PMID: 15979026. *Excluded: inadequate duration.*

Sjogren P, Gronbaek M, Peuckmann V, et al. A population-based cohort study on chronic pain: the role of opioids. Clin J Pain. 2010;26(9):763-9. PMID: 20842015. *Excluded: wrong outcome.*

Sjogren P, Thomsen AB, Olsen AK. Impaired neuropsychological performance in chronic nonmalignant pain patients receiving long-term oral opioid therapy. J Pain Symptom Manage. 2000;19(2):100-8. PMID: 10699537. *Excluded: wrong study design.*

Skinner MA, Lewis ET, Trafton JA. Opioid use patterns and association with pain severity and mental health functioning in chronic pain patients. Pain Med. 2012;13(4):507-17. PMID: 22497724. *Excluded: wrong outcome.*

Skurtveit S, Furu K, Borchgrevink P, et al. To what extent does a cohort of new users of weak opioids develop persistent or probable problematic opioid use? Pain. 2011;152(7):1555-61. PMID: 21450405. *Excluded: wrong population.*

Skurtveit S, Furu K, Bramness J, et al. Benzodiazepines predict use of opioids--a follow-up study of 17,074 men and women. Pain Med. 2010;11(6):805-14. PMID: 20624237. *Excluded: wrong outcome.*

Skurtveit S, Furu K, Kaasa S, et al. Introduction of low dose transdermal buprenorphine - did it influence use of potentially addictive drugs in chronic non-malignant pain patients? Eur J Pain. 2009;13(9):949-53. PMID: 19095476. *Excluded: wrong study design.*

Slatkin NE. Opioid switching and rotation in primary care: implementation and clinical utility. Curr Med Res Opin. 2009;25(9):2133-50. PMID: 19601703. *Excluded: wrong publication type.*

Sloan PA, Barkin RL. Oxymorphone and oxymorphone extended release: a pharmacotherapeutic review. J Opioid Manag. 2008;4(3):131-44. PMID: 18717508. *Excluded: wrong publication type.*

Sloots CE, Rykx A, Cools M, et al. Efficacy and safety of prucalopride in patients with chronic noncancer pain suffering from opioid-induced constipation. Dig Dis Sci. 2010;55(10):2912-21. PMID: 20428949. *Excluded: wrong intervention.*

Smith H. A comprehensive review of rapid-onset opioids for breakthrough pain. CNS Drugs. 2012;26(6):509-35. PMID: 22668247. *Excluded: systematic review or meta-analysis used only as a source document.*

Smith H, Bruckenthal P. Implications of opioid analgesia for medically complicated patients. Drugs Aging. 2010;27(5):417-33. PMID: 20450239. *Excluded: systematic review or meta-analysis used only as a source document.*

Smith HS. Morphine sulfate and naltrexone hydrochloride extended release capsules for the management of chronic, moderate-to-severe pain, while reducing morphine-induced subjective effects upon tampering by crushing. Expert Opin Pharmacother. 2011;12(7):1111-25. PMID: 21470065. *Excluded: wrong publication type.*

Smith HS, Kirsh KL, Passik SD. Chronic opioid therapy issues associated with opioid abuse potential. J Opioid Manag. 2009;5(5):287-300. PMID: 19947070. *Excluded: wrong publication type.*

Smith JB, Ridpath LC, Steele KM. A research protocol to determine if OMM is effective in decreasing pain in chronic paint patients and decreasing opiod use: brief report. AAO Journal. 2012;22(4):38-45. PMID: N/A. *Excluded: wrong publication type.*

Smith K, Hopp M, Mundin G, et al. Single- and multiple-dose pharmacokinetic evaluation of oxycodone and naloxone in an opioid agonist/antagonist prolonged-release combination in healthy adult volunteers. Clin Ther. 2008;30(11):2051-68. PMID: 19108793. *Excluded: wrong population.*

Smith MY, Irish W, Wang J, et al. Detecting signals of opioid analgesic abuse: application of a spatial mixed effect poisson regression model using data from a network of poison control centers. Pharmacoepidemiology & Drug Saf. 2008;17(11):1050-9. PMID: 18803336. *Excluded: wrong population.*

Smith MY, Kleber HD, Katz N, et al. Reducing opioid. analgesic abuse: models for successful collaboration among government, industry and other key stakeholders. Drug Alcohol Depend. 2008;95(1-2):177-81. PMID: 18484109. *Excluded: wrong publication type.*

Smith-Spangler CM, Asch SM. Commentary on Vickerman etal. (2012): Reducing hepatitis C virus among injection drug users through harm reduction programs. Addiction. 2012;107(11):1996-7. PMID: 23039752. *Excluded: wrong publication type.*

Smyth BP, Barry J, Keenan E, et al. Lapse and relapse following inpatient treatment of opiate dependence. Ir Med J. 2010;103(6):176-9. PMID: 20669601. *Excluded: wrong population.*

Snyder ML, Jarolim P, Melanson SEF. A new automated urine fentanyl immunoassay: technical performance and clinical utility for monitoring fentanyl compliance. Clin Chim Acta. 2011;412(11-12):946-51. PMID: 21281622. *Excluded: wrong outcome.*

Soderberg KC, Laflamme L, Moller J. Newly initiated opioid treatment and the risk of fall-related injuries. A nationwide, register-based, case-crossover study in Sweden. CNS Drugs. 2013;27(2):155-61. PMID: 23345030. *Excluded: wrong population.*

Soin A, Cheng J, Brown L, et al. Functional outcomes in patients with chronic nonmalignant pain on long-term opioid therapy. Pain Pract. 2008;8(5):379-84. PMID: 18844854. *Excluded: wrong study design.*

Solomon DH, Rassen JA, Glynn RJ, et al. The comparative safety of opioids for nonmalignant pain in older adults. Arch Intern Med. 2010;170(22):1979-86. PMID: 21149754. *Excluded: wrong population.*

Solomon DH, Rassen JA, Glynn RJ, et al. The comparative safety of analgesics in older adults with arthritis. Arch Intern Med. 2010;170(22):1968-76. PMID: 21149752. *Excluded: wrong population.*

Somerville S, Hay E, Lewis M, et al. Content and outcome of usual primary care for back pain: a systematic review. Br J Gen Pract. 2008;58(556):790-7, i-vi. PMID: 19000402. *Excluded: wrong intervention.*

Sorge J, Sittl R. Transdermal buprenorphine in the treatment of chronic pain: results of a phase III, multicenter, randomized, double-blind, placebo-controlled study. Clin Ther. 2004;26(11):1808-20. PMID: 15639693. *Excluded: inadequate duration.*

Soyka M. Buprenorphine and buprenorphine/naloxone soluble-film for treatment of opioid dependence. Expert Opin Drug Deliv. 2012;9(11):1409-17. PMID: 23013384. *Excluded: wrong intervention.*

Spano MS, Fadda P, Fratta W, et al. Cannabinoid-opioid interactions in drug discrimination and self-administration:

effect of maternal, postnatal, adolescent and adult exposure to the drugs. Curr Drug Targets. 2010;11(4):450-61. PMID: 20017729. *Excluded: wrong study design.*

Spector W, Shaffer T, Potter DE, et al. Risk factors associated with the occurrence of fractures in U.S. nursing homes: resident and facility characteristics and prescription medications. J Am Geriatr Soc. 2007;55(3):327-33. PMID: 17341233. *Excluded: wrong population.*

Spitz A, Moore AA, Papaleontiou M, et al. Primary care providers' perspective on prescribing opioids to older adults with chronic non-cancer pain: a qualitative study. BMC Geriatr. 2011;11:35. PMID: 21752299. *Excluded: wrong study design.*

Spoth R, Trudeau L, Shin C, et al. Longitudinal effects of universal preventive intervention on prescription drug misuse: three randomized controlled trials with late adolescents and young adults. Am J Public Health. 2013;103(4):665-72. PMID: 23409883. *Excluded: wrong population.*

Srivastava A, Kahan M, Jiwa A. Prescription opioid use and misuse: piloting an educational strategy for rural primary care physicians. Can Fam Physician. 2012;58(4):e210-6. PMID: 22611608. *Excluded: wrong study design.*

Stallvik M, Nordstrand B, Kristensen O, et al. Corrected qt interval during treatment with methadone and buprenorphine--relation to doses and serum concentrations. Drug Alcohol Depend. 2013;129(1-2):88-93. PMID: 23084592. *Excluded: wrong population.*

Stambaugh J, Drew J. A double-blind parallel evaluation of the efficacy and safety of a single dose of ketoprofen in cancer Pain. J Clin Pharmacol. 1988;28:S34-S9. PMID: 3072356. *Excluded: wrong intervention.*

Stambaugh JE, Jr. . Additive analgesia of oral butorphanol/acetaminophen in patients with pain due to metastaticcarcinoma. Curr Ther Res. 1982;31(3):386-92. PMID: N/A. *Excluded: wrong population.*

Stambaugh JE, Jr., Drew J. The combination of ibuprofen and oxycodone/acetaminophen in the management of chronic cancer pain. Clin Pharmacol Ther. 1988;44(6):665-9. PMID: 2461823. *Excluded: inadequate duration.*

Stanos S. Evolution of opioid risk management and review of the classwide REMS for extended-release/long-acting opioids. Phys Sportsmed. 2012;40(4):12-20. PMID: 23306411. *Excluded: wrong publication type.*

Stanos S. Continuing evolution of opioid use in primary care practice: implications of emerging technologies. Curr Med Res Opin. 2012;28(9):1505-16. PMID: 22937723. *Excluded: wrong publication type.*

Stanos SP, Bruckenthal P, Barkin RL. Strategies to reduce the tampering and subsequent abuse of long-acting opioids: potential risks and benefits of formulations with physical or pharmacologic deterrents to tampering. Mayo Clin Proc. 2012;87(7):683-94. PMID: 22766088. *Excluded: wrong publication type.*

Staquet M, Renaud A. Double-blind, randomized trial of piroxicam and codeine in cancer pain. Curr Ther Res Clin Exp 1993;53(4):435-40. PMID: N/A. *Excluded: inadequate duration.*

Staquet MJ. A double-blind study with placebo control of intramuscular ketorolac tromethamine in the treatment of cancer pain. J Clin Pharmacol. 1989;29(11):1031-6. PMID: 2689472. *Excluded: wrong intervention.*

Starrels JL, Becker WC, Alford DP, et al. Systematic review: treatment agreements and urine drug testing to reduce opioid misuse in patients with chronic pain. Ann Intern Med. 2010;152:712-20. PMID: 20513829. *Excluded: systematic review or meta-analysis used only as a source document.*

Starrels JL, Becker WC, Weiner MG, et al. Low use of opioid risk reduction strategies in primary care even for high risk patients with chronic pain. . J Gen Intern Med. 2011;26(9):958-64. PMID: 21347877. *Excluded: inadequate duration.*

Staud R. Pharmacological treatment of fibromyalgia syndrome: new developments. Drugs. 2010;70(1):1-14. PMID: 20030422. *Excluded: wrong publication type.*

Stauffer J, Setnik B, Sokolowska M, et al. Subjective effects and safety of whole and tampered morphine sulfate and naltrexone hydrochloride (ALO-01) extended-release capsules versus morphine solution and placebo in experienced non-dependent opioid users: a randomized, double-blind, placebo-controlled, crossover study. Clin Drug Investig. 2009;29(12):777-90. PMID: 19888784. *Excluded: inadequate duration.*

Stefaniak T, Vingerhoets A, Makarewicz W, et al. Opioid use determines success of videothoracoscopic splanchnicectomy in chronic pancreatic pain patients. Langenbecks Arch Surg. 2008;393(2):213-8. PMID: 17436011. *Excluded: wrong study design.*

Steigerwald I, Schenk M, Lahne U, et al. Effectiveness and tolerability of tapentadol prolonged release compared with prior opioid therapy for the management of severe, chronic osteoarthritis pain. Clin Drug Invest. 2013; 33(9): 607-19. PMID: 23912473. *Excluded: inadequate duration*

Stein C, Reinecke H, Sorgatz H. Opioid use in chronic noncancer pain: guidelines revisited. Curr Opin Anaesthesiol. 2010;23(5):598-601. PMID: 20585244. *Excluded: wrong publication type.*

Steiner D, Munera C, Hale M, et al. Efficacy and safety of buprenorphine transdermal system (BTDS) for chronic moderate to severe low back pain: a randomized, double-blind study. J Pain. 2011;12(11):1163-73. PMID: 21807566. *Excluded: inadequate duration.*

Steiner DJ, Sitar S, Wen W, et al. Efficacy and safety of the seven-day buprenorphine transdermal system in opioid-naive patients with moderate to severe chronic low back pain: An enriched, randomized, double-blind, placebo-controlled study. J Pain Symptom Manage. 2011;42(6):903-17. PMID: 21945130. *Excluded: inadequate duration.*

Stepanovic A, Pirc J, Lahajnar Cavlovic S. Clinical efficacy of OROS hydromorphone in patients suffering from severe chronic pain: a study undertaken in routine clinical practice. Wien Klin Wochenschr. 2011;123(17-18):531-5. PMID: 21710117. *Excluded: wrong comparator.*

Strand MC, Fjeld B, Arnestad M, et al. Can patients receiving opioid maintenance therapy safely drive? a systematic review of epidemiological and experimental studies on driving ability with a focus on concomitant methadone or buprenorphine administration. Traffic Inj Prev. 2013;14(1):26-38. PMID: 23259516. *Excluded: systematic review or meta-analysis used only as a source document.*

Sullivan MD, Edlund MJ, Fan M-Y, et al. Risks for possible and probable opioid misuse among recipients of chronic opioid therapy in commercial and medicaid insurance plans: the TROUP Study. Pain. 2010;150(2):332-9. PMID: 20554392. *Excluded: wrong population.*

Sunshine A, Olson NZ. Analgesic efficacy of ketoprofen in postpartum, general surgery, and chronic cancer pain. J Clin Pharmacol. 1988;28(12 Suppl):S47-54. PMID: 3072358. *Excluded: inadequate duration.*

Takkouche B, Montes-Martinez A, Gill SS, et al. Psychotropic medications and the risk of fracture: a meta-analysis. Drug Saf. 2007;30(2):171-84. PMID: 17253881. *Excluded: wrong population.*

Tassain V, Attal N, Fletcher D, et al. Long term effects of oral sustained release morphine on neuropsychological performance in patients with chronic non-cancer pain. Pain. 2003;104(1-2):389-400. PMID: 12855350. *Excluded: wrong study design.*

Taylor D, Galan V, Weinstein SM, et al. Fentanyl pectin nasal spray in breakthrough cancer pain. J Support Oncol. 2010;8(4):184-90. PMID: 20822038. *Excluded: wrong population.*

Taylor R, Pergolizzi JV, Raffa RB. Tapentadol extended release for chronic pain patients. Adv Ther. 2013;30(1):14-27. PMID: 23328938. *Excluded: systematic review or meta-analysis used only as a source document.*

Toscani F, Piva L, Corli O, et al. Ketorolac versus diclofenac sodium in cancer pain. Arzneimittelforschung. 1994;44(4):550-4. PMID: 8011010. *Excluded: wrong intervention.*

Tse DM, Sham MM, Ng DK, et al. An ad libitum schedule for conversion of morphine to methadone in advanced cancer patients: an open uncontrolled prospective study in a Chinese population. Palliat Med. 2003;17(2):206-11. PMID: 12701853. *Excluded: wrong population.*

Turnbull R, Hills LJ. Naproxen versus aspirin as analgesics in advanced malignant disease. J Palliat Care. 1986;1(2):25-8. PMID: 3450812. *Excluded: wrong intervention.*

Uberall MA, Mueller-Schwefe GH, Terhaag B. Efficacy and safety of flupirtine modified release for the management of moderate to severe chronic low back pain: results of SUPREME, a prospective randomized, double-blind, placebo- and active-controlled parallel-group phase IV study. Curr Med Res Opin. 2012;28(10):1617-34. PMID: 22970658. *Excluded: inadequate duration.*

Umbricht A, Hoover DR, Tucker MJ, et al. Opioid detoxification with buprenorphine, clonidine, or methadone in hospitalized heroin-dependent patients with HIV infection. Drug Alcohol Depend. 2003;69(3):263-72. PMID: 12633912. *Excluded: wrong population.*

Vaglienti RM, Huber SJ, Noel KR, et al. Misuse of prescribed controlled substances defined by urinalysis. W V Med J. 2003;99(2):67-70. PMID: 12874916. *Excluded: wrong population.*

Vainio A, Ollila J, Matikainen E, et al. Driving ability in cancer patients receiving long-term morphine analgesia. Lancet. 1995;346(8976):667-70. PMID: 7658820. *Excluded: wrong population.*

Ventafridda V, De Conno F, Panerai AE, et al. Non-steroidal anti-inflammatory drugs as the first step in cancer pain therapy: double-blind, within-patient study comparing nine drugs. J Int Med Res1990;18(1):21-9. PMID: 2185963. *Excluded: wrong intervention.*

Ventafridda V, Martino G, Mandelli V, et al. Indoprofen, a new analgesic and anti-inflammatory drug in cancer pain. Clin Pharmacol Ther. 1975;17(3):284-9. PMID: 47281. *Excluded: inadequate duration.*

Ventafridda V, Toscani F, Tamburini M, et al. Sodium naproxen versus sodium diclofenac in cancer pain control. Arzneimittelforschung. 1990;40(10):1132-4. PMID: 2291751. *Excluded: wrong intervention.*

Vestergaard P, Hermann P, Jensen JEB, et al. Effects of paracetamol, non-steroidal anti-inflammatory drugs, acetylsalicylic acid, and opioids on bone mineral density and risk of fracture: results of the Danish osteoporosis prevention study (DOPS). Osteoporos Int. 2012;23(4):1255-65. PMID: 21710339. *Excluded: wrong study design.*

Vestergaard P, Rejnmark L, Mosekilde L. Fracture risk associated with the use of morphine and opiates. J Intern Med. 2006;260(1):76-87. PMID: 16789982. *Excluded: wrong population.*

Von Korff M, Merrill JO, Rutter CM, et al. Time-scheduled vs. pain-contingent opioid dosing in chronic opioid therapy. Pain. 2011;152(6):1256-62. PMID: 21296498. *Excluded: wrong comparator.*

Von Korff MR. Long-term use of opioids for complex chronic pain. Best Pract Res Clin Rheumatol. 2013;27(5):663-72. PMID: 24315147. *Excluded: wrong publication type.*

Vondrackova D, Leyendecker P, Meissner W, et al. Analgesic efficacy and safety of oxycodone in combination with naloxone as prolonged release tablets in patients with moderate to severe chronic pain. J Pain. 2008;9(12):1144-54. PMID: 18708300. *Excluded: inadequate duration.*

Wallace M, Rauck RL, Moulin D, et al. Conversion from standard opioid therapy to once-daily oral extended-release hydromorphone in patients with chronic cancer pain. J Int Med Res2008;36(2):343-52. PMID: 18380946. *Excluded: inadequate duration.*

Wallace M, Thipphawong J. Open-label study on the long-term efficacy, safety, and impact on quality of life of OROS hydromorphone er in patients with chronic low back pain. Pain Med. 2010;11(10):1477-88. PMID: 21199302. *Excluded: wrong study design.*

Wallace MS, Charapata SG, Fisher R, et al. Intrathecal ziconotide in the treatment of chronic nonmalignant pain: A randomized, double-blind, placebo-controlled clinical trial. Neuromodulation. 2006;9(2):75-86. PMID: 22151630. *Excluded: wrong intervention.*

Wallace MS, Moulin D, Clark AJ, et al. A Phase II, multicenter, randomized, double-blind, placebo-controlled crossover study of CJC-1008--a long-acting, parenteral opioid analgesic--in the treatment of postherpetic neuralgia. J Opioid Manag. 2006;2(3):167-73. PMID: 17319450. *Excluded: inadequate duration.*

Wang H, Akbar M, Weinsheimer N, et al. Longitudinal observation of changes in pain sensitivity during opioid tapering in patients with chronic low-back pain. Pain Med. 2011;12(12):1720-6. PMID: 22082225. *Excluded: wrong population.*

Wasan AD, Ross EL, Michna E, et al. Craving of prescription opioids in patients with chronic pain: a longitudinal outcomes trial. J Pain. 2012;13(2):146-54. PMID: 22245713. *Excluded: wrong outcome.*

Watson CP, Babul N. Efficacy of oxycodone in neuropathic pain: a randomized trial in postherpetic neuralgia. Neurology. 1998;50(6):1837-41. PMID: 9633737. *Excluded: inadequate duration.*

Watson CP, Moulin D, Watt-Watson J, et al. Controlled-release oxycodone relieves neuropathic pain: a randomized controlled trial in painful diabetic neuropathy. Pain. 2003;105(1-2):71-8. PMID: 14499422. *Excluded: inadequate duration.*

Webster LR, Brewer R, Wang C, et al. Long-term safety and efficacy of morphine sulfate and naltrexone hydrochloride extended release capsules, a novel formulation containing morphine and sequestered naltrexone, in patients with chronic, moderate to severe pain. J Pain Symptom Manage. 2010;40(5):734-46. PMID: 21075272. *Excluded: wrong study design.*

Webster LR, Butera PG, Moran LV, et al. Oxytrex minimizes physical dependence while providing effective analgesia: a randomized controlled trial in low back pain. J Pain. 2006;7(12):937-46. PMID: 17157780. *Excluded: inadequate duration.*

Webster LR, Fine PG. Review and critique of opioid rotation practices and associated risks of toxicity. Pain Med. 2012;13(4):562-70. PMID: 22458884. *Excluded: systematic review or meta-analysis used only as a source document.*

Weingart WA, Sorkness CA, Earhart RH. Analgesia with oral narcotics and added ibuprofen in cancer patients. Clin Pharm. 1985;4(1):53-8. PMID: 3971683. *Excluded: inadequate duration.*

Weinstein SM, Shi M, Buckley BJ, et al. Multicenter, open-label, prospective evaluation of the conversion from previous opioid analgesics to extended-release hydromorphone hydrochloride administered every 24 hours to patients with persistent moderate to severe pain. Clin Ther. 2006;28(1):86-98. PMID: 16490582. *Excluded: inadequate duration.*

Weisner CM, Campbell CI, Ray GT, et al. Trends in prescribed opioid therapy for non-cancer pain for individuals with prior substance use disorders. Pain. 2009;145(3):287-93. PMID: 19581051. *Excluded: wrong study design.*

White AG, Birnbaum HG, Schiller M, et al. Analytic models to identify patients at risk for prescription opioid abuse. Am J Manag Care. 2009;15(12):897-906. PMID: 20001171. *Excluded: wrong study design.*

White AP, Arnold PM, Norvell DC, et al. Pharmacologic management of chronic low back pain: synthesis of the evidence. Spine. 2011;36(21 Suppl):S131-43. PMID: 21952185. *Excluded: systematic review or meta-analysis used only as a source document.*

White KT, Dillingham TR, Gonzalez-Fernandez M, et al. Opiates for chronic nonmalignant pain syndromes: can appropriate candidates be identified for outpatient clinic management? Am J Phys Med Rehabil 2009;88(12):995-1001. PMID: 19789432. *Excluded: wrong outcome.*

Whitehead AJ, Dobscha SK, Morasco BJ, et al. Pain, substance use disorders and opioid analgesic prescription patterns in veterans with hepatitis C. J Pain Symptom Manage. 2008;36(1):39-45. PMID: 18358690. *Excluded: wrong study design.*

Whittle SL, Richards BL, Buchbinder R. Opioid analgesics for rheumatoid arthritis pain. JAMA. 2013;309(5):485-6. PMID: 23385275. *Excluded: inadequate duration.*

Whittle SL, Richards BL, Husni E, et al. Opioid therapy for treating rheumatoid arthritis pain. Cochrane Database Syst Rev. 2011;(11)PMID: 22071805. *Excluded: inadequate duration.*

Wiedemer NL, Harden PS, Arndt IO, et al. The opioid renewal clinic: a primary care, managed approach to opioid therapy in chronic pain patients at risk for substance abuse. Pain Med. 2007;8(7):573-84. PMID: 17883742. *Excluded: wrong study design.*

Wiffen PJ. Evidence-based pain management and palliative care in Issue Three for 2007 of The Cochrane Library. J Pain Palliat Care Pharmacother. 2008;22(1):21-4. PMID: 17430832. *Excluded: wrong publication type.*

Wiffen PJ. Methadone for chronic noncancer pain (cncp) in adults. J Pain Palliat Care Pharmacother. 2013;27(2):180-. PMID: 23789850. *Excluded: wrong publication type.*

Wilsey BL, Fishman S, Li CS, et al. Markers of abuse liability of short- vs long-acting opioids in chronic pain patients: a randomized cross-over trial. Pharmacol Biochem Behav. 2009;94(1):98-107. PMID: 19660492. *Excluded: wrong study design.*

Wilsey BL, Fishman SM, Casamalhuapa C, et al. Documenting and improving opioid treatment: the Prescription Opioid Documentation and Surveillance (PODS) System. Pain Med. 2009;10(5):866-77. PMID: 19594846. *Excluded: wrong study design.*

Wilsey BL, Fishman SM, Casamalhuapa C, et al. Computerized progress notes for chronic pain patients receiving opioids; the Prescription Opioid Documentation System (PODS). Pain Med. 2010;11(11):1707-17. PMID: 21044261. *Excluded: wrong study design.*

Wilsey BL, Fishman SM, Tsodikov A, et al. Psychological comorbidities predicting prescription opioid abuse among patients in chronic pain presenting to the emergency department. Pain Med. 2008;9(8):1107-17. PMID: 18266809. *Excluded: wrong population.*

Wirz S, Wartenberg HC, Elsen C, et al. Managing cancer pain and symptoms of outpatients by rotation to sustained-release hydromorphone: a prospective clinical trial. Clin J Pain. 2006;22(9):770-5. PMID: 17057558. *Excluded: wrong study design.*

Witkin LR, Diskina D, Fernandes S, et al. Usefulness of the opioid risk tool to predict aberrant drug-related behavior in patients receiving opioids for the treatment of chronic pain. J Opioid Manag. 2013;9(3):177-87. PMID: 23771568. *Excluded: wrong comparator.*

Wolff RF, Aune D, Truyers C, et al. Systematic review of efficacy and safety of buprenorphine versus fentanyl or morphine in patients with chronic moderate to severe pain. Curr Med Res Opin. 2012;28(5):833-45. PMID: 22443154. *Excluded: systematic review or meta-analysis used only as a source document.*

Wool C, Prandoni P, Polistena P, et al. Ketorolac suppositories in the treatment of neoplastic pain: a randomized clinical trial versus diclofenac. Curr Ther Res Clin Exp. 1991;49(5):854-61. PMID: N/A. *Excluded: wrong intervention.*

Wu CL, Agarwal S, Tella PK, et al. Morphine versus mexiletine for treatment of postamputation pain: a randomized, placebo-controlled, crossover trial. Anesthesiology. 2008;109(2):289-96. PMID: 18648238. *Excluded: wrong population.*

Wu CL, Tella P, Staats PS, et al. Analgesic effects of intravenous lidocaine and morphine on postamputation pain: a randomized double-blind, active placebo-controlled, crossover trial. Anesthesiology. 2002;96(4):841-8. PMID: 11964590. *Excluded: wrong population.*

Wu LT, Ringwalt CL, Mannelli P, et al. Prescription pain reliever abuse and dependence among adolescents: a nationally representative study. J Am Acad Child Adolesc Psychiatry. 2008;47(9):1020-9. PMID: 18664996. *Excluded: wrong study design.*

Wu SM, Compton P, Bolus R, et al. The addiction behaviors checklist: validation of a new clinician-based measure of inappropriate opioid use in chronic pain. J Pain Symptom Manage. 2006;32(4):342-51. PMID: 17000351. *Excluded: wrong study design.*

Yalcin S, Gullu I, Tekuzman G, et al. Ketorolac tromethamine in cancer pain. Acta Oncol. 1997;36(2):231-2. PMID: 9140446. *Excluded: wrong intervention.*

Yalcin S, Gullu IH, Tekuzman G, et al. A comparison of two nonsteroidal antiinflammatory drugs (diflunisal versus dipyrone) in the treatment of moderate to severe cancer pain: a randomized crossover study. Am J Clin Oncol. 1998;21(2):185-8. PMID: 9537209. *Excluded: inadequate duration.*

Yarlas A, Miller K, Wen W, et al. A randomized, placebo-controlled study of the impact of the 7-day buprenorphine transdermal system on health-related quality of life in opioid-naive patients with moderate-to-severe chronic low back pain. J Pain. 2013;14(1):14-23. PMID: 23200931. *Excluded: inadequate duration.*

Ytterberg SR, Mahowald ML, Woods SR. Codeine and oxycodone use in patients with chronic rheumatic disease pain. Arthritis Rheum. 1998;41(9):1603-12. PMID: 9751092. *Excluded: inadequate duration.*

Yulug B, Ozan E. Buprenorphine: a safe agent for opioid dependent patients who are under the increased risk of stroke? J Opioid Manag. 2009;5(3):134. PMID: 19662922. *Excluded: wrong publication type.*

Zanis DA, McLellan AT, Randall M. Can you trust patient self-reports of drug use during treatment? Drug Alcohol Depend. 1994;35(2):127-32. PMID: 8055734. *Excluded: wrong population.*

Zedler B, Xie L, Wang L, et al. Risk factors for serious prescription opioid-related toxicity or overdose among veterans health administration patients. Pain Med. 2014. PMID: 24931395. *Excluded: wrong population*

Zenz M, Strumpf M, Tryba M. Long-term oral opioid therapy in patients with chronic nonmalignant pain. J Pain Symptom Manage. 1992;7(2):69-77. PMID: 1573287. *Excluded: wrong study design.*

Zerbini C, Ozturk ZE, Grifka J, et al. Efficacy of etoricoxib 60 mg/day and diclofenac 150 mg/day in reduction of pain and disability in patients with chronic low back pain: results of a 4-week, multinational, randomized, double-blind study. Curr Med Res Opin. 2005;21(12):2037-49. PMID: 16368055. *Excluded: inadequate duration.*

Ziedonis DM, Amass L, Steinberg M, et al. Predictors of outcome for short-term medically supervised opioid withdrawal during a randomized, multicenter trial of buprenorphine-naloxone and clonidine in the NIDA clinical trials network drug and alcohol dependence. Drug Alcohol Depend. 2009;99(1-3):28-36. PMID: 18805656. *Excluded: inadequate duration.*

Zin CS, Nissen LM, O'Callaghan JP, et al. A randomized, controlled trial of oxycodone versus placebo in patients with postherpetic neuralgia and painful diabetic neuropathy treated with pregabalin. J Pain. 2010;11(5):462-71. PMID: 19962354. *Excluded: inadequate duration.*

Zorba Paster R. Chronic pain management issues in the primary care setting and the utility of long-acting opioids. Expert Opin Pharmacother. 2010;11(11):1823-33. PMID: 20629606. *Excluded: wrong publication type.*

Appendix E. Data Abstraction Tables

Appendix Table E1. Uncontrolled Studies of Long-term Opioid Use and Abuse, Misuse, and Related Outcomes

Author, Year	Type of Study Setting Duration	Eligibility Criteria	Population Characteristics	Opioid Dose, Duration, and Indication	Method of Ascertaining and Defining Abuse/Misuse	Main Results	Quality
Banta-Green, 2009	Retrospective cohort Integrated group health system United States	Patients aged 21-79 with chronic opioid prescriptions over at least 3 years (filling ≥10 opioid prescriptions in a 12-month period or filling a prescription for at least a 120-day supply and ≥6 prescriptions in a 12-month period) Exclude: patients with cancers other than benign, nonmelanoma skin cancer	n=704 Mean age: 55 years Female sex: 62% Race: 89% White	Dose: mean 50 mg/day MED Duration: NR Indication: NR	Factor scores based on DSM-IV and PDUQ criteria UDT: not specified	Opioid dependence: 13% (91/704) Opioid abuse without dependence: 8% (56/704)	Fair
Boscarino, 2010	Cross-sectional study, outpatients from nine primary care (83%) and 3 specialty clinics (17%), based on 1 year of observation	≥4 physician orders for opioid therapy in past 12 mos., identified from E.H.R.; mean prescriptions=10.7 Exclude: cancer	n=705 Age: 18-64: 79% 65+: 21% Female sex: 61% White race: 98%	Dose: NR Duration: mean of 10.7 prescriptions over 1 year Indication: noncancer, otherwise not described	Diagnostic interview: CIDI; DSM-IV criteria for opioid dependence	25.8% (95% CI: 22.0-29.9) met criteria for current opioid dependence; 35.5% (95% CI: 31.1-40.2) met criteria for lifetime dependence Factors associated with dependence: Age <65 years (OR 2.3, 95% CI 1.6 to 3.5) History of opioid abuse (OR 3.8, 95% CI 2.6 to 5.7) History of high dependence severity (OR 1.8, 95% CI 1.4 to 2.5) History of major depression (OR 1.3, 95% CI 1.0 to 1.6), Current use of psychotropic medications (OR 1.7, 95% CI 1.2 to 2.5)	Fair

Author, Year	Type of Study Setting Duration	Eligibility Criteria	Population Characteristics	Opioid Dose, Duration, and Indication	Method of Ascertaining and Defining Abuse/Misuse	Main Results	Quality
Carrington Reid, 2002	Retrospective cohort Two primary care centers United States	Patients who received ≥6 months of opioid prescriptions during a 1- year period for noncancer pain and were not on methadone maintenance.	n=98 (50 at VA and 48 at urban primary care clinic) VA site vs. urban primary care site Median age: 54 vs. 55 years Female sex: 8% vs. 67% Race: 88% White, 12% Black vs. 52% White, 36% Black, 10% Hispanic Mean duration of pain: 10 vs. 13 years	VA site vs. urban primary care site Dose: NR Duration: NR Indication: 44% low back, 10% injury-related, 8% diabetic neuropathy, 16% degenerative joint disease, 4% headache, 10% spinal stenosis vs. 25% low back pain, 13% injury-related, 10% diabetic neuropathy, 13% degenerative joint disease, 13% headache, 4% spinal stenosis	Chart review for lost or stolen opioids, documented use of other sources to obtain opioids, and requests for ≥2 early refills UDT: not specified	VA site vs. urban primary care site Opioid abuse behaviors: 24% (12/50) vs. 31% (15/48) Median time of onset of abuse behaviors: 24 months Factors associated with decreased risk of opioid abuse behaviors: No history of substance use disorder (adjusted OR 0.72, 95% CI 0.45 to 1.1) Age (adjusted OR 0.94, 95% CI 0.94 to 0.99)	Fair
Compton, 2008	Prospective cohort VA pain clinic United States One year	Consecutive chronic nonmalignant pain patients receiving opioids Exclude: patients with diagnosed substance use disorder	n=135 Mean age: 53 years Female sex: 6% Race: NR Baseline VAS score: 6.75	Dose: NR Duration: NR Indication: 77% musculoskeletal, 19% neuropathic, 4% multicategory	Chart review for opioid discontinuation due to medication agreement violation (including for opioid misuse or abuse) UDT: not specified	Discontinuation due to medication agreement violation: 28% (38/135) Discontinuation due to specific problematic opioid misuse behaviors: 8% (11/135) Overdose deaths: none reported	Fair

Author, Year	Type of Study Setting Duration	Eligibility Criteria	Population Characteristics	Opioid Dose, Duration, and Indication	Method of Ascertaining and Defining Abuse/Misuse	Main Results	Quality
Cowan, 2003	Cross-sectional Pain clinic United Kingdom	Patients attending pain clinic and receiving controlled-release oral morphine sulfate or transdermal fentanyl	n=104 Mean age: 55.4 years Female sex: 39% Race: NR Mean duration of pain: 10.5 years	Dose: NR Duration: mean 14.1 months Indication: 34% degenerative disease, 24% failed back/neck surgery syndrome, 10% complex regional pain syndrome, 10% osteoarthritis	SUQ UDT: not specified	Self-reported addiction: 1.9% (2/104) Craving opioids: 2.9% (3/104) Has taken drugs to enhance the effect of opioids: 0.9% (1/104) Has used alcohol to enhance the effect of opioids: 0.9% (1/104)	Fair
Edlund, 2014	Retrospective HMO, PPO and point-of-service database review 2000-2005 United States	Patients age ≥18 years with a new chronic non-cancer pain diagnosis, no cancer diagnosis, and no opioid use or opioid use disorder diagnosis in prior 6 months	n=568,640 (197,269 prescribed opioids in first year; of these, 5.5% had chronic use (>90 days supply) Mean age not reported; 11% age 18-30, 20% age 31-40, 27% age 41-50, 30% age 51-64, 12% ≥age 65 Female sex: 58% Race: NR Mean duration of pain: all patients newly diagnosed	Dose: Among those with any opioid use, median = 36 mg/day MED. Daily MED categorized as none, low (1-36 mg), medium (36-120 mg), or high (≥120 mg). Duration: Mean NR; users identified as "chronic" had ≥91 days Indication: NR; inclusion criteria required newly diagnosed chronic non-cancer pain	Diagnosis of opioid abuse or dependence (ICD-9-CM code 304.00 or 305.50) within 18 months of first chronic non-cancer pain diagnosis	Opioid abuse or dependence - No opioid prescription: 0.004% (150/371,371) Low dose, chronic: 0.72% (50/6902) Medium dose, chronic: 1.28% (47/3654) High dose, chronic: 6.1% (23/378) Abuse or dependence, opioid use vs. no use - Low dose, chronic: aOR* 15 (95% CI 10 to 21) Medium dose, chronic: aOR 29 (95% CI 20 to 41) High dose, chronic: aOR 122 (95% CI 73 to 206) *Adjusted for age, sex, number of tracer pain sites, number of nonsubstance mental health disorders, previous substance abuse or dependence diagnosis, Charlson score.	Fair

Author, Year	Type of Study Setting Duration	Eligibility Criteria	Population Characteristics	Opioid Dose, Duration, and Indication	Method of Ascertaining and Defining Abuse/Misuse	Main Results	Quality
Fleming, 2007 See also: Saffier, 2007	Primary care practices of 235 physicians	Daily opioids over past 3 months; 96% had received opioids for 12 months Exclusions: cancer pain	n=801 Mean age: 48.6 Female sex: 68% Race: 75.6% White; 23.1% African American; 1% other Disability income: 48%	Mean daily dose: 92 MEQ/d Duration: ≥12 mos. For 96% Indication: Osteoarthritis: 24%; low back pain, herniated disc or stenosis: 25%; migraine 8%; neuropathy 5%	In person interviews with ASI; SDSS; Aberrant Behavior 12-item List UDT: collected at end of interview	Met DSM-4 criteria for opioid dependence: 3.1% Met DSM-4 criteria for opioid abuse: 0.6% Any illicit drug on UDS: 24% (mostly marijuana) Aberrant behaviors: purposely oversedated: 24% (186/785) Felt intoxicated from pain med: 33% (260/785) Requested early refills: 45% (359/785) Increased dose on own: 37% (288/785) Meds lost or stolen: 30% (236/785) Used opioid purpose other than pain: 16% (125/785) Drank alcohol to relieve pain: 20% (154/785)	Fair
Hojsted, 2010	Cross-sectional Pain clinic Denmark	Adults with chronic noncancer pain Exclude: patients suffering from cognitive dysfunction, in poor health due to other condition, or did not use any pain medication	n=253, of which 187 were receiving opioid therapy (207 total and 153 receiving opioids returned questionnaire) Mean age: 52 years Female sex: 64% Race: NR Mean pain score: NR Receiving opioids: 74% (187/253) Indication: 93% noncancer pain, 7% cancer pain	Dose: NR Duration: mean 6.8 years (among those who completed questionnaire, n=207) Indication: 28% nociceptive pain, 33% neuropathic pain, 39% mixed nociceptive and neuropathic	Addiction screening by physician and nurse (blinded to each other) using the ICD-10 and Portenoy's Criteria; a positive screen by either provider was considered positive UDT: not specified	Addiction to opioids or hypnotics, ICD-10: 11.1% (28/253) Addiction to opioids, ICD-10: 14.4% (27/187) Addiction to opioids or hypnotics, Portenoy's Criteria: 14.6% (37/253) Addiction to opioids, Portenoy's Criteria: 19.3% (36/187) Overdose deaths: NA	Fair

Author, Year	Type of Study Setting Duration	Eligibility Criteria	Population Characteristics	Opioid Dose, Duration, and Indication	Method of Ascertaining and Defining Abuse/Misuse	Main Results	Quality
Portenoy, 2007	Prospective registry study 35 pain clinics United States Three years (mean duration 23.8 months)	Adult patients who had participated in any of five previous CCTs of CR oxycodone for noncancer pain	n=227 Mean age: 56 years Female sex: 57% Race: 90% White BPI average pain score: 6.4	Dose: mean 52.5 mg/day Duration: mean 541.5 days Indication: 38% osteoarthritis, 31% diabetic neuropathy, 31% low back pain	Physician-completed brief questionnaire assessing problematic drug-related behavior with verification by an independent panel of experts UDT: not specified	Problematic drug-related behavior identified by physicians: 5.7% (13/227) Problematic drug-related behavior adjudicated by expert panel as positive and meeting DSM-IV criteria: 0 Problematic drug-related behavior adjudicated by expert panel as positive: 2.2% (5/227) Problematic drug-related behavior adjudicated by expert panel as possible: 0.4% (1/227) Problematic drug-related behavior adjudicated by expert panel as withdrawal: 0.4% (1/227) Problematic drug-related behavior adjudicated by expert panel as alleged: 2.2% (5/227) Problematic drug-related behavior adjudicated by expert panel as negative: 0.4% (1/227) Overdose deaths: 1 (phenylpropanolamine, oxycodone, and alcohol)	Fair

Author, Year	Type of Study Setting Duration	Eligibility Criteria	Population Characteristics	Opioid Dose, Duration, and Indication	Method of Ascertaining and Defining Abuse/Misuse	Main Results	Quality
Schneider, 2010	Chart review Single center pain clinic United States	Patients receiving opioid therapy for ≥1 year	n=197 Mean age: 49 years Female sex: 67% Race: NR	Dose: mean 180 mg/day MED (long acting), 49 mg/day MED (short acting) Duration: mean 4.7 years Indication: 51% back pain, 10% neck pain, 9% fibromyalgia, 8% other myofascial pain	UDT: immunoassay followed by confirmatory GC/MS	Positive UDT: 8.7% (14/161) Aberrant drug-related behaviors noted in chart: 15.7% (31/197)	Fair
Wasan, 2009	Cross-sectional 5 pain clinics United States	Patients with noncancer chronic pain receiving opioid therapy	n=622 Mean age: 50.4 years Female sex: 55% Race: 80% White Mean pain score: 5.96	Dose: NR Duration: mean 6.2 years Indication: 61% low back pain	POTQ, PUDQ, and UDT	Positive scores of ≥2 on POTQ: 24% (115/480) Score ≥11 on PDUQ: 29.1% (130/447) Positive UDT: 37.1% (134/356)	Fair

Note: The references are located in Appendix C.
ASI=Addiction Severity Index; CCT=case control trial; CR=case report; CI=confidence interval; CIDI= Composite International Diagnostic Interview; DSM-IV=Diagnostic and Statistical Manual of Mental Disorders, 4th edition; DSM-V=Diagnostic and Statistical Manual of Mental Disorders, 5th edition; GC/MS= Gas Chromatography with Mass Spectrometry confirmatory test; ICD-10=International Statistical Classification of Diseases and Related Health Problems, tenth revision; MED=morphine equivalent dose; MEQ/d=milliequivalent/hydrogen; NR=not relevant; PDUQ= Prescription Drug Use Questionnaire; POTQ=Prescription opioid therapy questionnaire; SDSS= Substance dependence severity scale; UDT=urine drug testing; VA=Veterans Administration; VAS= Visual Analog Scale

Appendix Table E2. Observational Studies of Long-Term Opioid Use and Overdose

Author, year	KQ	Type of study, setting	Eligibility criteria	Comparison groups	Population characteristics	Method for Assessing Outcomes and Confounders
Dunn, 2010	KQ2a, b	Retrospective cohort (Group Health) United States	Age > 18 years starting new episode of opioid use (no opioids in past 6 mos) from 1997-2005; having 3 or more opioid scripts filled in first 90 days of episode; diagnosis of chronic noncancer pain in 2 wks before first opioid script.	Morphine equivalent doses: A. 1-<20 mg/day B. 20-<49 mg/day C. 50-<99 mg/day D. >=100 mg/day	Mean (SD; range) age (years): 54 (16.8; 18-99) Female sex: 59.6% Race: NR Smoking: 29.5% Depression: 26.9% Substance abuse: 6.2% Charlson Score, mean (SD; range): 0.71 (1.48;0-14) Pain diagnosis: 37.9% back; 30.3% extremity, 12.7% osteoarthritis; 12.3% injury, contusion, or fracture;8.9% neck Opioid dose, mean (median): 13.3 mg (6.0 mg) Sedative-hypnotic use, any: 74.7% Muscle relaxant: 52.3% Benzodiazepine: 42.7% Opioid: Hydrocodone: 46.3% Oxycodone: 24.5% Codeine combination: 11.6% Long-acting morphine: 6.2% Any short acting opioid: 90.4% Any long-acting opioid: 9.6%	All patients in HMO meeting inclusion criteria

Author, year	Screened Eligible Enrolled Analyzed Loss to Followup	Adjusted Variables for Statistical Analysis	Main Results	Funding Source	Quality
Dunn, 2010	Screened: Not reproted Eligible: Not reported Enrolled: 9,940 Mean duration of follow-up (range): 42 mos (<1-119); Analyzed: All included in analysis Loss to followup: 61% had complete followup from cohort entry until end of study or event occurred; 32% left GHC during study; 7% died	Sedative-hypnotic use as time-varying covariate Age Sex Smoking Depression diagnosis Substance abuse diagnosis Index pain diagnosis Chronic disease comorbidity adjustors (RxRisk & Charlson)	51 patients with overdose events (148 per 100,000 person-years); 40 serious overdose events (116 per 100,000 person-years); 6 fatal overdose events (17 per 100,000 person-years) Rate of any overdose per 100,000 person-years (95% CI); HR (95% CI) No opioid: 36 (13-70); 0.31 (0.12-0.80); 6 overdose events A. (referent): 160 (100-233); 1.0 B. 260 (95-505); 1.44 (0.57-3.62) C. 677 (249-1317); 3.73 (1.47-9.5) D. 1791 (894-2995); 8.87 (3.99-19.72) Opioid dose, any: 256 (187-336); 5.16 (2.14-12.48); 45 overdose events HR, serious events (95% CI) No opioid: 0.19 (0.05-0.68); A. (referent): 1.0 B. 1.19 (0.4-3.6); C. 3.11 (1.01-9.51); D. 11.18 (4.8-26.03); Opioid dose, any: 8.39 (2.52-27.98)	National Institute of Drug Abuse and Wellcome Trust	Fair

Author, year	KQ	Type of study, setting	Eligibility criteria	Comparison groups	Population characteristics	Method for Assessing Outcomes and Confounders
Gomes, 2011	KQ2b	Case-Control Canada	Residents aged 15-64 with public drug coverage and an opioid for nonmalignant pain (1997-2006)	Cases: Died of an opioid-related cause (n=498 matched a control) Controls: received opioids (n=1714) A. 1-<20 mg/day B. 20-<50 mg/day C. 50-<100 mg/day D. 100-<200 mg/day E. >=200 mg/day	Total cohort n= 607,156 Mean age (years): 44.49 vs 44.72 Gender (not reported which one): 58.8% vs 58.0%	Controls matched on disease risk index (0.2 standard deviation caliper), age, gender, index year, and Charlson

Note: The references are located in Appendix C.

CI=confidence interval; EtOH=ethanol; GHC=Group Health Cooperative; HMO=Health Maintenance Organization; HR=hazard ratio; ICES= Institute for Clinical Evaluative Sciences; MOHLTC= Ontario Ministry of Health and Long-Term Care; NR=not relevant; RxRisk=drug index for prescription drugs

Author, year	Screened Eligible Enrolled Analyzed Loss to Followup	Adjusted Variables for Statistical Analysis	Main Results	Funding Source	Quality
Gomes, 2011	Screened: 1463 Eligible:1179 Primary-analysis: 593 with 498 matched Secondary-analysis: 873 with 781 matching	Opioid exposure categorized by Average Daily Dose: <20mg, 20-49mg, 50-99mg, 100-199mg, 200+mg. Logistic models adjusted for: duration, income, history of EtOH abuse, interacting prescription drugs, total number of different opioids dispensed, long-acting opioid used, number of physicians prescribing opioids, number of pharmacies dispensing opioids	Risk estimates reported as adjusted OR Risk of opioid overdose death A. 1 (reference) B. 1.32 (0.94-1.84) C. 1.92 (1.30-2.85) D. 2.04 (1.28-3.24) E. 2.88 (1.79-4.63) Secondary using 120-day exposure window risk of opioid overdose death A. 1 (reference) B. 0.93 (0.60-1.42) C. 1.31 (0.86-1.99) D. 1.47 (0.98-2.19) E. 2.24 (1.62-3.10)	MOHLTC Drug Innovation Fund and ICES, a nonprofit research institute sponsored by the Ontario MOHLTC	Good

Appendix Table E3. Observational Studies of Long-Term Opioid Use and Fractures

Author, year	KQ	Type of Study, Setting	Eligibility Criteria	Comparison Groups	Population Characteristics
Li, 2013	KQ2a	Nested case control United Kingdom	Cohort: Patients with non-cancer pain with at least 1 opioid prescription between 1/1/90 and 12/31/08 in the General Practice Research Database Cases (n=21,739): First-time diagnosed fracture of the hip, humerus, or wrist during 1990-2008, age 18-80 years, >2 years of medical history before index date; excluding patients with cancer, dementia, metabolic bone disease, Cushing syndrome, hyperparathyroidism, long-term immobiliation, or alcohol or drug abuse, fracture within 2 years, MVA within 90 days, osteoporosis diagnosis prior to index date Controls (n=85,326): Up to 4 controls without fracture selected for each case, matched on age, sex, index date, and general practice	A. Opioid nonuse B. Current cumulative opioid use 1 prescription C. 2-3 opioid prescriptions D. 4-5 opioid prescriptions E. 6-20 opioid prescriptions F. 21-50 opioid prescriptions G. 51-100 opioid prescriptions H. >100 opioid prescriptions 1. Opioid nonuse 2. Current use 3. Recent use 4. Past use	Mean age (years): 62 Female sex: 77% Race: NR Pain condition: NR Pain duration: NR Pain severity: NR Mean dose: NR Most commonly prescribed opioids: dihydrocodeine, codeine, propoxyphene, tramadol

Author, year	Method For Assessing Outcomes and Confounders	Screened Eligible Enrolled Analyzed Loss to Followup	Adjusted Variables For Statistical Analysis	Main Results	Funding Source	Quality
Li, 2013	Used General Practice Research Database, in which drug exposures and diagnoses (including fracture) have been validated	Screened: NR Eligible: NR Enrolled: NR Analyzed: 21,739 fracture cases and 85,326 controls Number not analyzable: NR	Smoking, BMI, number of general practice visits, recorded years before index date, opioid use (new vs. prevalent), comorbidities, comedications, types of pain, recent/past opioid use (matched on age, sex, index date, and general practice)	Adjusted OR for risk of hip, humerus, or wrist fracture A. 1 (reference) B. 2.70 (95% CI 2.34-3.13) C. 1.90 (95% CI 1.67-2.17) D. 1.44 (95% CI 1.22-1.69) E. 1.17 (95% CI 1.08-1.27) F. 1.06 (95% CI 0.98-1.15) G. 1.06 (95% CI 0.96-1.16) H. 1.12 (95% CI 0.99-1.25) 1. 1 (reference) 2. 1.27 (95% CI 1.21-1.33) 3. 1.05 (95% CI 0.99-1.13) 4. 0.96 (95% CI 0.92-1.01)	None	Good

Author, year	KQ	Type of Study, Setting	Eligibility Criteria	Comparison Groups	Population Characteristics
Saunders, 2010	KQ2a, b	Cohort, Group Health Cooperative United States	Age 60+, initiating opioids (no opioid prescriptions in prior 6 months) with 3+ prescriptions in 90 days and a diagnosis of non-cancer pain 2-3 weeks prior to the index prescription. Exclusions: Cancer, <270 days enrollment in health plan in the year prior to index.	Opioid dose per day (mg/day): A: Not currently using B: 1-<20 mg/day C: 20-<50 mg/day D: ≥50 mg/day E: Any use	Mean age (years): 73 Female sex: 66% Race: NR Depression diagnosis: 22% Substance abuse diagnosis: 3.8% Dementia diagnosis: 4.8% Prior fracture: 2.6% HRT/bisphosphonate use: 34% Rxrisk score, mean (SD): 4272 (2455) Charlson Index, mean (SD): 1.32 (2.0) Pain diagnosis at index visit 42% back pain, 4.8% neck pain, 25% osteoarthritis, 2.4% headache, 34% extremity pain, 5.3% abdominal pain/hernia, 0.6% menstrual/menopausal pain, 0.2% temporomandibular disorder pain Mean morphine equivalent daily dose (mg): (s.d.) 12.8 mg (17.0) Sedative hypnotic use: 60% Antidepressant use: 57% Opioid prescribed: Hydrocodone: 42% Oxycodone: 24% Codeine combination: 14% Long-acting morphine: 8.3%

Note: The references are located in Appendix C.

CI=confidence interval; HRT=hormone replacement therapy; ICD-9=International Classification of Diseases; KQ=key question; NR=not relevant; RxRisk= drug index for prescription drugs

Author, year	Method For Assessing Outcomes and Confounders	Screened Eligible Enrolled Analyzed Loss to Followup	Adjusted Variables For Statistical Analysis	Main Results	Funding Source	Quality
Saunders, 2010	Fractures initially identified by ICD-9 codes (800xx-804xx; 807xx-809xx; 810xx-829xx; 2000-2006, excluded vertebral fractures) and verified by medical record review; medication data from Group Health Cooperative automated pharmacy files (over 90% of prescriptions); covariates from automated health care data	Screened: ~500,000 Eligible, enrolled, and analyzed: 2,341 Loss to followup: Not reported Duration of followup (mean, person-months) (SD): 32.7 (21.3)	Age, sex, tobacco use, depression diagnosis, substance abuse diagnosis, dementia diagnosis, index pain diagnosis, chronic disease comorbidity adjustors, sedative-hypnotic use, antidepressant use, HRT/bisphosphonate use, and prior fractures.	Fracture rate: 5.0%/year Adjusted HRs for risk of fracture A: 1 (reference) B: 1.20 (95% CI 0.92, 1.56) C: 1.34 (95% CI 0.89, 2.01) D: 2.00 (95% CI 1.24, 3.24) E: 1.28 (95% CI 0.99, 1.64)	National Institute of Drug Abuse	Fair

Appendix Table E4. Observational Studies of Long-Term Opioid Use and Cardivascular Outcomes

Author, Year	KQ	Type of Study, Setting	Eligibility Criteria	Comparison Groups	Population Characteristics
Carman, 2011	KQ2a, b	Retrospective cohort United States	Claim submitted for dispensing of opioids or COX-2 inhibitors for ≥180 days from July 2002 to December 2005, patients aged ≥18 years; controls from general populations matched on age, sex, and cohort entry date Exclude: History of MI or revascularization, cancer	A. Opioids (n=148,657) B. Rofecoxib (n=44,236) C. Celecoxib (n=64,072) D. Valdecoxib (n=20,502) E. General population not using opioids or COX-2 inhibitors (n=148,657) 1. 0 to <1350 mg MED per 90 days 2. 1350 to <2700 mg MED per 90 days 3. 2700 to <8100 mg MED per 90 days 4. 8100 to <18,000 mg MED per 90 days 5. ≥18,000 mg MED per 90 days	**A vs. B vs. C vs. D vs. E** Age 18-29 years: 4.7% vs. 1.2% vs. 0.8% vs. 1.2% vs. 4.7% Age 30-39 years: 16.3% vs. 5.4% vs. 4.1% vs. 5.3% vs. 16.3% Age 40-49 years: 33.9% vs. 20.7% vs. 17.6% vs. 20.1% vs. 33.9% Age 50-64 years: 36.7% vs. 56.0% vs. 56.3% vs. 56.5% vs. 36.7% Age ≥65 years: 8.4% vs. 16.6% vs. 21.2% vs. 16.9% vs. 8.4% Female sex: 40.3% vs. 39.5% vs. 39.6% vs. 34.9% vs. 40.3% Diabetics: 11.7% vs. 10.2% vs. 12.4% vs. 11.1% vs. 4.1% Pain condition: NR Duration of pain: NR severity of pain: NR Opioids prescribed: NR

Appendix Table E4. Observational Studies of Long-Term Opioid Use and Cardiovascular Outcomes

Author, Year	Method For Assessing Outcomes and Confounders	Screened Eligible Enrolled Analyzed Loss to Followup	Adjusted Variables for Statistical Analysis	Main Results	Funding Source	Quality
Carman, 2011	All relevant claims in database during study period	Screened: NR Eligible, enrolled, analyzed: 426,124	Incidence rates adjusted for age and sex; incidence rate ratio adjusted for age sex, CV and other comorbidities, and use of concomitant medications	Adjusted incidence rate of MI, incidence rate ratio A: 5.93 (95% CI 5.58 to 6.30); IRR 2.66 (95% CI 2.30 to 3.08) B: 3.54 (95% CI 3.11 to 4.01); IRR 1.94 (95% CI 1.65 to 2.29) C: 3.53 (95% CI 3.15 to 3.94); IRR 1.79 (95% CI 1.53 to 2.10) D: 3.40 (95% CI 2.76 to 4.14); IRR 1.74 (95% CI 1.41 to 2.16) E: 1.58 (95% CI 1.40 to 1.78); IRR 1 (reference) Adjusted incidence rates of MI or revascularization, incidence rate ratio A. 11.91 (95% CI 11.40 to 12.43); IRR 2.38 (95% CI 2.15 to 2.63) B. 7.98 (95% CI 7.33 to 8.67); IRR 1.93 (95% CI 1.72 to 2.15) C. 7.94 (95% CI 7.36 to 8.54); IRR 1.81 (95% CI 1.62 to 2.01) D. 7.53 (95% CI 6.56 to 8.60); IRR 1.75 (95% CI 1.50 to 2.01) E. 3.38 (95% CI 3.12 to 3.67); IRR 1 (reference) Dosing Compared to a cumulative dose of 0 to 1350 mg MED over 90 days, the IRR for 1350 to <2700 was 1.21 (95% CI 1.02 to 1.45), for 2700 to <8100 mg was 1.42 (95% CI 1.21 to 1.67), for 8100 to <18,000 mg was 1.89 (95% CI 1.54 to 2.33), and for >18,000 mg was 1.73 (95% CI 1.32 to 2.26)	GlaxoSmithKline	Fair

Author, Year	KQ	Type of Study, Setting	Eligibility Criteria	Comparison Groups	Population Characteristics
Li, 2013	KQ2a	Case-Control UK General Practice Research Database United Kingdom	Cases (n=11,693): Age 18-80 years, 2 years of medical history data before index (onset of MI symptoms) Controls: (n=44,897): Up to 4 controls matched on age, gender, index date, and practice site using risk-set sampling Excluded: History of cancer, ischemic heart disease, heart failure, stroke, congenital heart disorders, heart transplat, arrhythmias, treated hypertension, diabetes, ETOH/Drug abuse, hepatic or renal disease before index, cardiac surgery in the 90 days prior to index.	A. Non-use B. Current (0-30 days from index) C. Recent (31-365 days out) D. Past Use (366-730 days out) Cumulative use (number of prescriptions): 1. 1-2 2. 3-10 3. 11-50 4. >50	Mean age (years): 61.8 vs. 61.6 Female sex: : 31.1% vs. 31.3% Current smoker: 38.6% vs. 23.3% Low BMI (<18.5): 1.2% vs. 1.2% Normal BMI: 25.8% vs. 28.9% Overweight: 31.7% vs. 30.2% Obese: 13.8% vs. 11.3% Arthritis: 25% vs. 24.2% Rheumatoid arthritis: 3.2% vs. 1.8% Fibromyalgia: 1.1% Duration or severity of pain: NR Codeine: 16% vs. 15% Dihydrocodeine: 9.6% vs. 8.1% Propoxyphene: 13% vs. 11%

Note: The references are located in Appendix C.
BMI=body mass index; CI=confidence interval; CV= cardiovascular; IRR=incidence rate ratio; KQ=key question; MI=myocardial infarction; NR=not relevant

Author, Year	Method For Assessing Outcomes and Confounders	Screened Eligible Enrolled Analyzed Loss to Followup	Adjusted Variables for Statistical Analysis	Main Results	Funding Source	Quality
Li, 2013	Used General Practice Research Database, which has been validated on drug exposure and diagnoses (including MI)	Screened: 1,700,000 Eligible: Not reported Enrolled: 11,693 cases and 44,897 controls Analyzed: 11,693 cases and 44,897 controls	Age, gender, smoking, body mass index, number of general practice visits, years of medical history, opioid new versus prevalent use, co-morbidities, concomitant medications, abdominal and pelvic pain and other pain	Risk of MI (adjusted OR) A. 1 (reference) B. 1.28 (95% CI 1.19–1.37) C. 1.17 (95% CI 1.10–1.24) D. 1.06 (95% CI 0.98–1.14) 1. 1.10 (95% CI 1.03–1.18) 2. 1.09 (95% CI 1.02–1.17) 3. 1.38 (95% CI 1.28–1.49) 4. 1.25 (95% CI 1.11–1.40)	None disclosed	Good

Appendix Table E5. Observational Studies of Long-Term Opioid Use and Endocrine Outcomes

Author,	KQ	Type of Study, Setting	Eligibility Criteria	Comparison Groups	Population Characteristics	Method For Assessing Outcomes and Confounders
Deyo, 2013	KQ2a, b	Cross-sectional Integrated healthcare United States	Ambulatory males aged ≥18 years with diagnoses associated with low back pain Exclude: patients with evidence of systemic disease or trauma	A. Patients prescribed medication for erectile dysfunction or testosterone replacement (n=909) B. Patients not prescribed medication for erectile dysfunction or testosterone replacement (n=10,418)	**A vs. B** Mean age (years): 55.7 vs. 48.0 Female sex: 0% Race: 89% White, 3% Black, 3% Asian/Pacific Islander, 1% American Indian, 3.9% other (among records with race/ethnicity data available, 59% of total sample) Sedative-hypnotic use: 24.4% vs. 15.6% Diagnosis of depression: 17.3% vs. 11.3%	Review of medical and pharmacy records

Note: The references are located in Appendix C.
KQ=key question; MED=morphine equivalent dose; NIH/NCRR=National Institutes of Health/National Center for Research

Author, year	Screened Eligible Enrolled Analyzed Loss to Followup	Adjusted Variables For Statistical Analysis	Main Results	Funding Source	Quality
Deyo, 2013	Screened: NR Eligible: 11,327 Enrolled: 11,327 Analyzed: 11,327	Age, comorbidity score, number of hospitalizations, sedative-hypnotic use, duration of opioid use, morphine dose at last dispensing, type of opioid (short- vs. long-acting), depression, and smoking status	No opioid use vs. short-term use vs. episodic use vs. long-term use Prescription for sildenafil, tadalafil, or vadenafil 6 months before or after index visit: 6.3% (294/4,655) vs. 6.9% (324/4,696) vs. 7.3% (12/164) vs. 11.3% (204/1,812); p<0.001 Testosterone replacement 6 months before or after index visit: 0.5% (25/2,655) vs. 0.6% (30/4,696) vs. 1.2% (2/164) vs. 2.4% (44/1,812); p<0.001 Testosterone replacement or erectile dysfunction treatment: 6.7% (312/4,655) vs. 7.4% (346/4,696) vs. 7.9% (13/164) vs. 13.1% (238/1,812); p<0.001; OR 1.5, 95% CI 1.1 to 1.9 Dosing Daily opioid dose of >120 mg MED/day associated with increased risk of use of medications for erectile dysfunction or testosterone replacement versus 0 to <20 mg MED/day (OR 1.6, 95% CI 1.0 to 2.4)	NIH/NCRR	Fair

Appendix Table E6. Observational Studies of Long-Term Opioid Use and Motor Vehicle Accidents

Author, year	KQ	Type of Study, Setting	Eligibility Criteria	Comparison Groups	Population Characteristics	Sampling Strategy
Gomes, 2013	KQ2b	Case-Control Canada	Residents aged 15-64 with public drug coverage and an opioid prescription (excluding methadone (2003-2011) at least 6 months of continuous eligibility for public drug coverage before their index date and at least 1 opioid prescription with a duration that overlapped their index date. Cases and controls were excluded if they had invalid patient identifiers, had missing information about age or sex, received palliative care services in the 6 months before their index date, lived in a long-term care home at the index date, or had a prescription for a nonstudy opioid with a duration that overlapped the index date.	Cases: ED with an external cause of injury related to road trauma (codes V00 to V89 from ICD-10) (n=5,300 matched a control) Controls: (n=5300) A. 1-<20 mg/day B. 20-<50 mg/day C. 50-<100 mg/day D. 100-<200 mg/day E. ≥200 mg/day	**Cases vs. Controls** Mean age (years): 45.76 vs 45.75 Female sex: 48.6% Urban resident: 83.75% vs. 83.98 Social Assistance:22% vs. 21% Disability support: 67.9% vs. 66.6% Duration of use (years): 7.09 vs. 6.84 <u>Charlson score</u> No hospitalization:61.7% vs. 62.3% 0: 23.4% vs. 22.4% 1: 6.85% vs. 6.32% ≥2: 7.96% vs. 8.49%	Incidence density sampling Cases were matched to controls by sex, age (within 3 years), index year (within 1 year), ED visit for road trauma in the past year, and disease risk index (within 0.2 SD). Cases with no matched controls were excluded from analyses.

Note: The references are located in Appendix C.
CI=confidence interval; ED=emergency department; ICD=International Classification of Diseases

Author, year	Screened Eligible Enrolled Analyzed Loss to Followup	Adjusted Variables For Statistical Analysis	Main Results	Funding Source	Quality
Gomes, 2013	Screened population: 549,878 Eligible Cases: 5300 Eligible Controls: 43,736 Controls matched 1:1	Logistic models adjusted for: age, past (3 years) hospitalization for alcoholism, past (1 year) ED visit for alcoholism, duration of opioid treatment, medication use in past 180 days (ie, selective serotonin reuptake inhibitors, other antidepressants, antipsychotics, benzodiazepines and other depressants of the central nervous system, separately), number of drugs dispensed in the past 180 days, and numbers of physician and ED visits in the past 1 year.	Risk estimates reported as adjusted OR Risk of motor vehicle crash A. 1 (reference) B. 1.09 (95% CI 0.97-1.21) C. 1.07 (95% CI 0.94-1.22) D. 1.08 (95% CI 0.93-1.24) E. 1.00 (95% CI 0.88-1.15) Dosing Relative to 1 to <20 mg MED/day, the odds of road trauma among drivers after adjustment for age, alcoholism history, concomitant medication use, total number of drugs, and number of physician and emergency department visits was 1.21 (1.02 to 1.42) for 20 to 49 mg, 1.29 (1.06 to 1.57) for 50-99 mg, 1.42 (1.15 to 1.76) for 100 to 199 mg, and 1.23 (1.02 to 1.49) for >200 mg	MOHLTC Drug Innovation Fund and ICES, a nonprofit research institute sponsored by the Ontario MOHLTC.	Good

Appendix Table E7. Trials of Different Methods for Initiating and Titrating Opioids

Author Year	Study design Duration	Setting Country	Eligibility Criteria	Interventions	Sample Characteristics	Screened Eligible Enrolled Analyzed Loss to Followup
Jamison, 1998	RCT 16 weeks	Single center Pain clinic United States	Chronic back pain >6 months duration, age 25 to 65 years, average pain intensify >40 on scale of 0 to 100, unsuccessful response to traditional pain treatment. Exclude: Cancer, acute osteomyelitis or acute bone disease, spinal stenosis and neurogenic claudication, non-ambulatory, significant psychiatric history, pregnancy, treatment for drug or alcohol abuse, clinically unstable systemic illness, acute herniated disc within 3 months	A. Long acting morphine + short-acting oxycodone (titrated doses) B. Short-acting oxycodone (set dose) + Naproxen C. Naproxen A vs. B vs. C Mean dose 41.1 mg vs. NR (max 20 mg oxycodone/day) vs. NR In all groups, max 1000 mg/day of naproxen 16 weeks	Mean age (years): 43 Female sex: 57% Race: NR Indication: 39% failed back syndrome, 25% myofascial pain syndrome, 19% degenerative spine disease, 14% radiculopathy, 3% discogenic back pain Prior opioid use: NR Mean pain duration: 79 months	Screened: 48 Eligible: NR Enrolled: 36 Analyzed: 36
Salzman, 1999	RCT 10 days	Multicenter Rheumatology clinics and others United States	18 years or older, chronic stable moderate to severe back pain despite analgesic therapy with or without opioids. Exclude: Contraindication to opioid history of substance abuse, unable to discontinue nonstudy narcotic, or current oxycodone dose >80 mg/day. Titration to 80 mg without achieving pain control	A: Sustained-release Oxycodone (titrated) B: Immediate-release Oxycodone (titrated) Titration comparison Mean dose A: 104 mg/day Mean dose B: 113 mg/day 10 days	Mean age (years): 56 Female sex: 54% Race: 87% White, 13% Hispanic Indication: Intervertebral disc disease, nerve root entrapment, spondylolisthesis, osteoarthritis, and other non-malignant conditions 84% (48/57) Pain duration: NR	Screened: NR Eligible: NR Enrolled: 57 Analyzed: 57

Note: The references are located in Appendix C.
NR=not reported; RCT=randomized control trial; SF=short form

Author Year	Outcomes Assessed	Results	Adverse Events and Withdrawals Due To Adverse Events	Sponsor	Quality
Jamison, 1998	Pain Intensity: timing not specified, Comprehensive Pain Evaluation Questionnaire Functional status: baseline and at end of treatment (SF-36) Symptom checklist: baseline and at end of treatment (Symptom Checklist-90) Weekly activity record at baseline and once a month Medication diary weekly Overall helpfulness during titration and at end of study (categorical scale, 0= no help, 10=extremely helpful)	A vs. B vs. C Average pain (means, 0-100 VAS): 54.9 vs. 59.8 vs. 65.5 Current pain (means, 0-100 VAS): 51.3 vs. 55.3 vs. 62.7 Highest pain (means, 0-100 VAS): 71.4 vs. 75.5 vs. 78.9 Anxiety (means): 11.2 vs. 15.0 vs. 31.6 Depression (means): 10.8 vs. 16.4 vs. 26.9 Irritability (means): 17.7 vs. 20.5 vs. 33.7 Level of activity (means, 0-100 scale): 49.3 vs. 49.3 vs. 51.5 Hours of sleep (means): 5.9 vs. 5.9 vs. 6.1	A vs. B Somnolence: 27% (8/30) vs. 37% (10/27) Nausea: 50% (15/30) vs. 33% (9/27) Vomiting: 20% (6/30) vs. 4% (1/27) Postural hypotension: 0% vs. 0% Constipation: 30% (9/30) vs. 37% (10/27) Pruritus: 30% (9/30) vs. 26% (7/27) Confusion: 3% (1/30) vs. 0% Dry mouth: 0% vs. 11% (3/27) Dizziness: 30% (9/30) vs. 22% (6/27) Nervousness: 0% vs. 7% (2/27) Asthenia: 7% (2/30) vs. 11% (3/27) Headache: 13% (4/30) vs. 26% (7/27) Withdrawal due to adverse events: 20% (6/30) vs. 7% (2/27)	Roxane Laboratories (maker of long-acting morphine and short-acting oxycodone). Not clear if authors employed by Roxane	Fair
Salzman, 1999	Pain Intensity: daily diary, categorical scale (0-3, none-severe) Study Medication Use: daily diary, amount used Rescue Drug Use: daily diary, amount used Achievement of Stable Pain Control: Stable pain control considered achieved if pain intensity rated as 1.5 or less for 48 hours with no more than 2 doses of rescue medication Time to Stable Pain Control: Days	A vs. B Mean decrease in pain intensity (0 to 3 scale): 1.1 vs. 1.3 (NS) Proportion achieving stable analgesia: 87% (26/30) vs. 96% (26/27) (p = 0.36) Time to stable pain control: 2.7 vs. 3.0 days (p = 0.90). Mean number of dose adjustments: 1.1 vs. 1.7 adjustments (p = 0.58)	A vs. B vs. C Withdrawal due to adverse events: 54% (29/54) vs. 34% (20/59) vs. 130% (6/54) (p=0.008 for A or C vs. B) Withdrawal due to nausea and/or vomiting: 46% (25/54) vs. 22% (13/59) vs. 22% (12/54) Any adverse event: 76% vs. 70% vs. 61% Dizziness: 7% vs. 7% vs. 7% Headache: 18% vs. 15% vs. 13% Dry mouth: 0% vs. 2% vs. 6% Constipation: 7% vs. 3% vs. 11% Diarrhea: 7% vs. 5% vs. 2% Vomiting: 18% vs. 12% vs. 7% Nausea: 54% vs. 42% vs. 33% Somnolence: 9% vs. 7% vs. 0% Pruritus: 4% vs. 2% vs. 7%	Purdue Pharma sponsored study 2 authors employees of Purdue Role not otherwise reported.	Fair

Appendix Table E8a. Head-to-Head Trials of Different Long-Acting Opioids

Author Year	Study design Duration	Setting Country	Eligibility criteria	Interventions	Sample Characteristics	Screened Eligible Enrolled Analyzed Loss to Followup	Outcomes Assessed
Allan, 2005	RCT 13 months	Europe Multicenter (number of sites not clear)	Adults with chronic low back pain requiring regular strong opioids Exclude: Receipt of more than 4 doses of strong opioids in a week in the 4 weeks before the study, high risk of ventilatory depression or intolerance to study drugs, prior alcohol or substance abuse, presence of other chronic pain disorders, or life-limiting illness	A: Transdermal fentanyl (titrated from 25 mcg/hr) (Mean dose 57 mcg/h) B: Sustained-release morphine (titrated from 30 mg q 12 hrs) (Mean dose: 140 mg)	Avg. 54.0 years, 61% female Race: not reported, Prior opioid use not reported 35% nociceptive, 4% neuropathic, 46% nociceptive and neuropathic, 3% nociceptive with psychologic factors, 4% neuropathic with psychologic factors, 83% mechanical low back pain, 8% inflammatory 39% trauma/surgery, 1% metabolic, 3% other Pain duration average 124.7 months	Number approached and eligible not reported 683 randomized (338 to transdermal fentanyl and 342 to sustained-release morphine, 3 group assignment not reported)	Pain score (mean, 0-100 VAS) Severe pain at rest Severe pain on movement Severe pain during the day Severe pain at night Rescue strong opioids use Quality of life (SF-36) Loss of working days Withdrawal due to lack of efficacy
Mitra, 2013	RCT 12 months	One site in Townsville, Australia	Inclusion: Patients > 18, reporting persistent pain for greater part of day and night for at least 1 year, opiood-naïve, appropriate for treatment with transdermal patches after medical assessment, with no comorbid psychiatric history.	A: TDB initial dose=-5 mcg/h, n=22; B: TDF initial dose=12.5 mcg/h, n=24; Both titrated to optimal doses over 4 weeks; increased doses beyond that given as clinically indicated	None reported by treatment group: Age, mean (range): 49 (22-80); Male: 48%; Back pain: 61%; Other types of pain: 39%; Duration of pain, mean (range): 11.7 yrs (6 mos to 50 yrs); Duration of follow-up: 3 mos (35%), 6 mos (13%), 12 mos (52%)	Considered for trial: 82; Enrolled: 46; Completed and analyzed at 12 mos: 30 (TDB-14 pts and TDF-16 pts)	SPAASMS: Activity & mobility: Rescue pain meds: GP/ED visits: Sleep quality: Side effects: Mood: Pain VAS: DASS21: PDI:

Author Year	Results	Adverse Events and Withdrawals Due To Adverse Events	Sponsor	Quality
Allan, 2005	Transdermal fentanyl (A) vs. sustained-release morphine (B): Pain score (mean, 0-100 VAS) at 56 weeks (N=608): 56.0 (A) vs. 55.8 (B) Severe pain at rest (per protocol analyses, N=248 and 162): 22/248 (9%) (A) vs. 20/162 (12%) (B), p=0.030 (no significant differences in ITT analysis, but data not provided) Severe pain on movement (per protocol): 70/248 (28%) (A) vs. 43/162 (27%) (B), p=0.61 Severe pain during the day (per protocol): 48/248 (19%) (A) vs. 40/162 (25%) (B), p=0.385 Severe pain at night (per protocol): 25/248 (10%) (A) vs. 26/162 (16%) (B), p=0.003 (no significant differences in ITT analysis, but data not provided) Rescue strong opioids use: 154/296 (52%) (A) vs. 154/291 (53%) (B). Quality of life (SF-36): No differences between interventions Loss of working days: No differences between interventions Withdrawal due to lack of efficacy: 18/335 (5%) vs.15/342 (4%)	Transdermal fentanyl (N=338) vs. sustained-release oral morphine (N=342) Any adverse event: 87% vs. 91% Constipation (ITT): 176/338 (52%) vs. 220/338 (65%) (p<0.05) Nausea: 54% vs. 50% Vomiting: 29% vs. 26% Somnolence: 17% vs. 30% Dizziness: 25% vs. 24% Fatigue: 17% vs. 14% Pruritus: 15% vs. 20% Application site reactions: 9% in transdermal fentanyl group. Deaths: None; Addiction: None reported. Use of laxatives: 177/336 (53%) vs. 221/336 (66%) (p<0.001) Use of antiemetics/anticholingergics:38% vs. 36% Use of antihistamines: 21% vs. 12% (p=0.002) Withdrawal (Overall): 52% (177/338) vs. 47% (162/342). Withdrawal (adverse events):125/335 (37%) vs. 104/337 (31%) (p=0.098)	Janssen Pharma-ceutica One author employed by Janssen	Fair
Mitra, 2013	12 month results: 16 of 46 patients continued for 12 mos and gained effective relief, SPAASMS: Score=13/28 possible in both groups at 12 mos (reading from Figure 5d) Activity & mobility: no numbers provided, groups look similar at 12 mos; Rescue pain meds: initially higher in TDF group; higher in TDB group near study end (no numbers provided); GP/ED visits: increase in visit frequency in TDB group near study end (no numbers provided); Sleep quality: No significant difference between groups (no numbers provided) Side effects: see Adverse event column Mood: TDB had relatively better score at 12 mos (no numbers provided); Pain VAS: 3-point (scale 1-10) reduction in pain in 11% in each treatment group (raw numbers not reported); DASS21: TDB had relatively better score at 12 mos (no numbers provided); PDI: looks similar in Figure 5b (no numbers provided)	Discontinued due to AEs or unsatisfactory relief (not separated by AEs only): A: TDB: 8/22 (41%); number patients with side effects at 12 mos≤1 (reading from Figure 4a); number patients with local skin reaction at 12 mos=1 (reading from Figure 4b); B: TDF: 8/24 (37.5%) number patients with side effcts at 12 mos≤1 (reading from Figure 4a); number patients with local skin reaction at 12 mos=0 (reading from Figure 4b)	Private Practice Research Fund of Townsville	Poor

Author Year	Study design Duration	Setting Country	Eligibility criteria	Interventions	Sample Characteristics	Screened Eligible Enrolled Analyzed Loss to Followup	Outcomes Assessed
Wild 2010	RCT 12 months	53 sites in North America; 36 sites in Europe	Inclusion: Men/ nonpregnant, nonlactating women ≥18 yrs, with diagnosis of moderate/ severe knee or hip osteo, or LBP of noncancer origin; ≥ 3 mo history pain prior to screening, dissatisfied with current analgesic; NRS score ≥4 (of 11) at baseline, after 3-7 day washout from previous anagesics. Exclusion: lifelong seizures; mild/moderate TBI, stroke, TIA, brain neoplasm within one year; severe TBI within 15 years; malignancy within 2 years; history of etoh/drug abuse; history of Hep B/C; HIV; allergy to oxycodone/ acetaminophen; participation in previous tapentadol studies; patients with reference joint or back surgery within 3 months or during study; hepatic or renal dysfunction, uncontrolled hypertension, significant pain with conditions other than osteo or LBP.	A. Tapentadol ER 100-250 mg BID (adjustable) (n=894; 413 completed 6 mos; 227 completed 12 mos) B. Oxycodone CR 20-50 mg BID (adjustable) (n=223; 78 completed 6 mos; 44 completed 12 mos)	A vs B Age, mean (SD): 56.8 (12.5) vs 58.1 (11.8); Age category: <65 72.6% vs 70%; Male: 42.4% vs 43.9%; Race: White:88.6% vs 91.0%, Black: 6.7% vs 5.8%, Hispanic: 2.9% vs 1.8%, Other: 1.8% vs 1.3%; BMI: 31.7 vs 31.8; Pain intensity, Mean (SD): 7.6 (1.5) vs 7.6 (1.62); Pain intensity category: Moderate: 10% vs 13%, Severe: 90% vs 87%; Prior opioids: No 47.1% vs 49.8%	Screened: 1123 Randomized: 1121 Received drug: 1117 Discontinued-A: 53.8%; 22.7% to AEs; Discontinued-B: 65.0; 36% to AEs%	AEs; vital signs; physical exams; labs; ECGs; PROs: PAC-SYM; COWS; SOWS; TEAEs

Note: The references are located in Appendix C.

AE=adverse event; ASA=aspirin; ECG=electrocardiogram; BID=twice daily; COWS=Clinical opiate withdrawal scale; DASS2= Depression Anxiety Stress Scale; GmbH=German liability company; GP/ED=general practitioner/emergency department; Hep B/C=Hepatitis B and/or C; HIV=human immunodeficiency virus; LBP=low blood pressure; NSAIDS=non-steroidal anti-inflammatory drug; PDI=physical disability index; ITT=intent to treat; PROs=patient reported outcomes; PAC-SYM=patient assessment of constipation syndrome; RCT=randomized controlled trial; SD=standard deviation; SE=standard error; SOWS=Subjective Opiate Withdrawal Scale; SPAASMS= score, physical, activity level, additional pain medication, additional physician/ER visits, sleep quality, mood, medication side-effects; TBI=traumatic brain injury; TDB=transdermal buprenorphine; TDF=transdermal fentanyl; VAS=visual analog scale; TEAC=treatment emergent adverse criteria; TEAEs=Treatment-Emergent Adverse Event; TIA=transient ischemic attack

Author Year	Results	Adverse Events and Withdrawals Due To Adverse Events	Sponsor	Quality
Wild 2010	Mean (SE) pain intensity score: decreased 4.4 (0.09) vs 4.5 (0.17); Global assessment, score of (very) much improved: 48.1% (394/819) vs 41.2% (73/177); Median duration of treatment (days): A: 268 (range 1-385) B: 59 (range 1-384); Mean (SD) total daily dose for study completers: A: 380.5 (102.43) mg B: 71.0 (22.89) mg Concomitant nonopioid analgesics (NSAIDS, ASA, acetaminophen): A: 19.9% (178/894) B: 17% (38/223)	Discontinued due to AEs: A: 22.7% B: 36.8%; At least one TEAC: A: 85.7% (766/894) B: 90.6% (202/223); A vs B: Constipation: 22.6% vs 38.6%; Nausea: 18.1% vs 33.2% Vomiting: 7.0% vs 13.5%; Pruritis: 5.4% vs 10.3%; Dizziness: 14.8% vs 19.3%; Serious TEACs: 5.5% vs 4.0%; No relevant AEs on labs, vitals, ECGs; No deaths; Mean change (SE) PAC-SYM: 0.3 (0.05) vs 0.5 (0.14); COWS,5 days post treatment, no withdrawal: 88% (145/166) vs 84% (42/50); Mean SOWS at 2-5 days post treatment - consistent with COWS	J & J; grunenthal GmbH	Fair

Appendix Table E8b. Observational Studies of Different Long-Acting Opioids

Author, Year	Type of Study, Setting	Eligibility Criteria	Comparison Groups	Population Characteristics	Method For Assessing Outcomes and Confounders
Hartung, 2007	Retrospective cohort Medicaid claims United States	Patients prescribed at least one ≥28-day supply of methadone, ER oxycodone, ER morphine, or transdermal fentanyl	A. Transdermal fentanyl (n=1,546) B. Methadone (n=974) C. ER oxycodone (n=1,866) D. ER morphine (n=1,298)	A vs. B vs. C vs. D Mean age: 70.6 vs. 51.1 vs. 57.4 vs. 58.5 years Female sex: 74% vs. 63% vs. 65% vs. 65% Race: 6.1% vs. 10.5% vs. 7.7% vs. 9.6% non-White Mean MED dose: 96 vs. 247 vs. 67 vs. 74 mg Cancer: 19.9% vs. 18.3% vs. 25.2% vs. 26.1% Osteoarthritis: 13.7% vs. 22.6% vs. 19.3% vs. 18.0% Back pain: 17.5% vs. 41.8% vs. 35.0% vs. 27.3%	Review of claims using ICD-9 codes

Author, Year	Screened Eligible Enrolled Analyzed Loss to Followup	Adjusted Variables For Statistical Analysis	Main Results	Funding Source	Quality
Hartung, 2007	Screened: NR Eligible: NR Enrolled: 5,684 Analyzed: 5,684	Age, sex, race, long-term care residence, number of unique prescribers, disease severity, concominant prescriptions known to interact with opioids, type of presumed pain diagnosis, history of abuse or dependence, enrollment in a substance abuse treatment program	A vs. B vs. C (reference: D) Mortality: adjusted HR 0.71 (95% CI 0.46 to 1.08) vs. HR 0.71 (95% CI 0.54 to 0.94) vs. 0.80 (95% CI 0.63 to 1.02) ED encounter or hospitalization involving an opioid-related adverse event (HR 0.45, 95% CI 0.26 to 0.77) Among patients with noncancer pain: Fentanyl associated with higher risk of ED encounters than sustained-release morphine (HR 1.27, 95% CI 1.02 to 1.59) Methadone associated with greater risk of overdose symptoms than sustained-release morphine (HR 1.57, 95% CI 1.03 to 2.40) No significant differences between methadone and long-acting morphine in risk of death (adjusted HR 0.71, 95% CI 0.46 to 1.08) or overdose symptoms	NR	Fair

Author, Year	Type of Study, Setting	Eligibility Criteria	Comparison Groups	Population Characteristics	Method For Assessing Outcomes and Confounders
Krebs, 2011	Retrospective cohort VA United States	New prescription for >= 28 days' supply of PO methadone or LA morphine tabs/caps from a VA outpatient pharmacy between 1/1/2000 and 12/31/2007. Preceded by 30 day window free of LA opioid prescriptions. Excluded: Liquid/IV forms of methadone/morphine; metastatic cancer, palliative care, receiving methadone for addiction; methadone 40 mg diskettes; < 17 or > 100 years of age; missing gender data.	A: Methadone (n=28,554) B: Long-acting morphine sulfate (MS) (n=79,938)	Mean (SD) daily LA MS dose: 67.5 mg (77.4); median (IQR) 46.7 (45); Mean (SD) daily methadone dose: 25.4 mg (25.8); median (IQR): 20 (20); 99th %ile MS: 360-7200 mg; 99th %ile methadone: 124-560 mg; A vs B: Age: mean (SD): 56 (12) vs 59 (13); Race: white: 40% vs 41%; nonwhite: 52% vs 49%; unknown: 8% vs 9%; MI: 9% vs 11%; CHF: 15% vs 19%; PVD: 17% vs 20%; CVD: 15% vs 17%; COPD: 35% vs 38%; Diabetes: 31% vs 33%; Malignancy: 15% vs 26%; Depression: 62% vs 54%; Bipolar: 10% vs 8%; Anxiety: 32% vs 27%; EtOH: 25% vs 22%; Drug disorderz: 25% vs 18%; Tobacco: 47% vs 42% Back pain: 85% vs 76%; Joint/limb pain: 86% vs 82%; Headache: 25% vs 21%; Neuropathic pain: 35% vs 29%	All patients meeting eligibility criteria

Note: The references are located in Appendix C.

CHF=congestive heart failure; CI=confidence interval; COPD=chronic obstructive pulmonary disease; CVD=cardiovascular disease; ER=extended release; EtOH=Ethyl alcohol; HR=hazard ratio; ICD-9=International Classification of Diseases; IQR=interquartile range; LA=long acting; MI=myocardial infarction; MS=morphine sulfate; PO=oral route; PVD=peripheral vascular disease SD=standard deviation; VA=Veterans Affairs; VISN=Veterans integrated service networks

Author, Year	Screened Eligible Enrolled Analyzed Loss to Followup	Adjusted Variables For Statistical Analysis	Main Results	Funding Source	Quality
Krebs, 2011	Screened: Not applicable; Eligible: 133,969; Enrolled: 108,492; Analyzed: 98,068; Loss to followup: 3,347 (died); 94,721 (censored)	Propensity score for receiving methadone was estimated with logistic regression model that included age, gender, race, geographic area (VISN), depression, anxiety, bipolar dx, schizophrenia, etoh, drug, tobacco disorders, back pain, joint/limb pain, headache, neuropathic pain; Medical comorbidities included via Romano adaptation of Charlson Comorbidity Score; Quintiles calculated and then used in Cox model; Interaction term consisting of propensity quintile and opioid group	All-cause mortality: Unadjusted: 3,347 (3.4%) patients died; highest mortality within 1st 30 days (1.2% in methadone and 3.7% in MS); raw death rates form MS higher than methadone for all 30-day intervals; Death rate: Quitile #1 (0.042 vs 0.133); Quintile #2 (0.034 vs 0.078); Quintile #3 (0.025 vs 0.053); Quintile #4 (0.022 vs 0.034); Quintile #5 (0.017 vs 0.020); Propensity adjusted mortality (HR): Overall risk of mortality lower with methadone than morphine (adjusted HR 0.56, 95% CI 0.51 to 0.62) Quintile #1: 0.36 (95% CI: 0.26, 0.49); Quintile #2: 0.46 (0.37, 0.56); Quintile #3: 0.50 (0.41, 0.61); Quintile #4: 0.66 (0.54, 0.81); Quintile #5: 0.92 (0.74, 1.16); Results robust in validation dataset	VA	Fair

Appendix Table E9. Trials of Opioid Dose Escalation Versus Dose Maintenance or Use of Maximum Dose Ceilings

Author Year	Study Design Duration	Setting Country	Eligibility Criteria	Interventions	Sample Characteristics	Screened Eligible Enrolled Analyzed Loss to Followup	Outcomes Assessed
Naliboff 2011	RCT 12 months	VA pain clinic U.S.	Patients referred to chronic pain clinic; nonmalignant chronic pain for at least 6 months; clinician determination that patient was eligible for long-term opioids. Excluded: anticipated surgery, post-op pain, pulmonary disease or CHF, current or history of substance abuse disorder, hospitalization for psych disorder in past 2 years	A. Escalating opioid dose; mean morphine equivalent 52 mg (n=67) B. Stable opioid dose; mean morphine equivalent 40 mg (n=73)	A vs B Mean age 53 vs 52 years 89% vs 99% male Race not reported Pain: -78% vs 77% musculoskeletal -19% vs 19% neuropathic -3% vs 4% complex Initial morphine equivalent 29.2 (SD 19.6) vs 32.3 (SD 23.1) mg Mean usual VAS 7.0 (SD 1.9) vs 6.7 (SD 1.8) Mean worst VAS 8.4 (SD 1.2) vs 8.0 (SD 1.7) Mean ABC score 1.5 (SD 2.0) vs 1.6 (SD 2.1) Mean ODI 48.6 (SD 12.6) vs 47.8 (SD 14.0)	Screened: not reported Eligible: 140 Enrolled: 140 Analyzed: 134 Loss to followup: 10/140 (7%)	Pain Functional disability Use of nonopioid medications

Note: The references are located in Appendix C.
CI=confidence interval, NSAID=nonsteroidal anti-inflammatory drug, ODI=Oswestry Disability Index, RCT=randomized controlled trial, SD=standard deviation, US=United States, VA=Veterans Affairs, VAS=Visual Analog Scale

Author Year	Results	Adverse Events and Withdrawals Due To Adverse Events	Sponsor	Quality
Naliboff 2011	A vs B Mean VAS usual pain at 12 months: 5.6 (SD 1.5) vs 6.2 (SD 1.5); p=0.11* Usual pain VAS decrease ≥1.5 points: 19/67 (28%) vs 15/73 (20%); RR 1.38; 95% CI 0.76 to 2.49 Mean VAS pain relief at 12 months: 6.0 (SD 1.7) vs 5.3 (SD 1.8); p=0.11* Increase in pain relief ≥1.5 points: 19/67 (29%) vs 11/73 (15%); RR 1.88; 95% CI 0.97 to 3.66 Worst pain VAS decrease ≥1.5 points: 9/67 (14%) vs 4/73 (6%); RR 2.45; 95% CI 0.79 to 7.59 Mean ODI at 12 months: 45.8 (SD 14.8) vs 45.0 (SD 19.4); p=0.85* ODI decrease ≥10 points: 19/67 (29%) vs 20/73 (23%); RR 1.04; 95% CI 0.61 to 1.76 Use of nonopioid treatments (A: n=64; B: n=70): -NSAID: 35/64 (55%) vs 42/70 (60%); RR 0.92; 95% CI 0.68 to 1.22 -Muscle relaxant: 10/64 (15%) vs 14/70 (20%); RR 0.78; 95% CI 0.37 to 1.63 -Anti-seizure: 40/64 (63%) vs 46/70 (66%); RR 0.95; 95% CI 0.74 to 1.23 -Anti-anxiety: 19/64 (29%) vs 24/70 (34%); RR 0.87; 95% CI 0.53 to 1.42 -Antidepressants: 45/64 (71%) vs 48/70 (69%); 1.03; 95% CI 0.82 to 1.28 -Topical: 11/64 (17%) vs 11/70 (16%); RR 1.06; 95% CI 0.49 to 2.28 -Injectable: 17/64 (26%) vs 25/70 (36%); RR 0.74; 95% CI 0.44 to 1.24 -Physical therapy: 31/64 (48%) vs 44/70 (63%); RR 0.77; 95% CI 0.57 to 1.05 *p-value calculated based on completers (A: n=34; B: n=32)	A vs B All-cause withdrawals: 33/67 (49%) vs 41/73 (56%); RR 0.88; 95% CI 0.64 to 1.20 Withdrawal due to opioid misuse: 16/67 (24%) vs 22/73 (30%); RR 0.79; 95% CI 0.46 to 1.38	Department of Veterans Affairs	Fair

Appendix Table E10. Trials of Different Strategies for Treating Acute Exacerbations of Chronic Pain in Patients on Long-term Opioid Therapy

Author year	Study Design Duration	Setting Country	Eligibility Criteria	Interventions	Sample Characteristics
Ashburn, 2011	RCT (crossover) Duration: up to 42 days total (two treatment periods of 10 breakthrough pain episodes each within 21 days)	46 centers United States	Patients aged 18 to 80 years with ≥3 months of chronic pain associated with diabetic neuropathy, postherpetic neuralgia, traumatic injury, complex regional pain syndrome, back pain, neck pain, fibromyalgia, chronic pancreatitis, osteoarthritis, or cancer; receiving ≥60 mg/day MED, with 1-4 episodes of breakthrough pain per day	A. Fentanyl buccal tablet (n=183) B. Oxycodone (n=183)	Mean age: 48.8 years Female sex: 62% Race: 92% White, 5% Black, 3% other Pain intensity in 24 hours prior to enrollment: 5.1 Indication (most common): 57% back pain, 11% osteoarthritis, 8% neck pain, 9% fibromyalgia, 4% traumatic injury, 4% complex regional pain syndrome
Davies, 2011	RCT (crossover) 3-21 days	35 cancer centers Europe and India	Patients with histologically confirmed cancer, receiving a fixed-schedule opioid regimen at a total daily dose equivalent ≥60 mg MED, with 1-4 episodes of breakthrough pain per day	A. Fentanyl pectin nasal spray (n=106 for safety and n=84 for efficacy) B. Immediate-release morphine sulfate (n=106 for safety and n=84 for efficacy)	Mean age: 55.9 years Female sex: NR Race: NR

Author year	Screened, Eligible, Enrolled, Analyzed Loss to Followup	Outcomes Assessed	Results	Adverse Events and Withdrawals Due To Adverse Events	Sponsor	Quality
Ashburn, 2011	Screened: 486 Eligible: 360 Enrolled: 323 (titration phase) Analyzed: 320 (safety), 183 (efficacy)	Pain intensity, pain relief, and total pain relief	A vs. B Pain intensity difference at 15 minutes: 0.82 vs. 0.60 ($p<0.001$) Pain relief at 15 minutes: 0.69 vs. 0.53 ($p<0.05$) Meaningful pain relief within 15 minutes: 16% vs. 12% of episodes ($p<0.05$)	A vs. B Any adverse event: 38% (106/281) vs. 31% (88/284); RR 1.22 (95% CI 0.97 to 1.53)	Cephalon, Inc.	Good
Davies, 2011	Screened: NR Eligible: NR Enrolled: 110 (titration phase) Analyzed: 106 (safety population), 84 (randomized after titration phase)	Pain intensity, pain relief, and total pain relief	A vs. B $\geq$2-point reduction in pain intensity at 10 minutes: 52.4% vs. 45.4% ($p<0.05$) $\geq$2 pain relief at 15 minutes: 60.2% vs. 53.4% ($p<0.05$) Total pain relief $\geq$33% at 15 minutes: 52.3% vs. 43.5% ($p<0.01$)	A vs. B Treatment-emergent adverse events resulting in discontinuation: 6 vs. 2	No financial support provided	Fair

Author year	Study Design Duration	Setting Country	Eligibility Criteria	Interventions	Sample Characteristics
Portenoy, 2007	RCT 3 weeks	Multicenter Clinic setting not described United States	18 to 80 years, chronic low back pain associated with osteoarthritis, degenerative disc disease, or spondylolisthesis resulting in functional disability for at least 3 months, receiving morphing average pain intensity scale in 24 hours prior to entry, duration of breakthrough pain less than 4 hours, use of an opioid to treat breakthrough pain described as at least somewhat effective Exclude: Uncontrolled or rapidly escalating pain, allergies or contraindications to study drug, cardiopulmonary disease that might affect safety, psychiatric or medical disease that might affect data collection, alcohol or substance abuse during the past 5 years, lactating, participated in an earlier fentanyl buccal tablet trial, or expected to have surgery during study	A: Buccal fentanyl 100 to 800 mcg for an episode of breakthrough pain B: Placebo Dose of buccal fentanyl: 800 mcg 56%; 600 mcg 24%; 400 mcg 15%; 200 mcg 5%	Not reported for randomization groups Mean age: 47 years Female gender: 55% Non-white race: 12% Baseline pain intensity: 5.1 (10 point scale) Primary etiology of low back pain degenerative disc disease: 68%

Author year	Screened, Eligible, Enrolled, Analyzed Loss to Followup	Outcomes Assessed	Results	Adverse Events and Withdrawals Due To Adverse Events	Sponsor	Quality
Portenoy, 2007	Screened: 124 Eligible: NR Enrolled: 105 (in open-label dose titration), 77 (in randomized phase; randomized to one of 3 treatment sequences consisting of 6 fentanyl buccal tablets and 3 placebo tablets in different orders)	Pain intensity: 0 to 10 scale Pain relief: 5-point scale (0 = none to 4 - complete) Onset time of "meaningful" pain relief	A vs. B Sum of the pain intensity differences from 5 through 60 minutes: 8.3 vs. 3.6 Proportion of breakthrough pain episodes with 'meaningful' pain reduction: 70% (289/413) vs. 30% (63/207) (p<0.0001) Proportion of breakthrough pain episodes with ≥33% reduction in pain intensity after 30 minutes: 42% (172/413) vs. 18% (18/207) (p≤0.0001) Proportion of breakthrough pain episodes with ≥50% reduction in pain intensity after 30 minutes: 30% (122/413) vs. 13% (27/207) (p≤0.0001) Proportion of breakthrough pain episodes with ≥33% reduction in pain intensity after 120 minutes: 65% (269/413) vs. 28% (57/207) (p≤0.0001) Proportion of breakthrough pain episodes with ≥50% reduction in pain intensity after 120 minutes: 48% (198/413) vs. 16% (33/207) (p≤0.0001)	All data reported only for buccal fentanyl Withdrawn due to adverse event: 1% (1/77) Serious adverse events: 3% (2/77) Nausea: 1% Dizziness: 4% Somnolence: 0% Dysgeusia: 8% Vomiting: 0% Dry mouth: 4%	Cephalon, Inc.	Good

Author year	Study Design Duration	Setting Country	Eligibility Criteria	Interventions	Sample Characteristics
Simpson, 2007	RCT (crossover) 3 weeks	Multicenter Clinic setting not described United States	18 to 80 years old, ≥3 months history of chronic neuropathic pain associated with diabetic peripheral neuropathy, postherpetic neuralgia, traumatic injury, or complex regional pain syndrome, on chronic opioids (at least 60 mg/day or morphine or equivalent), pain intensity <7 on a 0 to 10 scale, 1 to 4 daily episodes of breakthrough pain, use of opioid therapy for breakthrough pain described as at least partially effective; had to identify effective dose during dose-titration phase to be entered into randomized portion of trial Exclude: Unstable, uncontrolled, or rapidly escalating pain; allergies or other contraindications to study drug; alcohol or substance abuse in past 5 years; significant cardiopulmonary disease; significant medical or psychiatric disease; pregnancy or lactating	A: Buccal fentanyl 100 to 800 mcg for an episode of breakthrough pain B: Placebo Dose of buccal fentanyl: 800 mcg 54%; 600 mcg 19%; 400 mcg 18%; 200 mcg 5%, 100 mcg 5%	NR for randomization groups
Webster, 2013	RCT (crossover) Duration: up to 42 days total (two treatment periods of 10 breakthrough pain episodes each within 21 days)	42 sites Setting not described United States	Patients aged 18 to 80 years with >3 months of chronic pain associated with diabetic neuropathy, postherpetic neuralgia, traumatic injury, complex regional pain syndrome, back pain, neck pain, fibromyalgia, chronic pancreatitis, osteoarthritis, or cancer; receiving >60 mg/day MED, with and average pain intensity ≤6 and 1–4 episodes of breakthrough pain per day Exclude: recent history of substance abuse, positive UDT	A: Fentanyl buccal tablet (n=137) B: Oxycodone (n=137)	Mean age: 50.8 years Female sex: 58% Race: 91% White, 7% Black, 2% other Pain intensity in 24 hours prior to enrollment: 5.1

Note: The references are located in Appendix C.
CI=confidence interval; MED=morphine equivalent dose; NR=not relevant ; RCT=randomized controlled trial

Author year	Screened, Eligible, Enrolled, Analyzed Loss to Followup	Outcomes Assessed	Results	Adverse Events and Withdrawals Due To Adverse Events	Sponsor	Quality
Simpson, 2007	Screened: 129 Eligible: NR Enrolled: 103 (in open-label dose titration), 79 (in randomized phase; randomized to one of 3 crossover treatment sequences consisting of 6 fentanyl buccal tablets and 3 placebo tablets) Discontinued early: 2.5% (2/79)	Pain Intensity: 0 to 10 scale Sum of Pain Intensity differences from 5 through 60 minutes after administration of study drug	A vs. B Sum of the pain intensity differences from 5 through 60 minutes: 9.63 vs. 5.73 (p<0.001) Proportion of breakthrough pain episodes with 'meaningful' pain reduction: 69% vs. 36% (p<0.0001) Proportion of breakthrough pain episodes with ≥50% reduction in pain intensity after 15 minutes: 12% vs. 5% (p≤0.0001), p<0.0001 for each subsequent time point from 30 to 120 minutes Use of supplemental medication: 14% (59/432) vs. 36% (77/213) (OR=0.28, 95% CI 0.18 to 0.42)	All data reported only for buccal fentanyl: Withdrawn due to adverse event: 2.5% (2/79); 12% (12/103) withdrawn due to adverse events during open-label dose titration Nausea: 0% Dizziness: 1% Somnolence: 1% Vomiting: 0% Application site adverse event: 8% (8/103) during open-label dose titration	Cephalon, Inc.	Good
Webster, 2013	Screened: 307 Eligible: NR Enrolled: 213 (titration phase) Analyzed: 211 (safety), 137 (efficacy)	Pain intensity, pain relief, and total pain relief	A vs. B Pain intensity difference at 15 minutes: 0.88 vs. 0.76 (p<0.001) Pain relief at 15 minutes: 38% vs. 34% (p<0.05) Meaningful pain relief within 15 minutes: 17% vs. 16% (p=NS) Meaningful pain relief within 30 minutes: 46% vs. 38% (p<0.01)	A vs. B Any adverse event: 18% (25/138) vs. 14% (20/142); RR 1.29 (95% CI 0.75 to 2.20)	Teva Pharmaceuticals (formerly Cephalon, Inc.)	Good

Appendix Table E11. Trials of Decreasing Opioid Doses or of Tapering Off Opioids Versus Continuation of Opioids

Author year	Study design Duration	Setting Country	Eligibility criteria	Interventions	Sample Characteristics	Screened Eligible Enrolled Analyzed Loss to Followup
Cowan, 2005	RCT (crossover) 60 hours	Single center Pain clinic United Kingdom	>18 years, chronic noncancer pain on sustained-release oral morphine for ≥30 days, willing to abstain from morphine, able to give regular blood samples Exclude: Pain not adequately controlled by immobilization and alternative medication, patient may require a sudden change in opioid dose, pregnant or lactating	A: Continued sustained-release morphine for 60 hours B: Abrupt cessation of morphine for 60 hours	Mean age: 56 years Female gender: 40% Non-white race: Not reported Pain >5 years: 90% Duration of morphine use: mean 2.2 years Dose ≤60 mg/day: 90%	Screened: 33 Eligible: 11 Enrolled: 10 Analyzed: 10

Note: The references are located in Appendix C.
RCT=randomized controlled trial

Author year	Outcomes Assessed	Results	Adverse Events and Withdrawals Due To Adverse Events	Sponsor	Quality
Cowan, 2005	Effects of cessation of opioids: Unvalidated 19-item questionnaire Brief Pain Inventory Evaluation of physiologic parameters (heart rate, blood pressure, temperature, respiration, pupil size)	Continued sustained-release morphine vs. abrupt cessation Brief Pain Inventory, average pain in last 24 hours (0 to 10): 3.2 vs. 5.3 (p<0.026) Pain interference with general activity in last 24 hours (0 to 10): 0.2 vs. 4.3 (p<0.027) Physiologic parameters: No differences	Adverse events during cessation of opioids: 3/10 (30%) "Do you have any drug craving?": 0/10 after abrupt cessation of therapy	Janssen-Cilag Ltd., Napp Pharmaceuticals	Poor

Appendix Table E12. Nonrandomized Trials of Different Opioid Tapering Protocols and Strategies

Author Year	Study Design Duration	Setting Country	Eligibility Criteria	Interventions	Sample Characteristics
Ralphs, 1994	Non-randomized trial 6 months	Inpatient, single center United Kingdom	Patients referred to inpatient pain management, on opioids, chronic non-cancer pain, with any two of following: widespread disruption in activity due to pain, habitual over-activity leading to increased pain, regular use of analgesics and/or sedatives for >6 months, high affective distress, use of unnecessary aids, high levels of reported or observed pain behaviors, work reduced, impaired, or ceased owing to pain Exclude: Cannot use English, cannot climb stairs, current major psychiatric illness, unavailable for 4-week program, suitable for further physical treatments after medical examinations, pain of less than 1 year's duration, under 18 years old, currently using opioids for treatment of drug dependency	A: Patient-controlled reduction (patient discussed desired rate of reduction, aiming for abstinence by discharge, allowed to take longer if they wished, patients kept pills in room, plans adjusted as appropriate) B: Cocktail method (opioid mixed into a cocktail with dose gradually reduced, patient unaware of reduction schedule)	Mean age: 47 vs. 50 years Female gender: 49% vs. 71% Non-white race: Not reported Pain duration: 124 vs. 101 months Pain distress (0 to 100): 66 vs. 73 Mean opiate dose: 35.8 mg/day
Tennant, 1982	Non-randomized clinical trial 3 to 18 months	Single center Outpatient clinic United States	Patients on opioids who volunteered for outpatient treatment for withdrawing opioids	A: Detoxification/ counseling: Detoxification over 3 weeks with methadone, propoxyphene, clonidine, diphenoxylate, or sedative-hypnotics, followed by weekly psychotherapeutic counseling B: Detoxification/ maintenance: Detoxification as above, with maintenance on opioid if detoxification unsuccessful	Mean age: 33 vs. 44 years Female gender: 48% vs. 52% Nonwhite race: 19% vs. 14% Duration of opioid use: 7.2 vs. 9.2 years Proportion with chronic pain: 62% vs. 71% Back/spine disorder: 24% vs. 19% Use of codeine: 67% vs. 48%

Note: The references are located in Appendix C.
NR=not reported

Author Year	Screened Eligible Enrolled Analyzed Loss to Followup	Outcomes Assessed	Results	Adverse Events and Withdrawals Due To Adverse Events	Sponsor	Quality
Ralphs, 1994	Screened: 132 Eligible: NR Enrolled: 108 (63 to patient-controlled method and 45 to cocktail method) Analyzed: 108 Attrition: 24% (26/108)	Abstinent at discharge Abstinent at 6 month after discharge Use of other drugs, pain, or psychological variables at 6 months	Patient-controlled reduction versus cocktail method Abstinent at discharge: 68% vs. 89% (p<0.05) Abstinent 6 months after discharge: 54% (27/50) vs. 56% (18/32) Use of other drugs, pain, or psychological variables at 6 months: No differences between groups	NR	King Edwards Hospital Fund for London, Special Trustees of St. Thomas Hospital, and the South East Thames Regional Health Authority	Poor
Tennant, 1982	Screened: NR Eligible: NR Enrolled: 42 (21 to detoxification/ counseling and 21 to detoxification/ maintenance) Analyzed: 42	Proportion remaining in treatment past 3 weeks Proportion abstinent from opioids (as judged by history, negative urine test, and no further requests for opioids)	Detoxification/counseling vs. detoxification/maintenance Proportion remaining in treatment past 3 weeks: 24% (5/21) vs. 95% (20/21) Abstinent after 90 days: 10% (2/21) vs. 19% (4/21)	NR	NR	Poor

Appendix Table E13. Prospective Studies on Use of Screening Instruments To Predict the Risk of Aberrant Drug-Related Behaviors

Author, Year	Study Design	Eligibility Criteria	Population Characteristics	N	Instrument	Method of Administration	Reference Standard	True Positives (n)
Akbik 2006	Prospective cohort	Chronic pain patients attending one of two pain clinics	Mean age 43 years (SD 9.6) 33% female 86% White, other races not reported Pain: 39% back	n=155 (with reference standard, of 397 enrolled)	SOAPP	Self-report	Positive urine screening	SOAPP score ≥8: 30
Jones 2012 (Study 2)	Retrospective cohort	Consecutive pain clinic patients being evaluated for risk of opioid addiction prior to opioid initiation	Mean age 48 years (SD 13) 56% female 96% White, other races not reported Pain: 45% low back pain, 21% arthritis or fibromyalgia, 14% joint pain, 10% pelvic or abdominal pain, 7% neck or upper back pain	n=263	ORT PMQ SOAPP-R Clinician assessment	Self-report; clinician interview	Subsequent opioid discontinuation due to abuse	ORT score >4: 8 PMQ score >30: 13 SOAPP-R score >17: 20 Clinician assessment of high-risk: 27
Moore 2009	Retrospective cohort	New adult patients at a pain clinic	Mean age 44 years (SD 11) 60% female Race not reported Pain not reported	n=48	SOAPP DIRE ORT Clinician assessment	Self-report (SOAPP, DIRE, ORT); clinician interview	Subsequent opioid discontinuation due to abuse	SOAPP: 35 DIRE: 8 ORT: 21 Clinical interview: 37

Author, Year	False Positives (n)	True Negatives (n)	False Negatives (n)	Sensitivity	Specificity	Positive Likelihood Ratio	Negative Likelihood Ratio	AUROC	Quality
Akbik 2006	SOAPP score ≥8: 59	SOAPP score ≥8: 37	SOAPP score ≥8: 14	SOAPP score ≥8: 0.68 (95% CI 0.52 to 0.81)	SOAPP score ≥8: 0.39 (95% CI 0.29 to 0.49)	SOAPP score ≥8: 1.11 (95% CI 0.86 to 1.43)	SOAPP score ≥8: 0.83 (95% CI 0.52 to 1.31)	Not reported	Fair
Jones 2012 (Study 2)	ORT score >4: 19 PMQ score >30: 41 SOAPP-R score >17: 65 Clinician assessment of high-risk: 57	ORT score >4: 142 PMQ score >30: 134 SOAPP-R score >17: Clinician assessment of high-risk: 84	ORT score >4: 33 PMQ score >30: 25 SOAPP-R score >17: Clinician assessment of high-risk: 11	ORT score >4: 0.20 (95% CI 0.15 to 0.27) PMQ score >30: 0.34 (95% CI 0.20 to 0.51) SOAPP-R score >17: 0.39 (95% CI 0.26 to 0.54) Clinician assessment of high-risk: 0.71 (95% CI 0.54 to 0.84)	ORT score >4: 0.88 (95% CI 0.82 to 0.93) PMQ score >30: 0.77 (95% CI 0.69 to 0.80) SOAPP-R score >17: 0.69 (95% CI 0.63 to 0.75) Clinician assessment of high-risk: 0.60 (95% CI 0.51 to 0.68)	ORT score >4: 1.65 (95% CI 0.78 to 3.51) PMQ score >30: 1.46 (95% CI 0.87 to 2.45) SOAPP-R score >17: 1.27 (95% CI 0.86 to 1.90) Clinician assessment of high-risk: 1.76 (95% CI 1.32 to 2.34)	ORT score >4: 0.91 (95% CI 0.78 to 1.06) PMQ score >30: 0.86 (95% CI 0.68 to 1.08) SOAPP-R score >17: 0.88 (95% CI 0.70 to 1.10) Clinician assessment of high-risk: (0.49 (95% CI 0.29 to 0.81)	ORT 0.53 PMQ 0.57 SOAPP-R 0.54	Poor
Moore 2009	Not calculable	Not calculable	SOAPP: 13 DIRE: 40 ORT: 27 Clinical interview: 11	SOAPP score ≥6: 0.73 DIRE score <14: 0.17 ORT score >4: 0.45 Clinical interview assessment medium or high risk: 0.77	Not reported	Not reported	Not reported	Not reported	Poor

E-46

Author, Year	Study Design	Eligibility Criteria	Population Characteristics	N	Instrument	Method of Administration	Reference Standard	True Positives (n)
Webster 2005	Prospective cohort	New chronic pain patients at a pain clinic	Mean age 44 years (SD 13) 58% female Race not reported Pain: 45% back; 18% head; 16% neuropathic; 16% musculoskeletal; 5% visceral	n=185	ORT	Self-report	Documentation of aberrant behavior during followup	ORT score 1-3 (low risk): 1 ORT score 4-7 (moderate risk): 35 ORT score ≥8 (high risk): 40

Note: The references are located in Appendix C.
AUROC=area under receiver operating characteristic curve; CI=confidence interval; DIRE= Diagnosis, Intractability, Risk and Efficacy Inventory; ORT=Opioid Risk Tool; PMQ=Pain Medication Questionnaire; SOAPP-R= Revised Screener and Opioid Assessment for Patients with Pain

Author, Year	False Positives (n)	True Negatives (n)	False Negatives (n)	Sensitivity	Specificity	Positive Likelihood Ratio	Negative Likelihood Ratio	AUROC	Quality
Webster 2005	ORT score 1-3 (low risk): 17 ORT score 4-7 (moderate risk): 88 ORT score high (≥8): 4	ORT score 1-3 (low risk): 92 ORT score 4-7 (moderate risk): 21 ORT score high (≥8): 105	ORT score 1-3 (low risk): 75 ORT score 4-7 (moderate risk): 41 ORT score high (≥8): 36	ORT score ≥4: 0.99 (95% CI 0.92 to 0.999)	ORT score ≥4: 0.16 (95% CI 0.10 to 0.24)	ORT score ≥4: 1.17 (95% CI 1.07 to 1.27) ORT score 1-3 (low risk): 0.08 (95% CI 0.01 to 0.62) ORT score 4-7 (moderate risk): 0.57 (95% CI 0.44 to 0.74) ORT score ≥8 (high risk): 14.34 (95% CI 5.35 to 38)	ORT score ≥4: 0.08 (95% CI 0.01 to 0.65)	Not reported	Fair

Appendix F. Quality Assessment Tables

Appendix Table F1. Quality Assessment of Cohort Studies

Author, Year	KQ	Did the study attempt to enroll all (or a random sample of) patients meeting inclusion criteria (inception cohort)?	Were the groups comparable at baseline on key prognostic factors (e.g., by restriction or matching)?	Did the study maintain comparable groups through the study period?	Did the study use accurate methods for ascertaining exposures and potential confounders?	Were outcome assessors and/or data analysts blinded to the exposure being studied?	Did the article report attrition?	Is there important differential loss to followup or overall high loss to followup?	Did the study perform appropriate statistical analyses on potential confounders?	Were outcomes prespecified and defined, and ascertained using accurate methods?	Quality
Carman, 2011	KQ2a, b myocardial infarction	Yes	Yes	Yes	Yes	Unclear	No	Unclear	Yes	Yes	Fair
Dunn, 2010	KQ2a, b overdose	Yes	Unclear	Yes	Yes	Unclear	Yes	Yes	Yes	Yes	Fair
Edlund, 2014	KQ2a, b abuse	Yes	Unclear	Yes	Yes	Unclear	No	No	Yes	Yes	Fair
Hartung, 2007	KQ3c	Yes	No	Yes	Yes	Unclear	No	Unclear	Yes	Yes	Fair
Krebs, 2011	KQ3c	Yes	No	Yes	Yes	No	Yes	No	Yes	Yes	Fair
Saunders, 2010	KQ2a, b fractures	Yes	Unclear	Yes	Yes	Unclear	No	Unclear	Yes	Yes	Fair

Note: The references are available in Appendix C.
Based on United States Preventive Services Task Force Quality Assessment Criteria (see Methods section for details).
KQ=key question

Appendix Table F2. Quality Assessment of Cross-Sectional Studies

Author, Year	KQ	Did the study attempt to enroll all (or a random sample of) patients meeting inclusion criteria, or a random sample (inception cohort)?	Were outcome assessors blinded to patient characteristics?	Did the article report attrition?	Is there overall high loss to followup?	Were prespecified outcomes assessed in all patients?	Quality
Banta-Green, 2009	KQ2a abuse	Yes	Unclear	NA	NA	Yes	Fair
Boscarino, 2010	KQ2a abuse	Yes; random	No	NA	NA	No (high proportion of nonrespondents)	Fair
Carrington Reid, 2002	KQ2a abuse	Yes	No	NA	NA	Yes	Fair
Compton, 2008	KQ2a abuse	Yes; consecutive	No	No	Unclear	Yes	Fair
Cowan, 2003	KQ2a abuse	Yes	Unclear	NA	NA	Yes	Fair
Deyo, 2013	KQ2a , b endocrine	Yes	Unclear	NA	NA	Yes	Fair
Fleming, 2007 See also: Saffier, 2007	KQ2a abuse	Yes; all	No	NA	NA	Yes	Fair
Hojsted, 2010	KQ2a abuse	Unclear	No	NA	NA	Yes	Fair
Portenoy, 2007	KQ2a abuse	No (28% of eligible patients enrolled, not clear why most did not enroll)	No	Yes	Yes (Table 3)	Yes	Fair
Schneider, 2010	KQ2a abuse	Yes	No	NA	NA	No; UDT only in 82% of patients	Fair
Wasan, 2009	KQ2a abuse	Unclear	Yes	NA	NA	No	Fair

Note: The references are located in Appendix C.
Based on United States Preventive Services Task Force Quality Assessment Criteria (see Methods section for details).
KQ=key question; NA=not applicable; UDT=urine drug test

Appendix Table F3. Quality Assessment of Case Control Studies

Author, Year	KQ	Did the study attempt to enroll all or random sample of cases using predefined criteria?	Were the controls derived from the same population as the cases?	Were the groups comparable at baseline on key prognostic factors?	Were enrollment rates similar in cases and controls invited to participate?	Did the study use accurate methods for identifying outcomes?	Did the study use accurate methods for ascertaining exposures and potential confounders?	Did the study perform appropriate statistical analyses on potential confounders?	Quality
Gomes, 2011	KQ2b overdose	Yes	Yes	Yes	Unclear	Yes	Yes	Yes	Good
Gomes, 2013	KQ2b, motor vehicle accident	Yes	Yes	Yes	Unclear	Yes	Yes	Yes	Good
Li, 2013a	KQ2a fractures	Yes	Yes	Yes	Unclear	Yes	Yes	Yes	Good
Li, 2013b	KQ2a myocardial infarction	Yes	Yes	Yes	Unclear	Yes	Yes	Yes	Good

Note: The references are available in Appendix C.
Based on United States Preventive Services Task Force Quality Assessment Criteria (see Methods section for details).
KQ=key question

Appendix Table F4. Quality Assessment of Trials

Author, year	KQ	Random-ization	Concealed treatment allocation	Baseline group similarity	Patient blinded	Care provider blinded	Outcome assessor blinded	Cointer-ventions avoided or similar	Compli-ance accept-able in all groups	Attrition reported	Attrition accept-able	Timing of outcome assess-ment in all groups similliar	Intention to treat analysis	Avoid-ance of selective outcomes reporting	Quality
Allan, 2005	KQ3c	Yes	Yes	Yes	No	No	No	Yes	Yes	Yes	No	Yes	Yes	Yes	Fair
Ashburn, 2011	KQ3h	Yes	Yes	Yes	Yes	Yes	Unclear; probably yes	Yes	Yes	Yes	Yes	Yes	Yes	Yes	Good
Cowan, 2005	KQ3i	Yes	Unclear	Unclear	Yes	Yes	Unclear	Unclear	Yes	no	Unclear	Yes	Yes	Unclear	Poor
Davies, 2011	KQ3h	Unclear	Unclear	Yes	Yes	Yes	Unclear	Yes	Yes	Yes	Yes	Yes	Yes	Yes	Fair
Jamison, 1998	KQ3a	Unclear	Unclear	Unclear	No	No	No	No	Yes	Yes	Yes	Yes	Yes	Unclear	Fair
Mitra, 2013	KQ3c	Yes	No	Unclear	Unclear	No	Yes	Yes	No	Yes	No	Yes	No	No	Poor
Naliboff 2011	KQ3f	Yes	Yes	Yes	Yes	No	Unclear	Yes (similar in both groups)	Unclear	Yes	No	Yes	Yes	Yes	Fair
Portenoy, 2007	KQ3h	Yes	Yes	NA	Yes	Yes	Yes	Yes	Unclear	Yes	Yes	Yes	Yes	Yes	Good
Ralphs, 1994	KQ3j	No	No	No	No	No	No	yes	unclear	No	Unclear	yes	yes	unclear	Poor
Salzman, 1999	KQ3a	Unclear	Unclear	Yes	No	No	No	Yes	Yes	Yes	Yes	Yes	Yes	Unclear	Fair
Simpson, 2007	KQ3h	Yes	Unclear	NA	Yes	Yes	Yes	Yes	Yes	Yes	Yes	Yes	Yes	Yes	Good
Tennant, 1982	KQ3j	No	No	No	No	No	No	Unclear	Unclear	No	Unclear	Yes	Yes	Unclear	Poor
Webster, 2013	KQ3h	Yes	Yes	Yes	Yes	Yes	Unclear; probably yes	Yes	Yes	Yes	Yes	Yes	Yes	Yes	Good
Wild 2010	KQ3c	Yes	Yes	Yes	No	No	No	Yes	Yes	Yes	No	Yes	Yes	Yes	Fair

Note: The references are available in Appendix C.
Based on Cochrane Back Review Group Quality Assessment Methods (see Methods section for details).
KQ=key question

Appendix Table F5. Quality Assessment of Screening Instrument Studies

Author, year	Evaluates population other than the one used to derive the instrument	Avoided case-control design	Consecutive series of patients or a random subset	Describes severity of symptoms, opioid dose/duration and underlying conditions	Adequate descripton of screening instrument	Apprioriate criteria included in screening instrument	Adequate descripton of methods for identifying aberrant drug-related behaviors	Appropriate criteria used to identify aberrant drug related behaviors	Aberrant drug-related behaviors assessed in all enrollees	Blinded assessment of aberrant drug-related behaviors	Quality
Akbik, 2006	Yes	Yes	Yes	Yes	Yes	Yes	Yes	No	No	Unclear	Fair
Jones, 2012	Yes	No	No	Yes	Yes	Yes	Yes	No	No	Unclear	Poor
Moore, 2009	Yes	No	No	Yes	Yes	Yes	Yes	No	No	Unclear	Poor
Webster, 2005	Yes	Yes	Yes	Yes	Yes	Yes	No	Unclear	Unclear	Unclear	Fair

Note: The references are available in Appendix C.
Based on various methods sources (see Methods section for details).

Appendix G. Strength of Evidence Table

Key Question Outcome	Study Design Number of Studies (N)	Study Limitations	Consistency	Directness	Precision	Reporting Bias	Strength of Evidence Grade
1. Effectiveness and comparative effectiveness							
a. In patients with chronic pain, what is the effectiveness of long-term opioid therapy versus placebo or no opioid therapy for long-term (>1 year) outcomes related to pain, function, and quality of life?							
Pain, function, quality of life	No studies	-	-	-	-	-	Insufficient
b. How does effectiveness vary depending on: 1) the specific type or cause of pain (e.g., neuropathic, musculoskeletal [including low back pain], fibromyalgia, sickle cell disease, inflammatory pain, and headache disorders); 2) patient demographics (e.g., age, race, ethnicity, gender); 3) patient comorbidities (including past or current alcohol or substance use disorders, mental health disorders, medical comorbidities and high risk for addiction)?							
Pain, function, quality of life	No studies	-	-	-	-	-	Insufficient
c. In patients with chronic pain, what is the comparative effectiveness of opioids versus nonopioid therapies (pharmacological or nonpharmacological) on outcomes related to pain, function, and quality of life?							
Pain, function, quality of life	No studies	-	-	-	-	-	Insufficient
d. In patients with chronic pain, what is the comparative effectiveness of opioids plus nonopioid interventions (pharmacological or nonpharmacological) versus opioids or nonopioid interventions alone on outcomes related to pain, function, quality of life, and doses of opioids used?							
Pain, function, quality of life	No studies	-	-	-	-	-	Insufficient

Key Question Outcome	Study Design Number of Studies (N)	Study Limitations	Consistency	Directness	Precision	Reporting Bias	Strength of Evidence Grade
2. Harms and adverse events							
a. In patients with chronic pain, what are the risks of opioids versus placebo or no opioid on: 1) opioid abuse, addiction, and related outcomes; 2) overdose; and 3) other harms, including gastrointestinal-related harms, falls, fractures, motor vehicle accidents, endocrinological harms, infections, cardiovascular events, cognitive harms, and psychological harms (e.g., depression)?							
Abuse, addiction	1 cohort study (n=568,640)	Moderate	Unknown (1 study)	Direct	Precise	Undetected	Low
Abuse, addiction	10 uncontrolled studies (n=3,780)	High	Inconsistent	Direct	Precise	Undetected	Insufficient
Overdose	1 cohort study (n=9,940)	Moderate	Unknown (1 study)	Direct	Imprecise	Undetected	Low
Fractures	1 cohort study (n=2,341) and 1 case-control study (21,739 cases)	Moderate	Consistent	Direct	Precise	Undetected	Low
Myocardial infarction	1 cohort study (n=426,124) and 1 case-control study (11,693 cases)	Low	Consistent	Direct	Precise	Undetected	Low
Endocrine	1 cross-section study (n=11,327)	Moderate	Unknown (1 study)	Direct	Precise	Undetected	Low
Gastrointestinal harms, motor vehicle accients, infections, psychological harms, cognitive harms	No studies	-	-	-	-	-	Insufficient
b. How do harms vary depending on: 1) the specific type or cause of pain (e.g., neuropathic, musculoskeletal [including back pain], fibromyalgia, sickle cell disease, inflammatory pain, headache disorders); 2) patient demographics; 3) patient comorbidities (including past or current substance use disorder or at high risk for addiction)?							
Various harms	No studies	-	-	-	-	-	Insufficient

Key Question Outcome	Study Design Number of Studies (N)	Study Limitations	Consistency	Directness	Precision	Reporting Bias	Strength of Evidence Grade
b. How do harms vary depending on the dose of opioids used?							
Abuse, addiction	1 cohort study (n=568,640)	Moderate	Unknown (1 study)	Direct	Precise	Undetected	Low
Overdose	1 cohort study (n=9,940) and 1 case-control study (593 cases in primary analysis)	Moderate	Consistent	Direct	Precise	Undetected	Low
Fracture	1 cohort study (n=2,341)	Moderate	Unknown (1 study)	Direct	Imprecise	Undetected	Low
Myocardial infarction	1 cohort study (n=426,124)	Moderate	Unknown (1 study)	Direct	Precise	Undetected	Low
Motor vehicle accidents	1 case-control study (5,300 cases)	Low	Unknown (1 study)	Direct	Precise	Undetected	Low
Endocrine	1 cross-sectional study (n=11,327)	Moderate	Unknown (1 study)	Direct	Precise	Undetected	Low
3. Dosing strategies							
a. In patients with chronic pain, what is the comparative effectiveness of different methods for initiating and titrating opioids for outcomes related to pain, function, and quality of life; risk of overdose, addiction, abuse, or misuse; and doses of opioids used?							
Pain	2 randomized trials (n=93)	Moderate	Inconsistent	Direct	Imprecise	Undetected	Insufficient
Function, quality of life, outcomes related to abuse	No studies	-	-	-	-	-	Insufficient
b. In patients with chronic pain, what is the comparative effectiveness of short- versus long-acting opioids on outcomes related to pain, function, and quality of life; risk of overdose, addiction, abuse, or misuse; and doses of opioids used?							
Pain, function, quality of life, outcomes related to abuse	No studies	-	-	-	-	-	Insufficient

Key Question Outcome	Study Design Number of Studies (N)	Study Limitations	Consistency	Directness	Precision	Reporting Bias	Strength of Evidence Grade
c. In patients with chronic pain, what is the comparative effectiveness of different long-acting opioids on outcomes related to pain, function, and quality of life; and risk of overdose, addiction, abuse, or misuse?							
Pain and function	3 randomized trials (n=1,850)	Moderate	Consistent	Direct	Precise	Undetected	Low
Assessment of risk of overdose, addiction, abuse, or misuse	No studies	-	-	-	-	-	Insufficient
Overdose (as indicated by all-cause mortality)	1 cohort study (n=108,492)	Moderate	Unknown (1 study)	Direct	Precise	Undetected	Low
Abuse and related outcomes	1 cohort study (n=5,684)	Moderate	Unknown (1 study)	Direct	Imprecise	Undetected	Insufficient
d. In patients with chronic pain, what is the comparative effectiveness of short- plus long-acting opioids vs. long-acting opioids alone on outcomes related to pain, function, and quality of life; risk of overdose, addiction, abuse, or misuse; and doses of opioids used?							
Pain, function, quality of life, outcomes related to abuse	No studies	-	-	-	-	-	Insufficient
e. In patients with chronic pain, what is the comparative effectiveness of scheduled, continuous versus as-needed dosing of opioids on outcomes related to pain, function, and quality of life; risk of overdose, addiction, abuse, or misuse; and doses of opioids used?							
Pain, function, quality of life, outcomes related to abuse	No studies	-	-	-	-	-	Insufficient
f. In patients with chronic pain on long-term opioid therapy, what is the comparative effectiveness of dose escalation versus dose maintenance or use of maximum dose ceilings on outcomes related to pain, function, and quality of life?							
Pain, function, withdrawal due to opioid misuse	1 randomized trial (n=140)	Moderate	Unknown (1 study)	Direct	Imprecise	Undetected	Low

Key Question Outcome	Study Design Number of Studies (N)	Study Limitations	Consistency	Directness	Precision	Reporting Bias	Strength of Evidence Grade
g. In patients on long-term opioid therapy, what is the comparative effectiveness of opioid rotation versus maintenance of current opioid therapy on outcomes related to pain, function, and quality of life; and doses of opioids used?							
Pain, function, quality of life, outcomes related to abuse	No studies	-	-	-	-	-	Insufficient
h. In patients on long-term opioid therapy, what is the comparative effectiveness of different strategies for treating acute exacerbations of chronic pain on outcomes related to pain, function, and quality of life?							
Pain	5 randomized trials (n=802)	Moderate	Consistent	Direct	Precise	Undetected	Moderate
Function, quality of life, abuse and related outcomes	No studies	-	-	-	-	-	Insufficient
i. In patients on long-term opioid therapy, what are the effects of decreasing opioid doses or of tapering off opioids versus continuation of opioids on outcomes related to pain, function, quality of life, and withdrawal symptoms?							
Pain, function	1 randomized trial (n=10)	High	Unknown (1 study)	Direct	Imprecise	Undetected	Insufficient
j. In patients on long-term opioid therapy, what is the comparative effectiveness of different tapering protocols and strategies on measures related to pain, function, quality of life, withdrawal symptoms, and likelihood of opioid cessation?							
Opioid abstinence	2 nonrandomized trials (n=150)	High	Consistent	Direct	Imprecise	Undetected	Insufficient

Key Question Outcome	Study Design Number of Studies (N)	Study Limitations	Consistency	Directness	Precision	Reporting Bias	Strength of Evidence Grade
4. Risk assessment and risk mitigation strategies							
a. In patients with chronic pain being considered for long-term opioid therapy, what is the accuracy of instruments for predicting risk of opioid overdose, addiction, abuse, or misuse?							
Diagnostic accuracy: Opioid Risk Tool	3 studies of diagnostic accuracy (n=496)	Moderate	Inconsistent	Direct	Imprecise	Undetected	Insufficient
Diagnostic accuracy: Screening and Opioid Assessment for Patients with Pain version 1	2 studies of diagnostic accuracy (n=203)	High	Consistent	Direct	Imprecise	Undetected	Low
b. In patients with chronic pain, what is the effectiveness of use of risk prediction instruments on outcomes related to overdose, addiction, abuse, or misuse?							
Outcomes related to abuse	No studies	-	-	-	-	-	Insufficient
c. In patients with chronic pain prescribed long-term opioid therapy, what is the effectiveness of risk mitigation strategies, including 1) opioid management plans, 2) patient education, 3) urine drug screening, 4) use of prescription drug monitoring program data, 5) use of monitoring instruments, 6) more frequent monitoring intervals, 7) pill counts, and 8) use of abuse-deterrent formulations on outcomes related to overdose, addiction, abuse, or misuse?							
Outcomes related to abuse	No studies	-	-	-	-	-	Insufficient
d. What is the comparative effectiveness of treatment strategies for managing patients with addiction to prescription opioids on outcomes related to overdose, abuse, misuse, pain, function, and quality of life?							
Outcomes related to abuse	No studies	-	-	-	-	-	Insufficient